Relatedness, Self-Definition and Mental Representation

Over the course of a long and distinguished career, psychologist and psychoanalyst Sidney J. Blatt has made major contributions to cognitive-developmental theory, psychoanalytic object relations theory, applied psychoanalysis, and current research in the areas of psychopathology and psychotherapy. This book presents chapters by Dr. Blatt's many colleagues and students who address the key areas in which Dr. Blatt focuses his intellectual endeavours:

- Personality development
- Psychopathology
- Issues in psychological testing and assessment
- Psychotherapy and the treatment process
- Applied psychoanalysis and broader cultural trends

Relatedness, Self-Definition and Mental Representation explores Dr. Blatt's unique contributions within both psychoanalysis, where empirical research is often neglected, and clinical psychology, where psychoanalysis is increasingly ignored. It will be engaging reading for psychoanalysIs and clinical psychologists, as well as all those concerned with psychotherapy and personality theory and development.

John S. Auerbach, Professor, Department of Psychiatry and Behavioral Sciences, James H. Quillen College of Medicine, East Tennessee State University.
Kenneth N. Levy, Assistant Professor, Department of Psychology, Pennsylvania State University.
Carrie E. Schaffer, Clinical Assistant Professor of Psychiatric Medicine, University of Virginia School of Medicine.

Relatedness, Self-Definition and Mental Representation

Essays in honor of Sidney J. Blatt

Edited by John S. Auerbach,
Kenneth N. Levy, and Carrie E. Schaffer

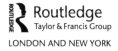

LONDON AND NEW YORK

First published 2005 by Routledge
2 Park Square, Milton Park, Abingdon, Oxfordshire OX14 4RN

Simultaneously published in the USA and Canada
by Routledge
711 Third Avenue, New York, NY 10017

Routledge is an imprint of the Taylor and Francis Group, an informa business

Typeset in Times by Garfield Morgan, Rhayader, Powys, UK
Cover design by Lou Page

British Library Cataloguing in Publication Data
A catalogue record for this book is available from the British Library

Library of Congress Cataloging in Publication Data
Relatedness, self-definition, and mental representation: essays in honor of
Sidney J. Blatt / edited by John S. Auerbach, Kenneth N. Levy, and Carrie E.
Schaffer.
       p.   cm.
   Includes bibliographical references and index.
   ISBN 1-58391-289-4 (alk. paper)
   1. Blatt, Sidney J. (Sidney Jules) 2. Clinical psychology. 3. Mental
representation. 4. Relatedness (Psychology) 5. Personality development. 6.
Psychoanalysis. 7. Psychotherapy. I. Blatt, Sidney J. (Sidney Jules) II.
Auerbach, John S. (John Samuel), 1958– III. Levy, Kenneth N. (Kenneth
Neil), 1963– IV. Schaffer, Carrie E. (Carrie Ellen), 1958– V. Title.

   RC467.R45 2004
   616.89–dc22

                                                      2004010647

ISBN 13: 978-1-58391-289-8 (hbk)
ISBN 13: 978-1-138-01193-9 (pbk)

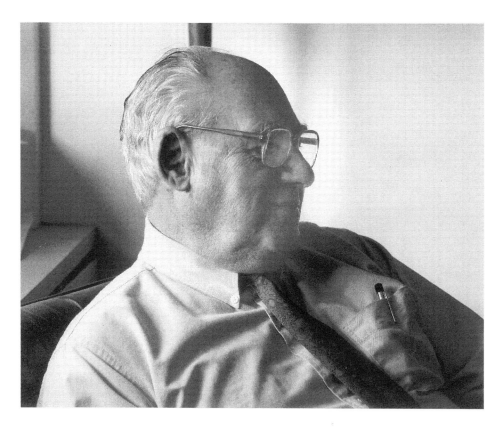

Sidney J. Blatt, Ph.D
Photograph by Braxton McKee

To Deborah, Kristen, and Taj

Contents

List of illustrations   x
List of contributors   xi
Foreword   xiv
Acknowledgments   xviii

1 Introduction: the contributions of Sidney J. Blatt   1
JOHN S. AUERBACH, KENNETH N. LEVY, AND CARRIE E. SCHAFFER

PART I
Personality development   21

2 A dyadic systems view of communication   23
BEATRICE BEEBE, JOSEPH JAFFE, AND FRANK LACHMANN

3 Representations in middle childhood: a dialogical perspective   43
BEATRIZ PRIEL

4 On spatialization: personal and theoretical thoughts   58
NORBERT FREEDMAN

PART II
Psychopathology   73

5 Dependency, self-criticism, and maladjustment   75
DAVID C. ZUROFF, DARCY SANTOR, AND MYRIAM MONGRAIN

6 Characterizing cognitive vulnerability in depression   91
NASREEN KHATRI AND ZINDEL V. SEGAL

7 The development of schizophrenia: a psychosocial and
biological approach   104
STEPHEN FLECK

8   Another "lens" for understanding therapeutic change: the
interaction of IQ with defense mechanisms   120
PHEBE CRAMER

PART III
Assessment   135

9   Sidney Blatt's contributions to the assessment of object
representations   137
BARRY RITZLER

10 Object relations and the Rorschach   154
HOWARD D. LERNER

11 The Rorschach method: a starting point for investigating
formal thought disorder   172
PHILIP S. HOLZMAN

PART IV
Psychotherapy and the treatment process   189

12 Some reflections on the therapeutic action of psychoanalytic
therapy   191
PETER FONAGY AND MARY TARGET

13 How often are relationship narratives told during
psychotherapy sessions?   213
LESTER LUBORSKY, TOMASZ ANDRUSYNA, AND LOUIS DIGUER

14 Research perspectives on the case study: single-case method   222
STANLEY B. MESSER AND LAURA MCCANN

PART V
Applied psychoanalysis   239

15 Greed as an individual and social phenomenon: an
application of the two-configurations model   241
PAUL L. WACHTEL

16 Narcissism as a clinical and social phenomenon   255
DIANA DIAMOND

17 Attachment and separateness and the psychoanalytic
     understanding of the act of faith   273
     RACHEL B. BLASS

18 The menace of postmodernism to a psychoanalytic psychology   288
     ROBERT R. HOLT

     Index   303

List of illustrations

Figures

5.1	A dynamic interactionist framework for studying dependency and self-criticism	77
7.1	The systems hierarchy	105
7.2	Development of schizophrenia	111
12.1	A schematic representation of the development of the experience of affect	196–7
12.2	The process of changing intersubjective representational shifts	198

Tables

11.1	TDI categories and levels of severity with selected examples	176–7
12.1	The three modes of psychic change	207
13.1	Gender differences in frequency of Relationship Episodes	217
13.2	Frequency of Relationship Episodes (REs) in relation to psychotherapy outcome	219

Contributors

Tomasz Andrusyna, B.A., Graduate Student, Northwestern University.

John S. Auerbach, Ph.D., Staff Psychologist and Coordinator, Post-Traumatic Stress Program, James H. Quillen Veterans Affairs Medical Center, Mountain Home, Tennessee; Professor, Department of Psychiatry and Behavioral Sciences, James H. Quillen College of Medicine, East Tennessee State University; Research Affiliate, Department of Psychiatry, Yale University School of Medicine; Private Practice, Johnson City, Tennessee.

Beatrice Beebe, Ph.D., Associate Clinical Professor of Medical Psychology in Psychiatry, College of Physicians and Surgeons, Columbia University; Faculty, New York University Postdoctoral Program in Psychotherapy and Psychoanalysis; Teaching Faculty, Parent–Infant Psychotherapy Program, Columbia University Center for Psychoanalytic Training and Research; Core Faculty, Institute for the Psychoanalytic Study of Subjectivity.

Rachel Blass, Ph.D., Associate Professor, Head of Clinical Psychology Program, The Hebrew University of Jerusalem; Candidate, Israel Psychoanalytic Institute.

Phebe Cramer, Ph.D., Professor of Psychology, Williams College.

Diana Diamond, Ph.D., Associate Professor, Clinical Psychology Doctoral Program, Graduate School and University Center, Department of Psychology, City College, City University of New York; Adjunct Assistant Professor of Psychology in Psychiatry, Joan and Sanford I. Weill Medical College of Cornell University.

Louis Diguer, Ph.D., Professor of Psychology, Laval University, Quebec, Canada.

Stephen Fleck, M.D. (deceased), Professor Emeritus, Departments of Psychiatry and Public Health, Yale University School of Medicine.

Peter Fonagy, Ph.D., F.B.A., Freud Memorial Professor of Psychoanalysis and Director of the Sub-Department of Clinical Health Psychology, University College London; Director, Menninger Center for Outcomes and Protocols; Director, Menninger Child and Family Center; Chief Executive Designate, Anna Freud Centre, London; Training and Supervising Analyst (child and adult analysis), British Psycho-Analytical Society.

Norbert Freedman, Ph.D., Professor, Department of Psychiatry, Downstate Medical Center, State University of New York; Training Analyst, Faculty, Director of Research, and Former President, Institute for Psychoanalytic Training and Research (IPTAR), New York, New York; Adjunct Professor, New York University Postdoctoral Program in Psychotherapy and Psychoanalysis.

Robert R. Holt, Ph.D., Emeritus Professor, Department of Psychology, New York University.

Philip S. Holzman, Ph.D. (deceased), Esther and Sidney R. Rabb Professor of Psychology, Emeritus, Harvard University; Training and Supervising Analyst, Boston Psychoanalytic Society and Institute, Boston, Massachusetts.

Joseph Jaffe, M.D., Professor of Clinical Psychiatry in Neurosurgery, College of Physicians and Surgeons, Columbia University; Chief, Department of Communication Sciences, New York State Psychiatric Institute.

Nasreen Khatri, Ph.D., Postdoctoral Fellow, Center for Addiction and Mental Health, Clarke Institute of Psychiatry, Section on Personality and Psychopathology, Toronto, Ontario.

Frank M. Lachmann, Ph.D., Core Faculty, Institute for the Psychoanalytic Study of Subjectivity; Training Analyst, Postgraduate Center for Mental Health, New York, New York.

Howard Lerner, Ph.D., Assistant Clinical Professor of Psychology, Department of Psychiatry, University of Michigan Medical School; Faculty, Michigan Psychoanalytic Institute, Farmington Hills, Michigan.

Kenneth N. Levy, Ph.D., Assistant Professor, Department of Psychology, Pennsylvania State University; Adjunct Assistant Professor, Psychology Section, Department of Psychiatry, Joan and Sanford I. Weill Medical College of Cornell University; Private Practice, State College, Pennsylvania.

Lester Luborsky, Ph.D., Professor of Psychology in Psychiatry, University of Pennsylvania School of Medicine; Faculty, Philadelphia Association for Psychoanalysis.

Laura McCann, M.A., Private Practice, Milltown, New Jersey.

Myriam Mongrain, Ph.D., Associate Professor, Department of Psychology, York University, Toronto, Canada.

Beatriz Priel, Full Professor in Clinical Psychology, Ben Gurion University, Beer Sheva, Israel.

Barry Ritzler, Ph.D., Professor, Department of Psychology, Long Island University, Brooklyn Campus, Brooklyn, New York.

Darcy Santor, Ph.D., Associate Professor, Departments of Psychology and Psychiatry, Dalhouise University, Halifax, Nova Scotia.

Carrie E. Schaffer, Ph.D., Clinical Assistant Professor of Psychiatric Medicine, University of Virginia School of Medicine, Charlottesville, VA; Private Practice, Charlottesville, Virginia; Research Associate, Institute for Psychoanalytic Training and Research (IPTAR) Research Program, New York, New York.

Zindel V. Segal, Ph.D., Associate Professor, Departments of Psychiatry and Psychology, University of Toronto; Head, Cognitive Behavior Therapy Unit, Center for Addiction and Mental Health, and Head, Psychotherapy Research, Psychotherapy Program, Department of Psychiatry, Clarke Institute of Psychiatry, Toronto, Canada.

Morris I. Stein, Ph.D., Emeritus Professor, Department of Psychology, New York University.

Mary Target, Ph.D., Senior Lecturer and Director of the M.Sc. in Theoretical Psychoanalytic Studies, University College London; Professional Director Designate and Academic and Research Organiser of the Doctorate in Child and Adolescent Psychotherapy, Anna Freud Centre, London; Associate Editor, Routledge New Library of Psychoanalysis and Joint Series Editor of the Whurr Series in Psychoanalysis.

Paul L. Wachtel, Ph.D., Distinguished Professor, Clinical Psychology Doctoral Program, Graduate School and University Center, and Department of Psychology, City College, City University of New York; Visiting Clinical Professor, Department of Psychology, New York University; Faculty, New York University Postdoctoral Program in Psychotherapy and Psychoanalysis.

David Zuroff, Ph.D., Professor of Psychology, Department of Psychology, McGill University.

Foreword

Among the various pleasures of an academic career, one stands out – that is, writing the foreword to a book dedicated to one's early graduate student. That is my pleasure now in writing about and for Professor Sidney ("Sid") Jules Blatt.

Sid received his Ph.D. in 1957, when I served as his dissertation chair in the Department of Psychology at the University of Chicago. He selected and developed his thesis, "An Experimental Study of the Problem-Solving Process." It involved a very difficult problem presented in a new apparatus built by John and Rimoldi (1955) and described later by Sid and me (Blatt and Stein 1959). From the very beginning of his work, Sid showed characteristics that would be evident throughout his grand career. First, Sid identified an important problem for his thesis and he approached it in an original and creative manner. Second, he searched the literature thoroughly to develop a proper background for the problem. He presented 101 references in five pages for a thesis that was 148 pages long. His earliest citation was *Science et Méthode* in French, published by Poincaré in 1908, followed by historical references to Titchener in 1909, Ruger in 1910, and Thorndike in 1911. He also integrated the 1945 contributions of Duncker and Wertheimer into his study of the problem-solving process. This was a masterful job. It always has been Sid's inclination to pursue difficult problems and to make them understandable and amenable to solution. This talent has been characteristic throughout his stellar career.

All this brings to mind the titles of the many papers Sid has published. One of these has a title that forewarns readers that they had better know their stuff before reading it. It is titled, "Internalization, Separation-Individuation and the Nature of Therapeutic Action"; another has a kind of poetic ring to it and is succinctly titled "A Cognitive Morphology of Psychopathology"; a third, the last for my purposes here is simply, or not so simply, titled, "Experiences of Depression in Normal Young Adults." In each of these articles one finds oneself immersed in a great deal of clinical sensitivity and wisdom that makes reading the article a great pleasure and a growth experience. In all of his papers, Sid demonstrates the value he places on clarity and significance of contribution to the field.

Within Professor Blatt's writings, one is always likely to come across a novel concept. Space allows only for two instances. In 1989 (reported in 1990), Professor Blatt received the Bruno Klopfer Award during the 50th anniversary of the Society for Personality Assessment. In his acceptance speech, Professor Blatt made a very important statement about "representational processes." He said,

> Interpretations of a Rorschach protocol as a perceptual test are still valid but they are insufficient. The use of the Rorschach . . . can be greatly enhanced if we also consider responses not just as a perceptual experience but as indicating cognitive representational processes . . . .

Then later in the same paragraph, Sid said,

> Most clinicians and clinical researchers would agree that the movement response is a mental representation – it is a result of meaning imposed on or created out of perceptual experiences. The movement response is often so remarkably informative because it is a representational variable.
>
> (Blatt 1990: 402)

In another major contribution, Sid

> conceptualized two primary sources of depression in adults – anaclitic and introjective. Anaclitic depression is related to issues of intense dependency on others for support and gratification, feelings of hunger and depletion, a vulnerability to feelings of deprivation, and difficulty in managing anger for fear of destroying the object and the satisfaction it provides. Introjective feelings of depression involve feelings of guilt, low self-esteem, excessively high standards and morality, a vulnerability to failure and criticism, and a tendency to assume blame and responsibility.
>
> (Blatt, D'Afflitti and Quinlan 1976: 387)

Both of the citations involve major contributions to our understanding of patients. There are so many others that I do not have the space to cover, but the reader would do well to be acquainted with them all. As I began writing this foreword, I reviewed a list of Sid's contributions to the field, and this is what I learned – keeping in mind that this is an incomplete list because Sid is still very actively involved in writing papers, books, talks, etc. Sid has authored or coauthored 10 books and monographs, with another book in press; 143 papers, with seven in press and five in review; eight reviews; and nine unpublished research manuals. It is therefore apparent that Sid is telling the truth when he said in one of his papers, that when his children were growing up, they "had to tolerate a father who was never without his briefcase on vacations" (Blatt 1990: 395). True, his children and his wife Ethel (who is coauthor with Sid on one of his books) had to tolerate this behavior, but it is we who are most fortunate that Sid wrote what he did, for we have learned so much of value from him.

After receiving a B.S. in 1950 and an M.S. in clinical psychology in 1952 from Pennsylvania State University, Sid went on to receive a Ph.D. from the Department of Psychology at the University of Chicago in 1957. In the department, Sid was influenced by Professors Carl Rogers, Joseph Wepman, Samuel Beck, William Henry, Hedda Bolgar, Donald Fiske, and me.

Two years later, he completed a United States Public Health Service postdoctoral fellowship in clinical psychology at the University of Illinois Medical School and the Michael Reese Hospital. In these institutions he studied and worked with Drs Alan Rosenwald, Sheldon Korchin, Erika Fromm, Sara Polka, Mary Engel, Joseph Kepecs, and Roy Grinker, Sr.

In the summer of 1960, as a new assistant professor, he joined the faculty of the Department of Psychology at Yale University, where he met and worked with Roy Schafer and Carl Zimet. In 1961, he began training at the Western New England Institute for Psychoanalysis (WNEIP), where in 1972 he received a certificate in psychoanalysis. He has also had teaching positions at the University of Chicago and in the psychology department of the Hebrew University in Jerusalem, where he held both the chair named in memory of Professor Sigmund Freud and the Alaya and Sam Zacks Professorship in the History of Art. More recently, he was visiting professor at University College London during summers from 1999 to 2003.

Currently, Sid is professor of psychiatry and psychology at Yale University. He is also chief of the Psychology Section at Yale University School of Medicine, and he is a faculty member of the WNEIP.

Not surprisingly, Sid has presented a great many papers at a host of national and international meetings. It is impossible to describe all of Professor Blatt's accomplishments. In his work, he is brilliantly imaginative yet systematic and organized. He is thorough and stays with a problem until he makes eminently good sense. When he concludes his work, it is known that he has made a significant contribution. He always provides a carefully organized bibliography as support for the work he has done. Sid has a great deal of energy that he puts to most effective use by writing about a wide range of important topics. When he presents his ideas to others, he chooses his terms carefully so that they are always to the point. He has built and used a language and a vocabulary that readers can comprehend easily.

I could go on and on describing Sid's ways of thinking and writing, but space is limited. Moreover, I fear that I would only be repetitious, with one positive adjective heaped on another and all well deserved.

In closing, I would like to recall some important events in Sid's life. As I stated previously, when Sid graduated from Pennsylvania State University, he left with a terminal master's degree. He came to Chicago, where he worked in a counseling center. The head of the center (William Gellman) was so impressed with him that he spoke to faculty in the Department of Psychology at the University of Chicago, where he was a graduate student, about arranging for Sid to be admitted to their graduate program. Sid, as we learned, got his Ph.D. there and then spent two years involved in clinical training. Now for the interesting part: Sid is offered a job in the psychology department at Yale. Shortly thereafter, he is accepted for psychoanalytic training at the WNEIP and receives a fellowship from the Foundations Fund for Research in Psychiatry to support his psychoanalytic training. The WNEIP is an unusual institute for the American Psychoanalytic Association because several of the founding members are psychologists (Brenman, Erikson, and Rapaport). Thus, when the American Psychoanalytic Association learns that it is unlawful to exclude psychologists from psychoanalytic training, Sid is now in a fabulous position. He continues his appointments in the psychiatry and psychology departments and is later appointed to the faculty of the WNEIP.

A fantastic career for a great psychologist – Professor Sidney ("Sid") Jules Blatt.

Morris I. Stein, Ph.D.
Professor Emeritus, Psychology
New York University

References

Blatt, S. J. and Stein, M. I. (1959) 'Efficiency in problem solving', *Journal of Psychology* 48: 193–213.

Blatt, S. J., D'Afflitti, J. P., and Quinlan, D. M. (1976) 'Experiences of depression in normal young adults', *Journal of Abnormal Psychology* 85: 383–9.

Blatt, S. J. (1990) 'The Rorschach: a test of perception or an evaluation of representation', *Journal of Personality Assessment* 55: 394–416.

John, E. R. and Rimoldi, H. J. A. (1955) 'Sequential observations of complex reasoning', *American Psychologist* 10: 470 (Abstract).

Acknowledgments

A book is always a collaboration, even when it has but a single author, and even more so when it is an edited collection with three editors. Thus, many people have helped us with this project, and we hope that we will have remembered all of them in this brief statement. If by chance we have forgotten anyone who has helped us along the way, we hope that those persons will forgive us if we fail to mention them. Also, before we turn to our words of thanks, we should say something about how this book came to be. In 1999, at the Annual Spring Meeting of the Division of Psychoanalysis (Division 39) of the American Psychological Association, held that year in New York, Carrie Schaffer and Ken Levy each independently came up with the idea of producing a Festschrift in honor of our mentor, Sidney J. Blatt. Sid had been Carrie's dissertation chair and had sat on Ken's dissertation committee; Ken had also worked for Sid as a research assistant in the 1990s and had continued to work with him on various publications since then, and Carrie had also worked with Sid on several projects besides her dissertation. The two of them approached John Auerbach regarding their proposal. John had worked for Sid as a research assistant in the 1980s and had continued to collaborate with Sid on various publications after his employment with him had ceased; John immediately agreed to participate in editing a Festschrift in Sid's honor. The three of us began work on the present volume in April 2000, with the naïve hope that we could finish the book rather quickly. We now know just exactly how long it actually takes to edit such a book, but that is of minor consequence to us. All three of us have been greatly enriched by our participation in this project. We have worked collaboratively on all aspects of the book and therefore have decided to list our names in alphabetical order to indicate the equality of our contributions.

We are grateful to the many people who have helped us in producing this Festschrift. First, we would like to thank our publisher; Brunner-Routledge, as well as our editor, Kate Hawes, and her editorial assistants, Dominic Hammond and Helen Pritt. This book could not have been completed without their efforts and warm guidance. We are also appreciative of Joan

Cricca and Beverly Abeshouse for their assistance with Dr. Stephen Fleck's manuscript and to Joan Cricca yet again for a variety of clerical matters too numerous to list. We, along with the publisher, would like to thank the following for their kind permission to reproduce copyrighted material: Analytic Press, Beatrice Beebe, Frank Lachmann, and Joseph Jaffe for Chapter 2 ('A Dyadic Systems View of Communication'); and Scandinavian University Press, Gyldendal Akademisk, and Stephen Fleck for Chapter 7 ('The Development of Schizophrenia: A Psychosocial and Biological Approach'). We must of course thank the many friends and colleagues who contributed chapters to this volume – without them, there could be no Festschrift – and the many friends and colleagues who kept this project a secret from Sid for two years while we designed the book and found contributors and a publisher. We are perhaps most thankful to the many people in our lives who put up with the long hours we spent editing this Festschrift.

In conjunction with this Festschrift, a symposium in Sid's honor was held on Saturday, 13 April 2002, at the 22nd Annual Spring Meeting of Division 39. We would like to thank the Psychoanalytic Research Society (Section VI) of Division 39 for sponsoring the symposium. In connection with this panel, special thanks are due to Stephen H. Portuges, who was then president of Section VI, and to the presenters that day: Diana Diamond and Paul Wachtel, as well as Morris Eagle, who graciously agreed to read Paul's paper when personal business necessitated Paul's being out of town. A reception followed the symposium, and we would like to thank the following organizations for their generous support: Sections I (Psychologist-Psychoanalyst Practitioners) and VI of Division 39, the Departments of Psychology and Psychiatry at Yale University, the Austen Riggs Center, the Connecticut Society for Psychoanalytic Psychology (CSPP), the Institute for Psychoanalytic Training and Research (IPTAR), the Society for Personality Assessment (SPA), the Sigmund Freud Center at the Hebrew University of Jerusalem, and the Western New England Psychoanalytic Society.

To Dr. Sidney Blatt, we owe our deepest gratitude. We have been fortunate to have a distinguished mentor in you, and we thankfully acknowledge your exceptional guidance, warm support, and invaluable advice. We are grateful to have had the opportunity to learn from your generous teachings and feel so very privileged to have worked with you. With warmth and an engaging style you have consistently provided incisive feedback on our work and invaluable advice about our careers. Over the years, you have acted as a mentor, through teaching and instruction, through encouragement and faith, but most of all through example. You have been a remarkable example of how to combine clinical insights with academic scholarship and, similarly, how to integrate research findings into clinical work and teaching. You have provided us with a model of the kind of psychologist we hope and strive to be. Your genuine interests and enthusiasm for psychology is infectious and inspiring, and your keen clinical insights have been a great inspiration for each of us in our own ways. In our work with you, we gained knowledge of a broad range of areas within psychology and came to recognize research as a way of answering critical questions regarding human experience. More importantly, for each of us, the experience of working with you contributed to a subtle, yet cumulatively powerful, evolution in our experiences of personal efficacy, our capacities for intimacy, and our abilities to parlay our interests into productive directions. Thank you for all that you have done on our behalf. We know we are not alone in our sentiments, but we are truly appreciative.

Chapter 1

Introduction

The contributions of Sidney J. Blatt

John S. Auerbach, Kenneth N. Levy, and Carrie E. Schaffer

Within the field the field of clinical psychology, contributors who are both psychoanalysts and leading empirical researchers are, epidemiologically speaking, increasingly rare, and contributors who are analysts, researchers, and leading personality theorists are rarer still. Yet one figure who has made extensive contributions as an analytic clinician, as a researcher, and as a theoretician is Sidney J. Blatt, professor of psychiatry and psychology at Yale University and, for more than 35 years now, chief of the Psychology Section in Yale University's Department of Psychiatry. In his long, distinguished career, Dr. Blatt (Sid, as we prefer to call him) has been a leading figure in both empirical psychology and psychoanalysis. In addition to being trained as a psychoanalyst, he has conducted extensive research on personality development, psychological assessment, psychopathology, and psychotherapeutic outcomes. He is considered an expert in the areas of mental representation (e.g., Blatt 1995b; Blatt, Auerbach and Levy 1997) and internalization (e.g., Behrends and Blatt 1985; Blatt and Behrends 1987), as well as on the Rorschach Inkblot Test (e.g, Allison, Blatt and Zimet 1968; Blatt 1990). He has studied extensively the differences between relational and self-definitional forms of depression (Blatt 1974; Blatt and Shichman 1983) and was doing so years before cognitive-behavioral theorist Aaron Beck (1983) proposed the similar distinction of sociotropy versus autonomy. Along with his many students and colleagues, he has developed several widely used measures, both self-report and projective, for assessing depressive style (i.e., relational versus self-definitional), self- and object representations, and boundary disturbances in thought disorder. Among these methods is a projective technique, the Object Relations Inventory (ORI), for collecting descriptions of self and significant others (Blatt *et al.* 1979).[1] Thus each year sees the completion of approximately 20 psychology dissertations in which his measures are used. A man of broad intellectual interests, he has also written a book on the implications of psychoanalytic and Piagetian developmental theories for art history (Blatt and Blatt 1984). In short, Sid has been a wide-ranging and productive scholar in a career of more than 40 years' duration, and throughout this career, he has been committed to the proposition that it is not only possible but also essential to investigate psychoanalytically derived hypotheses through rigorous empirical science. Equally important is that, in those 40 years, he has been committed to training students who also hold to the perspective that psychoanalytic ideas can be validated and refined through empirical test, and we, as editors of this volume, constitute a testament to that commitment. Indeed, it is particularly important that one of the contributors to this book, Paul Wachtel, was Sid's first dissertation student and that one of its editors, Carrie Schaffer, was his most recent.

For these many reasons, not least of which is his personal influence on all of us as a mentor and teacher, we believe that a volume honoring Sid Blatt's many contributions to both psychoanalysis and clinical psychology is long overdue. The present Festschrift volume is our attempt not only to honor these contributions but also to disseminate them more broadly within both psychoanalysis, where empirical research is increasingly neglected, and clinical psychology, where psychoanalysis is increasingly ignored.

Sidney J. Blatt: a biography in brief

A Philadelphia native and the oldest of three children, Sid was born October 15, 1928, to Harry and Fannie Blatt. Sid was raised in modest circumstances. He grew up in a Jewish family in South Philadelphia, where his father owned a sweet shop and where his family lived in the apartment upstairs. But this statement does not fully capture the nature of Sid's background. According to Sid, his father was the third child born to Sid's grandmother, but this woman died, perhaps in childbirth, when Sid's father was just three or four years old. Sid's grandfather then married a woman who had three children of her own by a previous marriage, and the new marriage in turn produced three more children. In consequence, Sid's father was raised in circumstances marked by maternal loss and economic poverty. He was forced, as the eldest son, to leave school after the sixth grade to help support his family, with its numerous half-siblings and step-siblings, although Sid recalls him as an intelligent man who worked hard, running his store seven days a week, 16 hours a day, and who read widely in the left-wing press.

One memory of his father was particularly important to Sid. He recalls that every year he would accompany his father to the cemetery where his grandmother, his father's mother, was buried, and there Sid would hold his father's hand and attempt to console him as his father wept over the grave. Sid also recalls that, at age 13, he accompanied his mother on a painful two-hour bus trip to New Jersey as she responded to an urgent phone call informing her that her father had just suffered a heart attack. He tried to reassure and console his mother during the trip while she, correctly anticipating her father's death, grieved his loss. Regarding these memories of his childhood, Sid says that it is no surprise that he eventually was to become interested in studying depressive experiences that focus on separation and loss. Another interesting facet of Sid's childhood is that, contrary to the (positive) stereotype about Jews and education, Sid was the only child of his parents to attend college. Sid was intellectually inclined from fairly early in life and recalls being moved when he saw Rodin's sculpture, *The Thinker*, at the Rodin Museum in Philadelphia. Nevertheless, his postsecondary education was not a foregone conclusion, given his family's difficult economic situation, but in addition, his parents were divided as to his academic ambitions. Sid recalls that his mother supported him in this goal but that his father was more skeptical. Indeed an emotional connection to his mother and a more distant relationship with his father may have been an important part of Sid's childhood. He recalls that, at age 9, he became disillusioned with his father for failing to support him in what he describes as some minor but symbolically important matter. Sid decided to run away from home. He defiantly packed his bags and walked out of the house. He had gone no more than a few blocks when he became aware that he could not remember what his mother looked like; he ran home in a panic. Sid says that this terrifying memory may be one of the roots of his lifelong interest in the mental representation of the important people in one's life.

Despite these childhood struggles, Sid eventually enrolled at the Pennsylvania State University in 1946. From that institution, he was to obtain both his bachelor's and his master's degrees. It was between his sophomore and junior years of college that he was introduced, by one of his fraternity brothers, to Ethel Shames, the woman who later became his wife. Sid recalls that his fraternity house provided cheap lodging and also a source of income; he washed dishes in the kitchen. In any case, he and Ethel dated for a few years and finally married on February 1, 1951, while he was in his master's program. He and Ethel were eventually to have three children, Susan (b. 1952), Judy (b. 1959), and David (b. 1963). Regarding the role that Ethel has played in his life, Sid also says that all of his professional accomplishments would have been impossible without her. He specifically mentions that, when they married, Ethel had been attending Temple University on a Senatorial Scholarship (i.e., a special academic scholarship for residents of Pennsylvania). When they married, she resigned her scholarship, left school, and went to work to support him. After the birth of their first child, she earned money by taking in typing jobs. Sid observes that Ethel would say that, when it came to career choices, he has always picked the one with the greatest opportunity and the least remuneration; this, Sid adds, is how he wound up at Yale. In any case, Sid says that, without Ethel's support, he never would have completed his Ph.D., and he adds that Ethel did not finish her own college education until 1976, when the children were finally old enough for her to return to school. She obtained a bachelor's degree in art history at Southern Connecticut State University

(SCSU) in Hamden, Connecticut, a suburb of New Haven. True to pattern, it was the discussions between Ethel and Sid regarding her college courses that led many years later to their book on cognitive-developmental theory and spatial representation in the history of art (Blatt and Blatt 1984).

Sid's interest in psychoanalysis began in high school with his reading of Freud's (1916–17) *Introductory Lectures on Psycho-Analysis*. Fascinated by Freud's descriptions of unconscious processes, Sid decided to become a psychiatrist and psychoanalyst and thus majored in chemistry and physics at Penn State, with a plan to apply to medical school. Unfortunately, Sid failed a double-credit organic chemistry course in his junior year at Penn State because of problems with a year-long laboratory project that he later learned, after he switched his major to psychology, were the result of red-green color blindness, a condition that, until then, he did not know he had. As a result, he had misperceived the color of his laboratory results. Despite this setback, Sid excelled as a psychology major and received A grades in all of the psychology courses that he took during his senior year.

Not surprisingly, it was as a psychology major at Penn State that Sid extended his earlier interests in psychoanalysis to an emerging interest in projective testing. But unfortunately, these emerging interests led to conflicts with some of the faculty there. For example, as an undergraduate, he took an abnormal psychology course taught by George Guthrie, a young faculty member who had recently earned his Ph.D. from the University of Minnesota. The professor gave a group Rorschach to the class with the intent of demonstrating how misguided the test was, but instead of rejecting the procedure, Sid was intrigued by how much his responses revealed about himself. Sid then had difficulty getting into the Penn State graduate program in psychology. While finishing his senior year, he applied twice for admission and twice was turned down. Then, with only a short time to go before the start of the 1950 academic year, he applied once again and this time was accepted. He surmises that a spot had come open at the last minute and that this was why the psychology department accepted him. In 1952, he was given a terminal master's degree, although he received honors for his thesis, a paper that was later published in *Archives of General Psychiatry* (Blatt 1959).

Sid then moved to Chicago, where he had taken a position as a counselor with the Jewish Vocational Service (JVS). At JVS, the facility director, William Gelman, who was attending the University of Chicago, thought that Sid would be a good student for the doctoral program. Sid called the psychology department and spoke to Charlotte Ellis, the graduate student adviser. He explained that he would be an atypical student who needed to work a few days a week, and she helped him to put together a schedule. From 1952 through 1954, Sid worked without vacation and accrued 66 days of leave. In 1954–5, therefore, he was able to take off two days each week, Tuesday and Thursday, from his job so that he could attend classes.

Unfortunately, in making this plan, he had not considered the cost of the tuition at the University of Chicago; whereas the cost of attending Penn State had been $40 for the year, it was $1000, a considerable sum of money in those days, to attend the University of Chicago. Sid recalls that he had to take a loan from the university that then took him years to repay. In 1955, he took his preliminary examination and earned a high enough score on the exam that he was awarded a fellowship from the National Institute of Mental Health (NIMH). With this fellowship and a research assistantship with Morris I. Stein, he was able to leave his job at JVS and go to school full time. His parents, he recalled, were furious that he, a married man with a child, had left his job to go to school full time, but with his fellowship and his research assistantship, Sid was able to complete his Ph.D. in 1957.

As regards his academic and intellectual development at the University of Chicago, Sid found the "U of C an intellectual paradise" where he maintained an ever increasing list of "must read books and articles." He did his predoctoral internship, in 1955 and 1956, under the supervision of Carl Rogers, whom he still describes 40 years later, even after his analytic training, as a profound influence on his psychotherapeutic approach. From Rogers, he learned the crucial importance of empathy – of understanding how his patients experienced the world and of framing his therapeutic interventions from the patient's standpoint. He also worked, as noted, as research assistant for Morris I. Stein, who had been a student of Henry Murray's at Harvard. Stein, who emphasized projective techniques in his research on creativity, eventually served as the chair of Sid's dissertation ("An Experimental Study of the Problem Solving Process"), completed in 1957 and eventually published in the *Journal of Psychology* (Blatt and Stein 1959). Additionally, Sid had the opportunity there to take testing courses from Samuel Beck. Sid's recollection was that Beck's knowledge of the Rorschach was in fact brilliant but that Beck often could not articulate the rationale for his conclusions and, when challenged about them, would eventually appeal simply to his clinical experience. These appeals to clinical experience left Sid distinctly unsatisfied because, as a beginner, he could not learn how to arrive at the same inferences himself.

In 1957, Sid began a postdoctoral fellowship at the University of Illinois Medical School and at Michael Reese Hospital's Psychiatric and Psychosomatic Institute (PPI), then headed by Roy Grinker, Sr. At the University of Illinois, Sid fell under the tutelage of Alan Rosenwald, a Sullivanian whom he considered a brilliant Rorschacher, and at PPI, he worked with Mary Engel and Sarah Kennedy Polka, both of whom had been trained in the Rapaport system at the Menninger Clinic, and also with Sheldon Korchin, who was chief psychologist. It was the Rapaport system that gave Sid the theoretical understanding of the Rorschach that Beck, only a few years earlier, simply could not give him at the University of Chicago, and it was Rapaport's ideas in general that gave Sid his first theoretical understanding of the workings of the mind, a way of linking motivation and cognition. Sid says that thoughout his graduate training he regarded Rapaport's (1951) *Organization and Pathology of Thought* as his academic Torah and Talmud.

After having finished his postdoctoral training, Sid worked as a staff psychologist at Michael Reese for a year, and then, when Sheldon Korchin left to go to NIMH, he was offered the job of chief psychologist. This was an offer that Sid decided he could not accept because it would mean supervising people who a year earlier had been his teachers. Instead, in 1960, he decided to leave Chicago and to join the Department of Psychology at Yale University as an assistant professor; he was also accepted for analytic training at the Western New England Institute for Psychoanalysis (WNEIP). Situated nowadays mainly in New Haven, the WNEIP at that time was centered in both Stockbridge, Massachusetts, and New Haven, and Sid hoped to have a chance to work directly with Rapaport, who had in 1948 moved east from the Menninger Clinic to the Austen Riggs Center and whose intellectual contributions Sid had come to admire enormously. Rapaport died suddenly on December 14, 1960. Although crestfallen at the loss of this opportunity, Sid had already established a relationship with Roy Schafer, his Yale faculty colleague, who in 1961 had completed his own analytic training at the WNEIP. From Schafer, who had coauthored Rapaport's magnum opus on psychological testing (Rapaport, Gill and Schafer 1945–6) and who had worked extensively with Rapaport at both the Menninger Clinic and Austen Riggs, Sid learned in greater depth the subtleties of Rapaport's thinking. In July 1963, after his friend and colleague Carl Zimet left New Haven for a faculty position in Colorado, Sid became chief of the psychiatry department's Psychology Section and had half of his time reassigned from the Department of Psychology to the Department of Psychiatry. Eventually, he would be spending almost all of his time in psychiatry, rather than psychology, and that is where he spends most of his time today.

From 1965 through 1968, Sid was also director of psychology at the newly established Connecticut Mental Health Center in the Department of Psychiatry at Yale University School of Medicine. Meanwhile, he continued his analytic training at the WNEIP. He recalls that his analyst, William Pious, was considered a maverick within the institution, and this reputation surely must have appealed to Sid, whose life history thus far had shown him to have a rebellious spirit and who, as a psychologist in an institute of the American Psychoanalytic Association, an organization at the time quite hostile to nonmedical analysts, must have felt himself to be a bit of an outsider. In addition, there was the considerable expense of analytic training with which to contend, but Sid was awarded a fellowship for psychoanalytic training by the Foundations Fund for Research in Psychiatry, and he supplemented this award by teaching evening courses at Southern Connecticut. In 1972, he completed his analytic training at the WNEIP.

Since then, Sid has had numerous professional honors. In 1973 and again in 1977 and in 1982, he was a visiting fellow at the Hampstead Child Therapy Clinic in London, England. His third stay there coincided, sadly, with the death of Anna Freud. In 1977, he was a visiting fellow at the Tavistock Centre, also in London, and that same year, he was in addition a visting scholar at the Warburg Institute of Renaissance Studies, at University College London, where he had the opportunity to work with Ernst Gombrich, and this relationship was crucial to the art history book that Sid and Ethel were later to write. From 1978 through 1989, he was a senior research associate at the Austen Riggs Center, and from this involvement came his book (Blatt and Ford 1994) on the process of change in long-term inpatient treatment. In 1988 and 1989, he was Sigmund Freud Professor at the Hebrew University of Jerusalem. At the Hebrew University of Jerusalem, he was also director of the Sigmund Freud Center for Psycho-analytic Study and Research, Ayala and Sam Zacks Professor of Art History, and a Fulbright Senior Research Fellow. In 1989, he was awarded the Society for Personality Assessment's Bruno Klopfer Award for Distinguished Contributions to Personality Assessment. Over the years, he has also served as a visiting professor at the Ben Gurion University of the Negev in Beer Sheva, Israel, the Nova Southeastern University in Fort Lauderdale, Florida, the Menninger Foundation in Topeka, Kansas, University College London, and the Catholic University of Leuven in Belgium. As Stein (this volume) records in the foreword to this Festschrift, he is the author or coauthor of more than 170 publications. In short, even in his mid-70s, Sid remains not only a renowned but a productive, generative, and creative psychologist, and this Festschrift is a testimony to his continuing influence, even in a biological and cognitive-behavioral age, as a psychoanalytic psychologist.

Sidney J. Blatt: intellectual contributions

When he arrived at Yale in the early 1960s, Sid, inspired by the pioneering efforts of Rapaport et al. (1945–6), focused his research efforts on psycho-dynamic interpretation of IQ testing (Blatt and Allison 1968). Although his Rapaportian approach to psychological testing (see Allison et al. 1968) reflected his interest in the relationship between cognitive processes and personality organization, as well as in the role of representational processes in both psychopathology and normal psychological functioning, the areas of work for which he was to become best known lay ahead. These were to include his model of representational development and psychopathology (Blatt 1991, 1995b; Blatt et al. 1997), his various unstructured techniques and rating scales for assessing representational aspects of object relations (e.g., Bers et al. 1993; Blatt, Brenneis et al. 1976; Blatt et al. 1979, 1988; Blatt, Bers and Schaffer 1992; Diamond et al. 1990, 1991), the two-configurations model of personality and psychopathology (Blatt 1974; Blatt and Blass 1992,

1996; Blatt and Shichman 1983), and the Depressive Experiences Questionnaire (Blatt, D'Afflitti and Quinlan 1976) for measuring the types of depression (anaclitic or relational and introjective or self-definitional). In essence, it may be said that underlying all of his thinking regarding personality development and psychopathology are two basic conceptual schemes, the cognitive-representational and two-configurations models. But although Sid's interest, influenced by Piaget and Werner, in the links between development and representation, was already evident in his early research, it was with his two-configurations approach to psychopathology, depression in particular, that he finally came into his intellectual own.

In 1972, as mentioned, Sid completed his psychoanalytic training, and his experiences with two of his control cases led him to formulate the anaclitic-introjective distinction (Blatt 1974). Although each of these two control cases at the WNEIP suffered from depression, one of them proved to be highly self-critical and guilt ridden, with much suicidal ideation, and the other emerged as highly dependent, wanting nurturance and desperately seeking emotional contact. From these clinical experiences, Sid proposed in 1974 that some depressed patients, whom he termed *introjective* because of their excessive superego introjects, are focused mainly on self-criticism, guilt, failure, and a need for achievement and that others, whom he termed *anaclitic* because of their need to lean on others for emotional support, are concerned mainly with loss, separation, abandonment, and a need for emotional contact. In later writings, Sid expanded this classification to apply to other forms of psychopathology (Blatt and Shichman 1983), as well as to normal personality development (Blatt and Blass 1990, 1992, 1996). As he expanded the scope of this model, he also became interested in attachment theory, primarily as a result of the influence of younger colleagues (see, e.g., Diamond and Blatt 1994; Levy, Blatt and Shaver 1998; Schaffer 1993), and his terminology shifted from anaclitic and introjective, both terms deriving from psychoanalytic theory, to the more inclusive distinction between *attachment* or *relatedness* on the one hand and *separateness* or *self-definition* on the other (e.g., Blass and Blatt, 1992, 1996; Blatt and Blass 1990, 1992, 1996; Blatt *et al.* 1997). Thus, this tension between relatedness and self-definition has been central to Sid's understanding of human life.

As he was formulating his theoretical ideas about the two-configurations model, Sid recognized that his theories needed grounding in empirical evidence. He and his colleagues developed the DEQ (Blatt *et al.* 1976), a self-report scale, and found that this structured questionnaire assesses the two types of depression, anaclitic (or dependent) and introjective (or self-critical), posited by his theories. The measure has now been validated in numerous studies (see Blatt 2004; Blatt and Zuroff 1992; Zuroff 1994; Zuroff, Quinlan and Blatt 1990), and an adolescent version of the measure has also been constructed (Blatt, Schaffer *et al.* 1992).

But although Sid is perhaps best known for his work on the two-configurations model, he has always developed his cognitive-representational understanding of personality and psychopathology in conjunction with his understanding of relatedness and self-definition, and this is evident even in the paper in which he first conceptualized the anaclitic-introjective distinction (1974). Much of that article is devoted to the delineation of a Piaget-influenced cognitive model of personality development. Briefly, in that article, Sid proposed that personality development proceeds from a sensorimotor-enactive stage, in which a person's object relations are dominated by concerns with need gratification and frustration, through a concrete perceptual stage, in which object relations are based on what the other looks like, an external iconic phase, in which object relations involve mainly what others do, an internal iconic phase, in which object relations involve mainly what others think and feel, and finally, a conceptual stage, in which all previous levels are integrated into a complex, coherent understanding of significant others. Sid was to use this model in developing the Conceptual Level (CL) scale for rating open-ended descriptions of parents and other significant figures. Sid linked these Piagetian ideas, together with concepts from Fraiberg (1969), A. Freud (1965), Jacobson (1964), and Mahler (e.g, 1968), in developing his views on boundary disturbances in Rorschach thought disorders. Specifically, he (Blatt and Ritzler 1974; Blatt, Wild and Ritzler 1975; Blatt and Wild 1976) argued, on the basis of research on disordered verbalization on the Rorschach, that thought disorder involves disturbances in the representation of psychological boundaries and that these disturbances are most severe in schizophrenia and less severe but still present in the diagnostic class that we have come to know as borderline personality organization. Sid and his colleagues (Blatt, Brenneis *et al.* 1976) used similar developmental concepts, mainly Werner's (1957; Werner and Kaplan 1963) ideas about differentiation, articulation, and integration in development, in the construction of the Concept of the Object Scale (COS) for Rorschach protocols. The theoretical assumptions underlying this scale, like those underlying the CL scale and Sid's work on boundary disturbances are that cognitive development and the development of object relations occur in parallel and that the emergence of psychopathology is closely linked to disturbances in the development of object relations and cognitive organization.

Gradually, therefore, Sid (Blatt 1974, 1991, 1995b; Blatt *et al.* 1997; Blatt and Blass 1990, 1992, 1996; Blatt and Shichman 1983) articulated a comprehensive, integrated model of personality development, psychopathology and therapeutic change. He referred to his model as a "cognitive morphology" (Blatt 1991) of normal and pathological development (see also Blatt 1995b; Blatt and Shichman 1983). In other words, using cognitive-developmental theory, psychoanalytic object relations theory, and, in his later work (e.g., Blatt 1995b; Blatt *et al.* 1997) attachment theory, Sid identified several central nodal points in the development of mental representations and delineated the relevance of these nodal points for personality development and psychopathology. Specifically, he proposed that, in the first three months of life, the chief psychological achievement is the formation of boundary constancy and that disruption of the establishment of intact cognitive-perceptual boundaries between independent objects is involved in many of the clinical features of schizophrenia. In the second six months of life, meanwhile, the primary psychological achievement is the formation of recognition constancy – i.e., the ability to recognize psychological objects, regardless of their emotional valence – and the emergence of this cognitive capacity at age 8 or 9 months, Sid theorizes, is an essential aspect of the development of interpersonal attachments. Then, in the second year of life, by age 16 to 18 months, the chief psychological achievement is the emergence of evocative constancy – the capacity to evoke the presence of a significant other in that other's absence. According to this model, severe disturbances in evocative constancy underlie borderline personality organization, and less severe disturbances in this capacity are linked to various levels of depressive psychopathology. In the third year of life, by approximately age 30 to 36 months, the child develops self and object constancy and therefore begins to understand the difference between the perspective of the self and the perspective of others. The consolidation of self and object constancy is, in this view, a precondition for the establishment, later in life, of a cohesive identity and mature object relations (see Blatt *et al.* 1996, 1998). In the fifth year of life, the child enters the world of concrete operational thought, and parallel to this cognitive achievement is the interpersonal ability to coordinate the perspectives of three participants in a triangular relationship; this capacity is necessary for the child's object relations to progress from preoedipal to oedipal configurations and, as regards psychopathology, underlies the classical neuroses. In early adolescence, formal operational thought emerges, and with it comes the capacity to appreciate the inner or psychological attributes of both self and other. Formal operational thought is necessary, per Erikson's (1963) theories, for identity formation and the development of the capacities for intimacy, generativity, and integrity, the adult stages of maturation.

What makes Sid's contribution here particularly powerful is that he uses this model to understand both normal and pathological psychological phenomena, and indeed his cognitive morphology underlies his analysis of the history of art (Blatt and Blatt 1984) as well. Furthermore, unlike many psychoanalytic thinkers, he does not use reductionistic concepts like fixation or developmental arrest to describe the developmental processes underlying psychopathology. Instead, using an epigenetic model derived from Bowlby (1973) and Waddington (1957), he recognizes that psychopathology arises from developmental deviations, in which maturation veers off from a central developmental line involving the integration of relational and self-definitional capacities and motivations, with pathology reflecting the overemphasis of one set of tendencies, as opposed to the other. Furthermore, following the ideas of Erikson (1963), Sid has extended his developmental model all the way from infancy to senescence, but recognizing that Erikson's model overemphasizes separation, individuation, and self-definition (i.e., autonomy versus shame and doubt, initiative versus guilt, industry versus inferiority, identity versus role diffusion, generativity versus stagnation, and integrity versus despair) at the expense of relatedness (trust versus mistrust, and intimacy versus isolation), he proposed interpolating another relational stage between those of initiative versus guilt and of industry versus inferiority in the Eriksonian model. In his first formulation of this idea, Sid termed this new stage mutuality versus competition (Blatt and Shichman 1983), and in his later writings, he referred to it as cooperation versus alienation (Blatt 1995b; Blatt and Blass 1990, 1992, 1996). His thinking here was that Freud's oedipal stage involved not only the fear of punishment for guilty wishes and competitive strivings but also the establishment of cooperative relationships in spite of relational conflict, not only self-definition but also relatedness.

In his most recent work (e.g., Blatt 1995b; Blatt *et al.* 1997; Blatt and Levy 2003; Diamond and Blatt 1994; Levy *et al.* 1998), Sid has reconceptualized his model of cognitive-affective development in terms of attachment theory. Thus, he has recognized that self-definitional forms of psychopathology most likely derive from avoidant forms of attachment and that relational forms of psychopathology derive from resistant forms of attachment (e.g., Blatt 1995a; Blatt and Levy 2003). Having already theorized that self-definitional and relational personality organizations have diverging cognitive styles, ideational and precise versus affective and global (Blatt and Shichman 1983), Sid has increasingly delineated connections between his model of cognitive-affective development and that proposed by Main (e.g., Main, Kaplan and Cassidy 1985) as a result of her work with the Adult Attachment Interview (see Blatt 1995a, 1995b; Blatt *et al.* 1997). Thus, he increasingly sees the cognitive styles associated with various forms of psychopathology as reflecting basic attachment processes, and he has come to view the construction of object representations as rooted in the development of intersubjectivity and of a theory of mind (e.g., Auerbach and Blatt 1996, 2001, 2002; Blatt *et al.* 1996, 1998; Diamond *et al.* 1990). From this perspective, psychological maturity involves the capacity fully to appreciate the thoughts, wishes, and feelings of intimate others without losing one's own autonomous perspective. In other words, maturity involves a dialectical and dynamic balance between relatedness and self-definition.

Finally, as regards Sid's professional career, the last several years have seen him contribute to the literature on psychotherapeutic processes and outcomes, and this is unusual because so much of his work is theoretical, focused on issues of personality, personality development, and psychopathology, rather than on concrete questions like what changes in treatment and how. Nevertheless, following from his argument that there are clear differences between persons focused on relational issues and those who emphasize self-definitional issues, Sid has attempted to demonstrate that relationally oriented and self-definitionally oriented persons have differential responses to psychotherapy. Thus, in his reanalysis of Wallerstein's (1986) Menninger Psychotherapy Research Project (Blatt 1992), Sid found that self-critical patients responded better to psychoanalysis, with its couch and its increased distance between patient and analyst, and that dependent patients responded better to psychotherapy, with the increased support provided by the face-to-face therapeutic relationship. Meanwhile, in his study of therapeutic change in long-term inpatient treatment at Austen Riggs (Blatt and Ford 1994), Sid found that dependent patients changed most with regard to interpersonal functioning while self-critical patients, who tend to be ideational, rather than affective, in their orientation to the world, showed change primarily through improved cognitive functioning and decreased thought disorder. Most important, however, has been a series of reanalyses by Sid and his colleagues (e.g., Blatt et al. 1995, 1996, 1998; Shahar et al. 2003, in press; Zuroff et al. 2000) of the NIMH Treatment of Depression Collaborative Research Program (TDCRP). Using the Dysfunctional Attitude Scale (DAS; Weissman and Beck 1978), Sid and his colleagues identified two factors in psychological functioning within the sample – perfectionism, which might otherwise be termed self-criticism, and need for approval, which might otherwise be termed dependence. They found that, regardless of the form of psychotherapy used (i.e., cognitive-behavioral, interpersonal, medication, and placebo), perfectionism had a negative effect on clinical outcome in short-term treatment of depression, presumably because patients with high standards were unlikely to resolve their problems after just 15 or 20 psychotherapy sessions. These findings prompted Blatt (1995a) to argue that one clinical group that would definitely need long-term treatment to effect change would be those he had identified as introjective or self-critical. In other words, these research findings suggested not only that personality differences are important in response to psychotherapy but also that the short-term treatments imposed on psychotherapy patients by managed care might have significant countertherapeutic effects on those patients who are high in perfectionism.

An overview of this book

In this volume, we present contributions from Sid's colleagues and students. In their various chapters, they address the main areas in which Sid has focused his intellectual endeavors: personality development, psychopathology, assessment, psychotherapy, and applied psychoanalysis. This book is therefore divided into five parts.

Part I of the book will focus on personality development. It was in his seminal 1974 paper, "Levels of Object Representation in Anaclitic and Introjective Depression," that Sid first articulated his theoretical position on personality development. In his writings, Sid posits that psychological development involves two primary maturational tasks: (a) the establishment of stable, enduring, mutually satisfying interpersonal relationships and (b) the achievement of a differentiated, stable, and cohesive identity. Normal maturation involves a complex reciprocal transaction between these two developmental lines throughout the life cycle. For instance, meaningful and satisfying relationships contribute to the evolving concept of the self, and a new sense of self leads, in turn, to more mature levels of interpersonal relatedness. Thus, Sid presents what he terms the *two-configurations model* of personality development. He also ties these two developmental lines to specific nodal points in the development of mental representations. The chapters in this part (by Beebe, Lachmann and Jaffe, by Priel, and by Freedman) will examine the implications of Sid's ideas for personality development and functioning. In their contribution, Beebe *et al.* describe mother–infant interaction, so crucial to psychological development, as a dyadic communicative system. They also review the research literature in support of their perspective. Priel reviews research documenting how object representations develop in middle childhood through children's interactions with their parents. She also discusses the role of adoption in the construction of children's object representations. Freedman, meanwhile, discusses the roles of space and spatialization in the development of object relations and representations. In arguing his case, he integrates research literature with his clinical experience.

Part II will focus on psychopathology. In his many writings, Sid explicates the relationship between the two lines of personality development described above and two corresponding types of depression: (a) an interpersonally oriented (anaclitic) depression characterized by dependency, fears of abandonment, and feelings of helplessness and (b) a self-evaluative (introjective) depression characterized by self-criticism and feelings of unworthiness. He also theorized that schizophrenia can be divided into nonparanoid and paranoid subtypes on the basis of the two-configurations model. During the past two decades, Sid's original formulations regarding anaclitic (dependent) and introjective (self-critical) lines of development and the role of impaired and distorted representations of self and others have been expanded into a broader model of psychopathology. Additionally, Sid has proposed that level of psychopathology is associated with cognitive developmental level, such that, for example, schizophrenia is associated with impaired boundary representation, borderline states are linked to disturbances in evocative constancy, and higher-level, neurotic disturbances require the establishment of self and object constancy. The chapters in this part (by Zuroff, Santor and Mongrain, by Khatri and Segal, by Fleck, and by Cramer) will examine the contributions of Sid's theoretical model for understanding psychopathology. Thus, Zuroff *et al.* present research evidence in support of the specificity hypothesis – i.e., that dependent persons become depressed in response to separation and loss and that self-critical persons become depressed in response to failures in achievement. In their contribution, Khatri and Segal compare and contrast Sid's personality typology (anaclitic or dependent versus introjective or self-critical) with Aaron Beck's (sociotropy versus autonomy) in the understanding of depression. Fleck's contribution is an attempt, in this age of biological psychiatry, to demonstrate the complex interaction of psychosocial and constitutional factors in the etiology of schizophrenia. His views are consistent with Sid's regarding the link between psychosocial factors and the underlying cognitive disturbances in schizophrenia. They are also consistent with Sid's views on the essential role of long-term psychosocial treatment in the care of severely disturbed patients. Cramer, meanwhile, reviews her research with Sid, part of the study of therapeutic change at Austen Riggs, on defense mechanisms in severe psychopathology and also presents data on how defense mechanisms interact with intelligence in predicting patients' responses to psychotherapeutic treatment.

Part III will focus on issues in psychological testing and assessment. Throughout his career, Sid has been a major contributor to the research, clinical, and theoretical literature on projective assessment. He views the Rorschach and other projective techniques as methods through which both clinicians and researchers could gain access to the unconscious mental representations that he regarded as central to both normal functioning and psychopathology. He is also particularly interested in the assessment of object relations, once again in both normal and pathological functioning, and in the assessment of thought disorder. The three chapters in this part therefore address the three topics that have been most central to Sid's concerns regarding the Rorschach: mental representations (Ritzler), object relations (Lerner), and thought disorder in schizophrenia (Holzman). Ritzler's main focus is on Sid's contributions to the use of projective instruments in the measurement of object representations. He summarizes a complex research literature in this area. Lerner's overlapping chapter discusses the theoretical and empirical literature pertaining to the implications of the Rorschach Inkblot Test for an understanding of object relations. Finally, in this part, Holzman discusses his research on the use of Rorschach thought disorder measures to differentiate among forms of psychosis, schizophrenic versus manic. He demonstrates that the Rorschach, an often maligned instrument, in fact provides a very effective means of differentiating among major classes of psychopathology.

Part IV will focus on psychotherapy and the treatment process. The main thrust of Sid's work in this area concerns two issues: (a) the implications of assessing mental representations and changes in representations for the study of the therapeutic process; and (b) the implications of the two-configurations model for current understandings of psychotherapeutic processes and outcomes. In this part, chapters by Fonagy and Target and by Luborsky, Andrusyna and Diguer will address issues of representations in the psychotherapeutic process. Fonagy and Target argue that psychotherapy and psychoanalysis have their action through a complex interaction between relational and representational factors, between the therapeutic relationship and therapeutic insight. Luborsky *et al.*, meanwhile, present some empirical findings pertaining to a topic that has received much theoretical attention in psychoanalysis – the role of narrative in the psychotherapeutic process. The chapter by Messer and McCann pertains to a subject that has informed Sid's entire career – the extent to which the study of psychoanalysis can be placed on an adequate empirical footing. They demonstrate how single-case methodology can be used to capture the complexity and richness of the psychoanalytic encounter while maintaining adequate empirical rigor.

Part V will focus on the links between psychoanalysis and broader cultural trends. In his work, Sid applied his representational and two-configurations models to developments in art history, the culture of narcissism, and developments in the history of science. In the spirit of Sid's contributions in these areas, two of the chapters will discuss the implications of the two-configurations model for an understanding of sociocultural phenomena. Wachtel's chapter demonstrates how the two-configurations model can be used to illuminate the psychodynamics of greed. Blass's chapter discusses religious faith in terms of the interacting developmental lines of attachment and separation. Another chapter in this part, that by Diamond, compares and contrasts psychoanalytic theories of narcissism with the social theories posited by members of the Frankfurt School. Diamond discusses how narcissism is both a psychological and a social problem. In the final chapter of the book, Holt discusses, from an empirical-scientific viewpoint similar to that embraced by Sid, the implications of postmodernism for psychoanalysis. Holt's concern is to uphold psychoanalysis as a scientific discipline, one that depends on empirical research if it is to advance, while at the same time disputing the argument, often advanced by postmodern thinkers, that a scientific approach is necessarily reductionistic.

Note

1 The ORI is sometimes also referred to as the Object Representation Inventory (Diamond, Kaslow, Coonerty and Blatt 1990; Gruen and Blatt 1990). The original technique (Blatt, Wein, Chevron and Quinlan 1979) asked participants to write brief prose descriptions of each of their parents; it was used in a nonclinical sample and was known as Parental Description. When the technique was adapted for use with psychiatric patients, it was administered in the form of an interview, and participants were asked to describe a significant other, a pet, self, and ther-

apist, as well as, per the original procedure, mother and father. This unstructured interview was called the ORI.

References

Allison, J., Blatt, S. J. and Zimet, C. N. (1968) *The Interpretation of Psychological Tests*. New York: Harper and Row.

Auerbach, J. S. and Blatt, S. J. (1996) 'Self-representation in severe psychopathology: the role of reflexive self-awareness', *Psychoanalytic Psychology* 13: 297–341.

—— and —— (2001) 'Self-reflexivity, intersubjectivity, and therapeutic change', *Psychoanalytic Psychology* 18: 427–50.

—— and —— (2002) 'The concept of the mind: a developmental analysis', in R. Lasky (ed.) *Symbolization and Desymbolization: essays in honor of Norbert Freedman*, New York: Other Press, pp. 75–117.

Beck, A. T. (1983) 'Cognitive therapy of depression: new perspectives', in P. J. Clayton and J. E. Barrett (eds) *Treatment of Depression: old controversies and new approaches*, New York: Raven, pp. 265–90.

Behrends, R. S. and Blatt, S. J. (1985) 'Internalization and psychological development throughout the life cycle', *Psychoanalytic Study of the Child* 40: 11–39.

Bers, S. A., Blatt, S. J., Sayward, H. K. and Johnston, R. S. (1993) 'Normal and pathological aspects of self-descriptions and their change over long-term treatment', *Psychoanalytic Psychology* 10: 17–37.

Blass, R. B. and Blatt, S. J. (1992) 'Attachment and separateness: a theoretical context for the integration of self psychology with object relations theory', *Psychoanalytic Study of the Child* 47: 189–203.

—— and —— (1996) 'Attachment and separateness in the experience of symbiotic relatedness', *Psychoanalytic Quarterly* 65: 711–46.

Blatt, S. J. (1959) 'Recall and recognition vocabulary: implications for intellectual deterioration', *Archives of General Psychiatry* 1: 473–6.

—— (1974) 'Levels of object representation in anaclitic and introjective depression', *Psychoanalytic Study of the Child* 29: 107–57.

—— (1990) 'The Rorschach: a test of perception or an evaluation of representation', *Journal of Personality Assessment* 54: 236–51.

—— (1991) 'A cognitive morphology of psychopathology', *Journal of Nervous and Mental Disease* 179: 449–58.

—— (1992) 'The differential effect of psychotherapy and psychoanalysis on anaclitic and introjective patients: the Menninger Psychotherapy Research Project revisited', *Journal of the American Psychoanalytic Association*, 40: 691–724.

—— (1995a) 'The destructiveness of perfectionism: implications for the treatment of depression', *American Psychologist* 50: 1003–20.

—— (1995b) ' Representational structures in psychopathology', in D. Cicchetti and S. Toth (eds) *Rochester Symposium on Developmental Psychopathology, vol. 6, emotion, cognition, and representation*, Rochester, NY: University of Rochester Press, pp. 1–33.

—— (2004) *Experiences of Depression*, Washington, DC: American Psychological Association.

Blatt, S. J. and Allison, J. (1968) 'The intelligence test in personality assessment', in A. I. Rabin (ed.) *Assessment with Projective Techniques: a concise introduction*, New York: Springer, 1981, pp. 187–232.

—— Auerbach, J. S. and Aryan, M. (1998) 'Representational structures and the therapeutic process', in R. F. Bornstein and J. M. Masling (eds) *Empirical Studies of Psychoanalytic Theories, vol. 8, empirical studies of the therapeutic hour*, Washington, DC: American Psychological Association, pp. 63–107.

—— —— and Levy, K. N. (1997) 'Mental representations in personality development, psychopathology, and the therapeutic process', *Review of General Psychology* 1: 351–74.

—— and Behrends, R. S. (1987) 'Internalization, separation-individuation, and the nature of therapeutic action', *International Journal of Psychoanalysis* 68: 279–97.

—— Bers, S. A. and Schaffer, C. (1992) *The Assessment of Self*, unpublished research manual, Yale University, New Haven, CT.

—— and Blass, R. B. (1990) 'Attachment and separateness: a dialectic model of the products and processes of psychological development', *Psychoanalytic Study of the Child* 45: 107–27.

—— and —— (1992) 'Relatedness and self-definition: two primary dimensions in personality development, psychopathology, and psychotherapy', in J. Barron, M. Eagle and D. Wolitsky (eds) *Interface of Psychoanalysis and Psychology*, Washington, DC: American Psychological Association, pp. 399–428.

—— and —— (1996) 'Relatedness and self definition: a dialectic model of personality development', in G. G. Noam and K. W. Fischer (eds) *Development and Vulnerabilities in Close Relationships*, Hillsdale, NJ: Erlbaum, pp. 309–38.

—— and Blatt, E. (1984) *Continuity and Change in Art: the development of modes of representation*, Hillsdale, NJ: Erlbaum.

—— Brenneis, C. B., Schimek, J. G. and Glick, M. (1976) 'The normal development and psychopathological impairment of the concept of the object on Rorschach', *Journal of Abnormal Psychology* 85: 364–73.

—— Chevron, E. S., Quinlan, D. M., Schaffer, C. E. and Wein, S. J. (1988) *The Assessment of Qualitative and Structural Dimensions of Object Representations* (rev. ed.), unpublished research manual, Yale University, New Haven, CT.

—— D'Afflitti, J. P. and Quinlan, D. M. (1976) 'Experiences of depression in normal young adults', *Journal of Abnormal Psychology* 85: 383–9.

—— and Ford, R. (1994) *Therapeutic Change: an object relations perspective*, New York: Plenum.

—— and Levy, K. N. (2003) 'Attachment theory, psychoanalysis, personality development, and psychopathology', *Psychoanalytic Inquiry* 23: 104–52.

—— Quinlan, D. M., Chevron, E. S. McDonald, C. and Zuroff, D. (1982) 'Dependency and self-criticism: psychological dimensions of depression', *Journal of Consulting and Clinical Psychology* 50: 113–24.

—— —— Pilkonis, P. A. and Shea, T. (1995) 'Impact of perfectionism and need for approval on the brief treatment of depression: the National Institute of Mental Health Treatment of Depression Collaborative Research Program revisited', *Journal of Consulting and Clinical Psychology* 63: 125–32.

—— and Ritzler, B. A. (1974) 'Thought disorder and boundary disturbances in psychosis', *Journal of Consulting and Clinical Psychology* 42: 370–81.

—— Schaffer, C. E., Bers, S. A. and Quinlan, D. M. (1992) 'Psychometric properties of the Adolescent Depressive Experiences Questionnaire', *Journal of Personality Assessment* 59: 82–98.

Blatt, S. J. and Shichman, S. (1983) 'Two primary configurations of psychopathology', *Psychoanalysis and Contemporary Thought* 6: 187–254.

—— Stayner, D., Auerbach, J. and Behrends, R. S. (1996) 'Change in object and self representations in long-term, intensive, inpatient treatment of seriously disturbed adolescents and young adults', *Psychiatry* 59: 82–107.

—— and Stein, M. I. (1959) 'Efficiency in problem solving', *Journal of Psychology* 48: 193–213.

—— Wein, S. J., Chevron, E. S. and Quinlan, D. M. (1979) 'Parental representations and depression in normal young adults', *Journal of Abnormal Psychology* 88: 388–97.

—— and Wild, C. M. (1976) *Schizophrenia: a developmental analysis*, New York: Academic Press.

—— —— and Ritzler, B. A. (1975) 'Disturbances in object representation in schizophrenia', *Psychoanalysis and Contemporary Science* 4: 235–88.

—— Zohar, A. H., Quinlan, D. M., Zuroff, D. C. and Mongrain, M. (1995) 'Subscales within the dependency factor of the Depressive Experiences Questionnaire', *Journal of Personality Assessment*, 64: 319–39.

—— and Zuroff, D. C. (1992) 'Interpersonal relatedness and self-definition: two prototypes for depression', *Clinical Psychology Review* 12: 527–62.

Bowlby, J. (1973) *Attachment and Loss, vol. 2, separation: anxiety and anger*, New York: Basic Books.

Diamond, D. and Blatt, S. J. (1994) 'Internal working models and the representational world in attachment and psychoanalytic theories', in M. B. Sperling and W. H. Berman (eds) *Attachment in Adults: clinical and developmental perspectives*, New York: Guilford Press, pp. 72–97.

—— —— Stayner, D. and Kaslow, N. (1991) *Self-other Differentiation of Object Representations*, unpublished research manual, Yale University, New Haven, CT.

—— Kaslow, N., Coonerty, S. and Blatt, S. J. (1990) 'Change in separation-individuation and intersubjectivity in long-term treatment', *Psychoanalytic Psychology* 7: 363–97.

Erikson, E. H. (1963) *Childhood and Society* (2nd edn), New York: Norton.

Fraiberg, S. (1969) 'Libidinal object constancy and mental representation', *Psychoanalytic Study of the Child* 24: 9–47.

Freud, A. (1965) *Normality and Pathology in Childhood: assessments of development*, New York: International Universities Press.

Freud, S. (1916–17) 'Introductory Lectures on Psycho-Analysis', in J. Strachey (ed. and trans.) *The Standard Edition of the Complete Psychological Works of Sigmund Freud*, vols 15 and 16, London: Hogarth Press.

Gruen, R. and Blatt, S. J. (1990) 'Change in self and object representation during long-term dynamically oriented treatment', *Psychoanalytic Psychology* 7: 399–422.

Jacobson, E. (1964) *The Self and the Object World*, New York: International Universities Press.

Levy, K. N., Blatt, S. J. and Shaver, P. (1998) 'Attachment styles and parental representations', *Journal of Personality and Social Psychology* 74: 407–19.

Mahler, M. S. (1968) *On Human Symbiosis and the Vicissitudes of Individuation: infantile psychosis*, New York: International Universities Press.

Main, M., Kaplan, N. and Cassidy, J. (1985) 'Security in infancy, childhood and adulthood: a move to the level of representation', in I. Bretherton and E. Waters (eds) *Growing Points in Attachment Theory and Research, Monographs of the Society for Research in Child Development* 50 (1–2, Serial No. 209): 66–104.

Rapaport, D. (ed. and trans.) (1951) *Organization and Pathology of Thought*, New York: Columbia University Press.

—— Gill, M. M. and Schafer, R. (1945–6) *Diagnostic Psychological Testing*, 2 vols, Chicago: Year Book Publishers.

Schaffer, C. E. (1993) 'The role of attachment in the experience and regulation of affect', unpublished doctoral dissertation, Yale University, New Haven, CT.

Shahar, G., Blatt, S. J., Zuroff, D. C., Krupnick, J. and Sotsky, S. M. (in press) 'Perfectionism impedes social relations and response to brief treatment of depression', *Journal of Social and Clinical Psychology*.

—— Blatt, S. J., Zuroff, D. C. and Pilkonis, P. A. (2003) 'Role of perfectionism and personality disorder features in response to brief treatment for depression', *Journal of Consulting and Clinical Psychology* 71: 629–33.

Waddington, C. H. (1957) *The Strategy of the Genes*, London: Allen and Unwin.

Wallerstein, R. S. (1986) *Forty-Two Lives in Treatment: a study of psychoanalysis and psychotherapy*, New York: Guilford Press.

Weissman, A. N. and Beck, A. T. (1978, August-September) 'Development and validation of the Dysfunctional Attitudes Scale: a preliminary investigation', paper presented at the 86th Annual Convention of the American Psychological Association, Toronto.

Werner, H. (1957) *Comparative Psychology of Mental Development*, rev. edn, G. Murphy (ed.) and E. B. Garside (trans.), New York: International Universities Press.

—— and Kaplan, B. (1963) *Symbol Formation: an organismic-developmental approach to language and the expression of thought*, New York: Wiley.

Zuroff, D. C. (1994) 'Depressive personality styles and the five factor model of personality', *Journal of Personality Assessment* 63: 453–72.

—— Blatt, S. J., Sotsky, S. M., Krupnick, J. L., Martin, D. J., Sanislow, C. A. and Simmens, S. (2000) 'Relation of therapeutic alliance and perfectionism to outcome in brief outpatient treatment of depression', *Journal of Consulting and Clinical Psychology* 68: 114–24.

—— Quinlan, D. M. and Blatt, S. J. (1990) 'Psychometric properties of the Depressive Experiences Questionnaire in a college population', *Journal of Personality Assessment* 55: 65–72.

Part I

Personality development

Chapter 2

A dyadic systems view of communication[1]

Beatrice Beebe, Joseph Jaffe, and Frank Lachmann

Although psychoanalysis has developed a rich understanding of the self and the object, we suggest that the dyad as a system of communication is less well conceptualized. The dyad has always been of interest to psychoanalysis, but not until recently has it begun to be recognized as central to an understanding of development and of psychoanalytic theory and practice. A dyadic systems view of communication can elucidate the nature of interpersonal process and interactive regulation in the dyad. It has implications for our concepts of psychic structure and its formation and can facilitate an integration of one-person and two-person psychology models.

Historically, dyadic systems and the process of interpersonal influence have been of major concern to psychoanalysts (Sullivan 1953), social psychologists (Cottrell 1942), cognitive psychologists (Vygotsky 1978), philosophers (Simmel 1950; Mead 1934), biological systems theorists (von Bertalanffy 1952; Weiss 1973) and ethologically oriented observers (Bowlby 1980; Blurton Jones 1972; McGrew 1972). Much of the early work was programmatic, even poetic, and devoid of operational definitions that might enable quantitative studies. In the time domain, the analysis of dyadic systems has been given methodological sophistication by researchers employing the method of "interaction chronometry" (Chapple 1970, 1971; Matarazzo and Wiens 1972; Cappella 1991a; Condon and Sander 1974; Jaffe and Feldstein 1970; Warner 1987). Interpersonal process in the dyadic system has also been one of the central themes in the literature on mother–infant interaction that has burgeoned in the last 20 years.

We use Bloom's (1983) distinctions to define communication in two senses. One refers to the linguistic content of messages, including wishes and fantasies. This chapter does not address communication in this sense. The second refers to the way communication has most often been studied in infant social interactions: "a framing of the interaction – a 'getting into sync' – that involves a process in which persons act in ways that are responsive to the actions of those with whom they are in communication" (p. 84). This aspect of communication, often out of awareness, conveys "the affective quality of the relationship, . . . through observation of rhythm sharing, body movement, timing of speech, and silences" (p. 84). Although psychoanalysis tends to focus on the linguistic content of communication, it is important to note that the paralinguistic aspect of communication is a "necessary frame . . . for communication with language" to occur (Bloom 1983, p. 84).

Altmann (1967, p. 326) defines social communication as "a process by which the behavior of an individual affects the behavior of others." We conceive of communication as the mutual modification of two ongoing streams of behavior of two persons. Each person has his own likelihood (probability) of behaving. At any particular moment, the behavior of an individual is not a determined process. Communication occurs when each person affects the probability distribution of the other's behavior. We believe that when such communication occurs, cognitive and affective changes also occur.

Historical background of dyadic systems

In describing the interactive model informing much of infant research, Tronick (1980) reviewed the contributions of a number of philosophers and scientists who all, in various ways, articulated a dyadic systems view of communication (Mead 1934; Ryan 1974; Lashley 1951; Bruner 1977; Habermas 1979). He noted that, using such terms as a system of mutuality, a system of reciprocal relations and reciprocal obligations, mutual recognition, and a shared set of rules, they converged in their views regarding how interactions are structured. Exemplifying a profoundly dyadic view of communication, Habermas (1979) suggested that the primary task in communication is to understand the messages of the other while at the same time modifying one's own action in accord both with the other's intentions and with one's own (see also Tronick 1980). This formulation implicitly takes into account both the self-regulatory and the interactive dimensions of interaction that we spell out later.

Vygotsky (1978) also proposed the dyad as the irreducible unit of study. He considered that all higher functions originate as actual relations between individuals. He wrote, "Any function in the child's development appears . . . first on the social level, and later on the individual level; first between people . . . and then inside the child . . ." (p. 57). Ruesch and Bateson (1951) also used the term mutual influence and emphasized the dyadic nature of communication.

> The mutual recognition of having entered into each other's field of perception equals the establishment of a system of communication . . . . The perception of the perception . . . is the sign that a silent agreement has been reached by the participants, to the effect that mutual influence is to be expected.
>
> (p. 23)

Purely verbal conversation, as on the telephone, requires turntaking, since it is difficult to speak and listen at the same time (Jaffe 1978). When two people smile at each other, however, they are simultaneously sending and receiving information. In a face-to-face dyadic system, unlike in telephone communication, there can be simultaneous transmission of information between continuously adjusting organisms. Such nonverbal communication provides the most extreme example of simultaneous transmission of information where the information-processing limitations of verbal exchange are absent. It requires a continuous control model, where sending and receiving are concurrent and reciprocally evoked (Jaffe 1962). In his conceptualizations of the evolution of dialogue and the derailment of dialogue, Spitz (1983) also conceptualized a process where sending and receiving were simultaneous.

Bidirectional model of influence

Although the ideas underlying a dyadic systems view have been conceptually influential for decades, only more recently have they been operationalized sufficiently for quantitative research to be done. This quantitative emphasis has been particularly strong in the research on mother–infant interaction where bidirectional influences have now been extensively documented and a systems model of the dyad has been richly elaborated. In his study of adaptation in the early weeks of life, Sander (1977, 1985) has suggested that the organization of behavior be viewed primarily as a property of the mother–infant system rather than as a property of the individual. The dyad, rather than the individual, is treated as the system. Nevertheless, the individuals are the components, each with his or her own range of self-regulatory capacities. Within this model, mother and infant should no longer be studied as two isolated entities, each sending the other discrete messages as if one person provides the "stimulus" and the other the "response" (Condon and Sander 1974). Rather, they should be studied as a system of "shared organizational forms," such as shared rhythms, or shared affective directions. Using this model, it is also no longer possible to conceptualize either partner as "activated by the other." Rather, each brings to the exchange his or her own intrinsic motivation (Berlyne 1966; Hunt 1965; Piaget 1937) and primary endogenous activity. Sander (1977) emphasizes the primary activity characteristic of all living organisms:

> In the process of adaptation between the components (organism and environment), one is not activated by the other, but the two, already complexly organized and actively generating behavior, must be interfaced with each other to reach an enduringly harmonious coordination . . . . That is, both mother and infant are seen as inherently in states of

readiness or reactivity; these become synchronized or coordinated one with each other.

(p. 136)

A remarkable body of research, both experimental and naturalistic, now exists with which to further define Sander's claim that the infant brings an inherent readiness to the interactive exchange. A body of research on perceptual capacities documents the infant's ability to detect and expect order in the environment and to react with distress to violations of expected order (DeCasper and Carstens 1980; Fagen, Morrongiello, Rovee-Collier and Gekoski 1984; Watson 1985; Spelke and Cortelyou 1981). Haith (cited in Emde 1988a) suggests that "the infant is biologically prepared to engage in visual activity in order to stimulate its own brain" and is "self-motivated to detect regularity, to generate expectancies, and to act upon these expectancies" (p. 29). The work on perturbations of naturalistic exchanges extends the conclusions of the experimental perception work into the naturalistic domain (Tronick, Als, Adamson, Wise and Brazelton 1978; Cohn and Tronick 1983; Murray and Trevarthen 1985). These studies all demonstrate that in the naturalistic social exchange infants bring a similar inherent readiness to behave. They have the capacity to detect order and to react with distress to violated expectancies. Finally, Sander's (1977) suggestion that these inherent states of reactivity in both partners must become coordinated has been borne out by two decades of work on the naturalistic social exchange documenting many patterns of mutually regulated coordination to be described later.

These dyadic systems concepts have influenced infant researchers and helped to generate a bidirectional model of mutual influence. In his seminal paper, Bell (1968) opened the question of direction of influence. He argued that most of the literature to date had emphasized parental influence upon children, a one-way influence model, to the relative exclusion of the child's influence on the parent.

Interest in the contribution of the infant was paralleled by a growing body of evidence that infants are both active and socially effective (Lewis and Rosenblum 1974). With increasing recognition of the infant's social competence, researchers became interested in a bidirectional, or mutual, model of influence. Informally, the most romantic extremes of this theorizing seemed to verge upon a notion of adult–infant symmetry. The mutual influence model, however, does not assume that each partner influences the other in equal measure or like manner. The mother obviously has a greater range, control, and flexibility of behavior than the infant. Rather, the basic assumption is that each partner's behavior can be shown to be predictable from that of the other, regardless of the particular content of the behavior, which may indeed be age- or experientially specific. Thus, when we speak of dyadic symmetry, we mean something more abstract, in the sense that both partners actively contribute to the regulation of the exchange. This notion is beautifully illustrated by the analyses of communicative timing using the method of interaction chronometry and time-series analysis to be discussed.

There is a dynamic interplay between mother and infant, and each affects the other's actions, perception, affect, and proprioceptions to create a great variety of mutual regulatory patterns. With development, both infant and caretaker are continuously influenced and altered by the other in systematic ways. Although the bidirectional model of influence points to the import- ance of the dyad in conceptualizing the organization of individual behavior, this model is incomplete without the additional specification of the individual's self-regulatory contribution.

The integration of mutual regulation and self-regulation

Various research traditions, each with its own methods and literature spanning development across the lifespan, have tended to focus either on self-regulation or interactive regulation to the relative exclusion of the other. Such traditions as psychophysiology, cybernetic models, endocrinol- ogy, and maturational approaches to development have examined self- regulation by addressing such issues as arousal; rhythmicity; organization of cycles of sleep-wake, REM sleep, breathing, and feeding; and various pathological patterns of autonomic reactivity. In contrast, ethology and social psychology have focused on dyadic regulation and examined such issues as eye contact, proxemics, conversational rhythms, games, and signaling. These approaches to dyadic regulation construe the dyad as the critical unit of organization. The dyad is seen as a system of joint partici- pation in shared organizational forms, such as shared rhythms or affective displays (Condon and Sander 1974). Some research approaches, however, have explicitly integrated the self-regulatory and the interactive approaches (see, e.g., Hofer 1984, 1987; Sander 1977, 1985; Brazelton, Kozlowski and Main 1974; Lichtenberg 1983; Gianino and Tronick 1988).

Similarly, in the infant literature on the development of psychic structure and the self, some authors emphasize self-regulation as the key organizing principle (see, e.g., Emde 1981; Stechler and Kaplan 1980). Others empha- size mutual interactive regulation (Beebe and Lachmann 1988; Stern, 1971, 1977) or an integration of the two (Demos 1983, 1984; Gianino and Tronick 1988; Hofer 1984, 1987; Lachmann and Beebe 1992; Beebe and Lachmann 1990; Lichtenberg 1983; Sander 1977, 1985). Sander's view that organization is a property of the dyadic system, rather than solely of the individual, explicitly integrates the simultaneous influences of self and mutual regulation. A theory of interactive behavior must specify how each person is affected by his own behavior – self-regulation – as well as that of the partner – interactive regulation (Thomas and Martin 1976).

The study of self-regulation can begin with the fetus. Brazelton (1973, 1992) has shown that the fetus regulates its level of arousal and responsivity as a function of the nature of the stimulation provided. For example, when the experimenter shone a very bright light on the mother's belly, the fetus changed its state, dampened its arousal, and eventually put itself to sleep to cope with aversive stimulation. When the light was changed to a more moderate level, the fetus again changed state and now showed patterns of approaching the stimulus. Thus, the fetus continued to monitor the nature of incoming stimulation and regulate its own state in relation to the nature of this stimulation.

Newborns differ in temperament and in their capacity to regulate their states, modulate their arousal levels, and in general to organize their behaviors predictably. The importance of the initial intactness of the organism's capacity to tolerate and use stimulation alerts us to the enormous contribution of normal self-regulatory capacities that are prerequisite to engaging with the environment. This capacity can be compromised to varying degrees, for example, in premature infants or in autistic children. The Brazelton (1973) Neonatal Assessment Scale was specifically designed to evaluate the joint contribution of self- and mutual regulation. It assesses the infant's self-regulatory capacity, for example, to dampen his state in response to aversive stimuli. At the same time, it assesses how much help from the partner is required and can be utilized by the infant to stabilize his state after stress and to maintain engagement with the environment.

The integration of mutual and self-regulation has a direct bearing on the development of representations and psychic structure as organized through the dyad. The current concept that self and object and their representations are rooted in relationship structures (Fast 1985, 1987; Kegan 1982; Stern 1985; Wilson and Malatesta 1989) holds true only so long as relationship structures are broadly construed to include an integration of self-regulatory with mutual regulatory processes. To posit the dyadic interaction alone as the source of psychic structure formation omits the crucial contribution of the organism's own self-regulatory capacities (Beebe and Lachmann 1990).

Individual stability of responsivity versus emergent properties of the dyad

To what degree can interpersonal responsivity be conceptualized as a stable characteristic of a person, and to what degree can a person's responsivity be conceptualized as unique to a particular partner? These two factors always operate, but the balance between them may shift in different dyadic systems. For example, in a pathological mother–infant dyad, the difficulty may be seen as a relatively stable characteristic of either partner. That is, the baby may be intrinsically hard to reach, or the adult partner may actually be producing difficulty in the baby. Alternatively, the nature of relatedness may be seen as an emergent property of the unique dyadic system, that is, unique to this particular dyad, and not attributable to stable characteristics of either partner. An integration of these factors provides a view of the dyadic system as organized *both* by stable characteristics of the participants (a one-person psychology model) and by emergent dyadic properties (a two-person psychology model).

Consistency of responsiveness across partners is one way of defining the degree to which a person's responsivity is a stable characteristic. This question is ideally addressed using a "round robin" design, in which each person interacts with every other person, yielding interactions between all possible dyads in the group. For each individual in the round robin design, a range of interpersonal environments can be studied, and each person can be evaluated both as actor and as partner. For example, if persons A, B, C, and D interact, it is possible to evaluate whether person A (the actor) is consistent in responding to partners B, C and D. This is known as the "actor effect" (B → A, C → A, D → A). It is also possible to evaluate whether A is consistent in eliciting responsivity from partners B, C, and D. This is known as the "partner effect" (A → B, A → C, A → D). The same procedure can be followed with each of B, C, and D as the target person. Finally, it is possible to evaluate the degree to which each dyad matches level of responsivity, that is, whether A's responsivity to B is similar to B's responsivity to A. This is known as the "relationship effect."

Cappella (1991b) used this round-robin design to evaluate the coordination of vocal timing in eight adults. He did not find much consistency in either actor effects or partner effects. He did, however, find high relationship effects. Each dyad reached some kind of match of responsivity that was specific to that particular interaction. Although this work needs to be replicated with a larger sample, it suggests that each person does not necessarily have a generalized level of responsivity or stimulus value that he carries with him into various interactions. Instead, each dyad generates its own unique system in which both participants adjust their level of responsivity to each other in ways they do not necessarily display with other partners.

Transactional approaches propose that systems that function together are changed by their mutual activity; that is, they generate emergent properties (Sameroff 1983). Cappella's (1991b) findings illustrate the concept that the dyad is a system with emergent properties, with its own tendency to match level of responsivity, which is not easily predictable from knowing either partner separately. This work suggests that a one-person psychology model, in which each person "has" a relatively stable or consistent personality, measured here as the disposition to respond in a predictable way, does not do justice to the complexity of human relatedness. Nevertheless, stable characteristics of the person (see Ryle 1949), the contribution of the one-person model, still play a role.

It is possible that the concept of emergent properties of the dyad may help conceptualize the nature of therapeutic action in psychoanalysis. What emerges from the therapeutic dyad is something generative that could not be completely predicted from the patient alone or from the analyst alone. Transference and countertransference can also be conceptualized as emergent dyadic properties. That is, knowing both the patient's and the analyst's self-regulatory and interactive patterns prior to the analysis will not completely or even adequately predict the specific nature of the match that the dyad will generate. This view of transference differs from that of a one-person model, in which transference is defined as a pattern that the patient brings to the interaction, as a stable characteristic of the individual. Rather, we conceptualize transference as a complex product of both the stable characteristics of the patient and analyst individually, as well as of the emergent properties of the dyad (see also, e.g., Lachmann and Beebe 1990, 1992; Atwood and Stolorow 1984; Gill 1982; Racker 1968).

More generally, in attempting to conceptualize the dyadic system, we suggest that there is always a complex integration between some part of the variance that is accounted for by the stability of each individual's behavior and some that is accounted for by the particular nature of the interactive regulatory match. Still remaining for empirical investigation are which aspects of behavior and representations are more stable and which are more subject to interpersonal influence, under what conditions, and their respective relevance to structure formation and transformation.

Dyadic rules of regulation

A basic empirical concern in a dyadic systems approach to communication is to discern the structure of the mutual regulatory system. What are the dyadic rules that create order? What are the potential shared organizational forms? What are the ways of conceptualizing and measuring dyadic regulation? Stern (1971, 1977) addresses this issue by documenting the rules for initiating, maintaining, terminating, or avoiding dyadic states. Tronick (1980, 1982) discusses the regulation of joint exchanges as a shared set of generative communicative rules. These rules generate predictions in each partner about the other's behavior. The rules are probabilistic, in the sense that particular dyadic sequences are significantly different from chance (Ryle 1949). These dyadic sequences are defined by the predictability of one partner's behavior from that of the other. That is, each partner's behavior is contingent on that of the other. Tronick (1980) considers the basis of joint regulation to be the mutual matching of communicative acts and predictions, that is, the continuous confirmation and disconfirmation of predictions of the partner's behavior. In a well-coordinated interaction, each participant's communicative act conforms to the partner's prediction.

Perhaps the central contribution of infant research on the structure of social interaction has been the rich documentation of many patterns of rules for the regulation of joint action, thus defining the complexity of early dyadic communication. We refer to these patterns of rules as "interaction structures" (Beebe and Lachmann 1988). These rules have been shown to be mutually regulated by both mother and infant. The rules begin to define the ways in which the dyad jointly constructs patterns of order, variously termed resonance, synchrony, coordination, or relatedness. Using experimental perturbations of ongoing interactions, research has also begun to demonstrate ways in which these patterns can be disrupted and repaired (Tronick *et al.* 1978; Cohn and Tronick 1983; Murray 1991; Beebe and Lachmann 1990). Researchers have documented various phenomena of mutual regulation that have been variously termed synchronization (Stern 1971, 1977), behavioral dialogue (Bakeman and Brown 1977), echo (Trevarthen 1977, 1979), tracking (Kronen 1982), protoconversation (Beebe, Stern and Jaffe 1979), accommodation (Jasnow and Feldstein 1986), reciprocity (Brazelton, Tronick, Adamson, Als and Wise 1975), mutual dialogues (Tronick, Als and Brazelton 1980), reciprocal and compensatory mutual influence (Cappella 1981), and coordinated interpersonal timing (Crown 1991; Beebe, Jaffe, Feldstein, Mays and Alson 1985; Jaffe, Feldstein, Beebe, Crown and Jasnow 1991). These researchers share a method of quantitative analysis of the organization of two ongoing naturalistic streams of behavior (one for mother, one for infant) and their interrelation. However, the behavioral categories used, the statistical methods that document the interrelation of the two streams of behavior, and the metaphors used to describe these interrelations differ widely from study to study.

The measurement of dyadic rules of regulation

The problem of how to conceptualize interpersonal process and dyadic regulation sufficiently well to measure it has plagued infant research for the last two decades. Generous borrowing from other fields, such as econometrics, has given us a kit of statistical tools that yield quantitative statements about interpersonal influence and self-regulation. At the root of all these measures is the concept of predicting the behavior of each partner in the dyad from that of the other.

Time series regression techniques are one approach to the analysis of interaction structures (Gottman 1981; Gottman and Ringland 1981). Time series regression (TSR) addresses the central issues that have preoccupied infancy research in its attempt to define the organization of interpersonal process in mother–infant interactions. This method preserves the entire moment-to-moment behavioral stream; statistically controls for "autocorrelation," a self-regulatory component; determines, by lag correlation, who influences whom; and identifies the sign of the influence. A positive sign indicates that the behaviors of the two partners are similar; for instance, when one partner elongates the duration of a vocalization, the other partner does also. A negative sign indicates that the behaviors of the two partners are systematically dissimilar; when one person elongates the duration of vocalization, the other partner shortens the duration.

To demonstrate that an infant and caregiver may influence, or be influenced by, each other, autocorrelational effects must first be identified and statistically "removed" (Gottman and Ringland 1981). Autocorrelation refers to the influence of each partner's past behavior on his own current behavior and has been termed "self-influence" (Thomas and Martin 1976). Large cross-covariances can be totally spurious; that is, the apparent covariation of two processes that are actually uncorrelated may be the result of a large autocorrelation within each process (Gottman and Ringland 1981). Once autocorrelation is controlled, time series regression provides separate indices of each interactant's influence on the other ("lag correlation"). Influence is defined by the degree to which either partner's behavior can be predicted by the other's. By separately addressing the effects of autocorrelation and lagged correlation, TSR explicitly integrates the contributions of a self-regulatory component with interactive regulation in its strategy of analysis.

For example, if we find that the daily closing prices on the Tokyo and Wall Street stock exchanges are correlated, we have no idea of which is influencing the other. But if we realize that the closing is earlier in Tokyo than in New York, we can infer that the influence is going from Tokyo to New York. The lag in time defines the direction of influence. Similarly, TSR first lags one person's stream of behavior relative to that of the other and then reverses this procedure. Thus, the possibility that either person influences the other can be assessed. These assessments are lag correlations. This model does not yield causality but does imply that one stream of behavior can predict the other. In bidirectional influence, where each partner's behavior predicts that of the other, neither has "caused" the other. Rather, both are seen as jointly constructing the pattern of regulation.

The time series regression model has been used to demonstrate bidirectional influence in the mother–infant facial-visual exchange, with each partner matching the direction of affective change second-by-second (Cohn and Tronick 1988), and fraction-of-second-by-fraction-of-second (Cohn and Beebe 1990). Time series regression has demonstrated bidirectional influence in the timing of vocal exchanges between mother and infant and between stranger and infant (Jaffe et al. 1991), with each partner tracking and matching the durations of vocalizations and pauses of the other. This vocal dialogue model was translated into the mother–infant kinesic system, where time series analysis demonstrated a similar bidirectional tracking of the durations of "movements" and "holds" in the changes of facial expression and direction of gaze (Beebe *et al.* 1985). Time series regression has also been used to investigate the affective exchange between depressed mothers and their infants. In some samples, the bilateral influence process was shown to be intact (Cohn, Campbell, Matias and Hopkins 1990) and in other samples it broke down (Cohn and Tronick 1989). This same time-series regression model has been used to demonstrate bilateral influence in the timing of adult vocal interactions (Crown 1991; Cappella 1991a, 1991b; Jaffe *et al.* 1991; Warner 1987).

Interpersonal involvement and empathy are associated with similarity or matching of adult communicative behaviors (Feldstein and Jaffe 1963; Jaffe and Feldstein 1970; Feldstein and Welkowitz 1978). In adult conversation, to the degree that the partners match timing patterns of their speech, they rate each other as warmer and more similar (Welkowitz and Kuc 1973; Feldstein and Welkowitz 1978). In mother–infant interaction, the various findings of time-series analysis documenting bilateral influence show that each partner is sensitive to the affective direction or temporal pattern of the other's behavior. These findings provide a behavioral basis for each partner to perceive and enter into the temporal world and feeling state of the other (Beebe *et al.* 1985; Beebe and Lachmann 1988).

We now have evidence that the timing of the adult communicative process is very similar to that of the infant–adult process. For example, in both the durations of vocal pauses are matched, the degree of control of various vocal rhythms is matched, and there is bidirectional influence where each partner's vocal durations are predictable from the other's (Beebe *et al.* 1985; Crown 1991; Jaffe *et al.* 1991). These striking similarities suggest that there are important continuities in the timing of the communicative process across the life span. The timing of the communicative process affects what it feels like to be with the other and contributes to the representation of self and other at every developmental level. Although much of our own work has focused on the timing of communication, similar organizational coherence has begun to be documented in other communicative modalities, such as the facial-visual exchange (Cohn and Tronick 1988; Cohn and Beebe 1990; Kronen 1982; Stern 1971, 1977, 1983).

The representation of interaction structures

The dyad provides the route to predictability in development (Zeanah, Anders, Seifer and Stern 1990; Emde 1988a, 1988b; Sameroff 1983; Sameroff and Chandler 1976; Sander 1983, 1985; Sroufe 1979; Sroufe and Fleeson 1986). Many authors note the relative failure of predicting development from the individual alone. Sameroff argues that difficulty in prediction stems from using oversimplified models of development. It is not possible to predict from the organism alone, nor from the environment alone. Prediction is based on the transaction between organism and environment and the transaction's regular restructurings (Sameroff and Chandler 1976). Zeanah *et al.* (1990) argue that continuity in development as documented in the empirical infant literature is at the level of relationship structures. Stern (1989) argues that a relationship pattern resides in the interaction, in the dyad, not in the individual.

Thus, our concept of the interactive organization of experience and of psychic structure is based on a dyadic systems view of communication. Mother and infant jointly construct the rules of negotiating social relatedness. These rules guide the management of attention, turntaking, participating in discourse, and affect sharing. These rules are represented, are "internalized," and define the initial organization of psychic structure (Beebe and Stern 1977; Beebe and Lachmann 1988, 1990).

The model of representation that we employ is a process model. We claim that it is an interactive process, or a patterned sequence of movements between two people, that is represented by the infant (Beebe 1986). Stern (1977, 1983; Beebe and Stern 1977) employs a similar process model, which defines representation in the social sphere as the internalization of an intercoordination of dynamic interpersonal schemes of action. A schema of being with another person is a memory of a dynamic series of events. We conceptualize these as "interactive representations" in which the pattern of interplay of the interactive behaviors is represented.

In Piaget's (1937) framework, action schemes provide the infant with a way of knowing about the object. These action schemes are interiorized in the first mental representations. We suggest that the detailed knowledge of infant action schemas in relation to the mother's and their interactive regulation provide a way of assessing the nature of the object relation that is constructed and represented. The dominant modes of the ongoing relationship, based on detailed analysis of the mutual regulation of the dyadic system and of self-regulation processes, will prevail in the representation of the relationship. Piaget has shown that the internalization of the object does not proceed independently of the child's actions with reference to the object. We suggest, then, that what is initially represented is not an object per se, but an object relation: actions of self in relation to actions of partner and their pattern of dyadic regulation (Beebe and Stern 1977; Beebe and Lachmann 1988). These representations of self and object are simultaneously constructed in relation to each other. Thus, what is represented by the infant is an emergent dyadic phenomenon not residing in either partner alone. This initial representation will proceed through the nonverbal representation system and may or may not be later translated into the verbal representation system. Bucci (1985) suggests that such a translation is one task of adult psychoanalysis.

Modell (1993) has recently reviewed the use of the terms self and object representations in psychoanalysis. He points out that the origins of these terms in 18th-century philosophers such as Locke and Mill have tended to influence their usage in psychoanalysis toward a discrete, static, atomistic image of self and object. He notes that Sandler and Rosenblatt (1962) did not view representations as passive or atomistic. Instead, they influenced the usage of the terms toward a more fluid creation of the child. The idea of the representation of the interactive process emerging out of the infant research further elaborates Sandler and Rosenblatt's formulations and substantially changes the use of the terms away from their discrete, atomistic origins. The interaction is represented in relation to the self-regulatory system as each alters the other. Zelnick and Buchholz (1990), in reviewing the concept of mental representations in the light of recent infant research, come to a conclusion similar to that of Modell, that these early interactions constitute unconscious organizing structures or unconscious memory structures.

Therapeutic action and transference

The mutual and self-regulation processes documented in the infant literature can provide analogues to two-person and one-person psychology perspectives. A one-person psychology model emphasizes the intrapsychic organization of experience as primary. Experience is shaped initially according to one's needs, one's biologically based urges, and, later wishes, although certainly the environment plays a role. A two-person psychology view emphasizes the original interactive organization of experience. Psychoanalysis has tended to use one or the other of these models in addressing the question of the primary organizational principles structuring experience. One- and two-person psychology perspectives are presented as though they were dichotomies, as though either endogenously organized and elaborated structures or relational, interactively organized structures were primary. The considerable polarization around these "mutually exclusive" theories in adult analysis has been detailed by Greenberg and Mitchell (1983). Similar polarizations exist in the infant literature.

Both self- and mutual regulations are organized at birth and play a crucial role from the beginning of life. The necessity for integrating these two regulatory organizations in infancy argues for integrating them in a psychoanalytic theory of adult treatment as well (see Ghent 1989; Gianino and Tronick 1988; Tronick 1989; Lichtenberg 1983; Beebe and Lachmann 1990; Lachmann and Beebe 1990; Stolorow and Atwood 1992). Both the one- and the two-person psychology views, each without recognition of the other, contain serious drawbacks. If one takes an exclusively two-person view of structure formation, how can one distill a sense of individuality, a sense of one's own self, as distinct from the dyad? If one takes an exclusively one-person view, the contributions of the partner and the environment are underestimated. The research we have cited in illustrating a dyadic systems model depicts the dyad as a more complex organization than is usually recognized by either the one- or the two-person psychology view.

The contrasts between one-and two-person psychologies are nowhere more evident than in our understandings of the transference. Is the analyst required to function as a "screen" upon which the patient displays his life, past and present? Or is the analyst an active participant in the construction of the treatment relationship and the transference? We propose a model of transference and structuralization in adult treatment that integrates the simultaneous contributions of the patient–analyst interaction (the two-person psychology perspective) and the enduring structures from the patient's past that the patient has retained, rigidified, or diminished through his own subjective, personal elaborations (the one-person psychology perspective). Both sources operate interactively and concurrently through-out treatment, regardless of the origins of the pathology (Lachmann and Beebe 1990, 1992). A consideration of both perspectives opens many more paths for intervention.

Our overview of the research documenting the negotiation of mother–infant interaction suggests two consequences for our understanding of the analytic dyad. First, the "rules" that the patient has internalized through the experiences of joint constructions between patient and analyst will contribute to the organizing principles in the transference. Second, the manner in which the relatedness is constructed will bear the stamp of both participants. Each influences the process through his own self-regulatory range, as well as through specific contributions to the pattern of interaction.

In development, the organizing principles of psychic structure are an emergent dyadic phenomenon. In the adult, the capacity to generate these principles, their availability, and their specific content is both generalized from past relationships and also partially specific to the particular current dyadic system. In this sense, the psychic structure of an individual may only be completely definable in the context of a specific dyad.

Note

1 This chapter was first published in N. J. Skolnick and S. C. Warshaw (1992) (eds) *Relational Perspectives in Psychoanalysis*, Hillsdale, NJ: Analytic Press, pp. 61–81. It is reprinted here with minor editorial corrections and revisions.

The authors wish to thank Stanley Feldstein, Ph.D., Cynthia Crown, Ph.D., Michael Jasnow, Ph.D., Kenneth Feiner, Psy.D., Sarah Hahn-Burke, Nancy Freeman, and Marina Koulomzin. We acknowledge the support of NIMH grant 41675-03.

References

Altmann, S. (1967) 'The structure of primate communication', in S. Altmann (ed.) *Social Communication among Primates*, Chicago: University of Chicago Press, pp. 325–62.

Atwood, G. and Stolorow, R. (1984) *Structures of Subjectivity*, Hillsdale, NJ: Analytic Press.

Bakeman, R. and Brown, J. V. (1977) 'Behavioral dialogues: an approach to the assessment of the mother-infant interaction', *Child Development* 48: 195–203.

Beebe, B. (1986) 'Mother-infant mutual influence and precursors of self- and object representations', in J. Masling (ed.) *Empirical Studies of Psychoanalytic Theories*, vol. 2, Hillsdale, NJ: Analytic Press, pp. 27–48.

—— Jaffe, J., Feldstein, S., Mays, K. and Alson, D. (1985) 'Interpersonal timing: the application of an adult dialogue model to mother-infant vocal and kinesic interactions', in T. Field and N. Fox (eds) *Social Perception in Infants*, Norwood, NJ: Ablex, pp. 217–47.

—— and Lachmann, F. (1988) 'Mother-infant mutual influence and precursors of psychic structure', in A. Goldberg (ed.) *Frontiers in Self Psychology: progress in self psychology*, vol. 3, Hillsdale, NJ: Analytic Press, pp. 3–26.

—— and —— (1990) 'The organization of representations in infancy: three principles of salience', paper presented at the 10th Annual Spring Meeting, Division of Psychoanalysis, American Psychological Association, New York, NY.

—— and —— (1992) 'The contributions of mother-infant mutual influence to the origins of self- and object representations', in N. J. Skolnick and S. C. Warshaw (eds) *Relational Perspectives in Psychoanalysis*, Hillsdale, NJ: Analytic Press, pp. 61–81.

—— and Stern, D. (1977) 'Engagement-disengagement and early object experiences', in N. Freedman and S. Grand (eds) *Communicative Structures and Psychic Structures*, New York: Plenum, pp. 35–55.

—— and Jaffe, J. (1979) 'The kinesic rhythm of mother-infant interactions', in A. W. Siegman and S. Feldstein (eds) *Of Speech and Time: temporal patterns in interpersonal contexts*, Hillsdale, NJ: Erlbaum, pp. 23–34.

Bell, R. Q. (1968) 'A reinterpretation of the direction of effects in studies of socialization', *Psychological Review* 75: 81–95.

Berlyne, D. (1966) 'Curiosity and exploration', *Science* 153: 25–33.

Bertalanffy, L. von. (1952) *Problems of Life: an evaluation of modern biological thought*, New York: Wiley.

Bloom, L. (1983) 'Of continuity and discontinuity and the magic of language development', in R. Gollinkoff (ed.) *The Transition from Prelinguistic to Linguistic Communication*, Hillsdale, NJ: Erlbaum, pp. 79–92.

Blurton Jones, N. (1972) *Ethological Studies of Child Behaviour*, Cambridge, England: Cambridge University Press.

Bowlby, J. (1980) *Attachment and Loss, vol. 3, loss*, New York: Basic Books.

Brazelton, T. B. (1973) 'Neonatal Behavioral Assessment Scale', *Clinics in Behavioral Medicine* 50, Spastics International Medical Publications, London: Heinemann Medical Books.

—— (1992) 'Touch and the fetus', paper presented at the Touch Research Institute, Miami, FL.

Brazelton, T. B., Kozlowski, B. and Main, M. (1974) 'The origins of reciprocity', in M. Lewis and L. Rosenblum (eds) *The Effect of the Infant on its Caregiver*, New York: Wiley-Interscience, pp. 49–76.

—— Tronick, E., Adamson, L., Als, H. and Wise, S. (1975) 'Early mother-infant reciprocity', in M. A. Hofer (ed.) *The Parent-Infant Relationship*, New York: Elsevier, pp. 137–54.

Bruner, J. (1977) 'Early social interaction and language acquisition', in H. R. Schaffer (ed.) *Studies in Mother-Infant Interaction*, New York: Norton. pp. 271–89.

Bucci, W. (1985) 'Dual coding: a cognitive model for psychoanalytic research', *Journal of the American Psychoanalytic Association* 33: 571–608.

Cappella, J. N. (1981) 'Mutual influence in expressive behavior: adult and infant-adult dyadic interaction', *Psychological Bulletin* 89: 101–32.

—— (1991a) 'The biological origins of automated patterns of human interaction', *Communication Theory* 1: 4–35.

—— (1991b) 'Individual consistency in temporal adaptation in nonverbal behavior in conversations: high and low expressive dyads', paper presented at the meeting of the International Communication Association.

Chapple, E. (1970) *Culture and Biological Man: explorations in behavioral anthropology*, New York: Holt, Rinehart & Winston.

—— (1971) 'Toward a mathematical model of interaction: some preliminary considerations', in P. Kay (ed.) *Explanations in Mathematical Anthropology*, Cambridge, MA.: MIT Press, pp. 141–78.

Cohn, J. and Beebe, B. (1990) 'Sampling interval affects time-series regression estimates of mother-infant influence', abstracts of papers presented at the International Conference on Infant Studies, Montreal, Quebec, Canada, April 1990, *Infant Behavior and Development* 13: 317.

—— Campbell, S., Matias, R. and Hopkins, J. (1990) 'Face-to-face interactions of post-partum depressed and nondepressed mother-infant pairs at 2 months', *Developmental Psychology* 26: 15–23.

—— and Tronick, E. (1983) 'Three-month-old infants' reaction to simulated maternal depression', *Child Development* 54: 185–93.

—— and —— (1988) 'Mother-infant face-to-face interaction: influence is bidirectional and unrelated to periodic cycles in either partner's behavior', *Developmental Psychology* 24: 386–92.

—— and —— (1989) 'Specificity of infants' response to mothers' affective behavior', *Journal of the American Academy of Child and Adolescent Psychiatry* 28: 242–8.

Condon, W. and Sander, L. (1974) 'Synchrony demonstrated between movements of the neonate and adult speech', *Child Development* 45: 456–62.

Cottrell, L. S. (1942) 'The analysis of situational fields in social psychology', *American Sociological Review* 7: 370–82.

Crown, C. (1991) 'Coordinated interpersonal timing of vision and voice as a function of interpersonal attraction', *Journal of Language and Social Psychology* 10: 29–46.

DeCasper, A. and Carstens, A. (1980) 'Contingencies of stimulation: effects on learning and emotion in neonates', *Infant Behavior and Development* 4: 19–36.

Demos, V. (1983) 'Discussion of papers by Drs. Sander and Stern', in J. Lichtenberg and S. Kaplan (eds) *Reflections on Self Psychology*, Hillsdale, NJ: Analytic Press, pp. 105–12.

Demos, V. (1984) 'Empathy and affect: reflections on infant experience', in J. Lichtenberg, M. Bornstein and D. Silver (eds) *Empathy*, vol. 2, Hillsdale, NJ: Analytic Press, pp. 9–34.

Emde, R. (1981) 'The prerepresentational self and its affective core', *Psychoanalytic Study of the Child* 36: 165–92.

—— (1988a) 'Development terminable and interminable: 1. innate and motivational factors', *International Journal of Psycho-Analysis* 69: 23–42

—— (1988b) 'Development terminable and interminable: 2. recent psychoanalytic theory and therapeutic considerations', *International Journal of Psycho-Analysis* 69: 283–96.

Fagen, J. W., Morrongiello, B. A., Rovee-Collier, C. and Gekoski, M. J. (1984) 'Expectancies and memory retrieval in three-month-old infants', *Child Development* 55: 936–43.

Fast, I. (1985) *Event Theory: a Piaget-Freud integration*, Hillsdale, NJ: Erlbaum.

Fast, I. (1987) 'Interaction schemes in the establishment of psychic structure and therapeutic change', unpublished manuscript, University of Michigan, Ann Arbor, MI.

Feldstein, S. and Jaffe, J. (1963) 'Language predictability as a function of psychotherapeutic interaction', *Journal of Consulting Psychology* 27: 123–6.

Feldstein, S. and Welkowitz, J. (1978) 'A chronography of conversation: in defense of an objective approach', in A. W. Siegman and S. Feldstein (eds) *Nonverbal Behavior and Communication*, Hillsdale, NJ: Erlbaum, pp. 329–77.

Ghent, E. (1989) 'Credo: the dialectics of one-person and two-person psychologies', *Contemporary Psychoanalysis* 26: 169–211.

Gianino, A. and Tronick, E. (1988) 'The mutual regulation model: the infant's self and interactive regulation and coping and defensive capacities', in T. Field, P. McCabe and N. Schneiderman (eds) *Stress and Coping*, Hillsdale, NJ: Erlbaum, pp. 47–68.

Gill, M. (1982) *The Analysis of Transference, vol. 1, theory and technique, Psychological Issues*, Monograph 53, New York: International Universities Press.

Gottman, J. (1981) *Time Series Analysis*, Cambridge, England: Cambridge University Press.

—— and Ringland, J. (1981) 'Analysis of dominance and bidirectionality in social development', *Child Development* 52: 393–412.

Greenberg, J. and Mitchell, S. (1983) *Object Relations in Psychoanalytic Theory*, Cambridge, MA: Harvard University Press.

Habermas, J. (1979) *Communication and the Evolution of Society*, Boston, MA: Beacon Press.

Hofer, M. (1984) 'Relationships as regulators: a psychobiological perspective on bereavement', *Psychosomatic Medicine* 46: 183–97.

—— (1987) 'Early social relations: a psychobiologist's view', *Child Development* 58: 633–47.

Hunt, J. McV. (1965) 'Intrinsic motivation and its role in psychological development', in D. Levine (ed.) *Nebraska Symposium on Motivation*, vol. 13, Lincoln, Nebraska: University of Nebraska Press, pp. 189–282.

Jaffe, J. (1962) 'Dyadic analysis', unpublished manuscript.

Jaffe, J. (1978) 'Parliamentary procedure and the brain', in A. W. Siegman and S. Feldstein (eds) *Nonverbal Behavior and Communication*, Hillsdale, NJ: Erlbaum.

—— and Feldstein, S. (1970) *Rhythms of Dialogue*, New York: Academic Press.

—— —— Beebe, B., Crown, C. L., Jasnow, M., Fox, H., Anderson, S. W. and Gordon, S. (1991) *Interpersonal Timing and Infant Social Development*, final report for NIMH Grant No. MH41675.

Jasnow, M. and Feldstein, S. (1986) 'Adult-like temporal characteristics of mother-infant vocal interactions', *Child Development* 57: 754–61.

Kegan, R. (1982) *The Evolving Self*, Cambridge, MA: Harvard University Press.

Kronen, J. (1982) 'Maternal facial mirroring at four months', doctoral dissertation, Yeshiva University, New York.

Lachmann, F. M. and Beebe, B. (1990) 'On the formation of psychic structure: transference', paper presented at the 10th Annual Spring Meeting, Division of Psychoanalysis, American Psychological Association, April, New York, NY.

—— and —— (1992) 'Reformulations of early development and transference: implications for psychic structure formation', in J. Barron, M. Eagle and D. Wolitzky (eds) *Interface of Psychoanalysis and Psychology*, Washington, DC: American Psychological Association, pp. 133–53.

Lashley, K. S. (1951) 'The problem of serial order in behavior', in L. A. Jeffress (ed.) *Cerebral Mechanisms in Behavior*, New York: Wiley, pp. 112–46.

Lewis, M. and Rosenblum, L. (eds) (1974) *The Effect of the Infant on its Caregiver*, New York: Wiley.

Lichtenberg, J. D. (1983) *Psychoanalysis and Infant Research*, Hillsdale, NJ: Analytic Press.

Matarazzo, J. D. and Wiens, A. N. (1972) *The Interview: research on its anatomy and structure*, Chicago: Aldine-Atherton.

McGrew, W. C. (1972) *An Ethological Study of Children's Behavior*, New York: Academic Press.

Mead, G. H. (1934) *Mind, Self and Society*, Chicago: University of Chicago Press.

Modell, A. (1993) *The Private Self*, Cambridge, MA: Harvard University Press.

Murray, L. (1991) 'Intersubjectivity, object relations theory, and empirical evidence from mother-infant interactions', *Infant Mental Health Journal* 12: 219–232.

—— and Trevarthen, C. (1985) 'Emotion regulation of interactions between 2 month old infants and their mothers', in T. Field and N. Fox (eds) *Social Perception in Infants*, New Jersey: Ablex, pp. 137–54.

Piaget, J. (1937) *The Construction of Reality in the Child*, trans. M. Cook, New York: Basic Books, 1954.

Racker, H. (1968) *Transference and Countertransference*, New York.: International Universities Press.

Ruesch, J. and Bateson, G. (1951) *Communication: the social matrix of psychiatry*, New York: Norton.

Ryan, J. (1974) 'Early language development', in M. P. M. Richards (ed.) *The Integration of a Child into a Social World*, Cambridge, England: Cambridge University Press.

Ryle, G. (1949) *The Concept of Mind*, London: Hutchinson.

Sameroff, A. (1983) 'Developmental systems: contexts and evolution', in W. Kessen (ed.) *Mussen's Handbook of Child Psychology*, vol.1, New York: Wiley, pp. 237–94.

Sameroff, A. and Chandler, M. (1976) 'Reproductive risk and the continuum of caretaking casualty', in F. D. Horowitz (ed.) *Review of Child Development Research*, vol. 4, Chicago: University of Chicago Press, pp. 187–244.

Sander, L. (1977) 'The regulation of exchange in the infant-caretaker system and some aspects of the context-content relationship', in M. Lewis and L. Rosenblum (eds) *Interaction, Conversation, and the Development of Language*, New York: Wiley, pp. 133–56.

—— (1983) 'Polarity, paradox, and the organizing process in development', in J. D. Call, E. Galenson and R. Tyson (eds) *Frontiers of Infant Psychiatry*, New York: Basic Books, pp. 315–27.

—— (1985) 'Toward a logic of organization in psycho-biological development', in H. Klar and L. Siever (eds) *Biologic Response Styles: clinical implications*, Clinical Insights Monograph, Washington, DC: American Psychiatric Press.

Sandler, J. and Rosenblatt, B. (1962) 'The concept of the representational world', *Psychoanalytic Study of the Child* 17: 128–45.

Simmel, G. (1950) *The Sociology of Georg Simmel*, ed. and trans. K. H. Wolff, Glencoe, IL: Free Press.

Spelke, E. S. and Cortelyou, A. (1981) 'Perceptual aspects of social knowing', in M. Lamb and L. Sherrod (eds) *Infant Social Cognition*, Hillsdale, NJ: Erlbaum, pp. 61–84.

Spitz, R. (1983) 'The evolution of dialogue', in R. Emde (ed.) *Rene A. Spitz: dialogues from infancy: selected papers*, New York: International Universities Press, pp. 179–95.

Sroufe, L. A. (1979) 'The ontogenesis of emotion', in J. Osofsky (ed.) *Handbook of Infant Development*, New York: Wiley, pp. 462–516.

—— and Fleeson, J. (1986) 'Attachment and the construction of relationships', in W. Hartup and Z. Rubin (eds) *Relationships and Development*, New York: Cambridge University Press, pp. 51–71.

Stechler, G. and Kaplan, S. (1980) 'The development of the self', *Psychoanalytic Study of the Child* 35: 85–105.

Stern, D. (1971) 'A microanalysis of the mother-infant interaction', *Journal of the American Academy of Child Psychiatry* 10: 501–507.

—— (1977) *The First Relationship*, Cambridge, MA: Harvard University Press.

—— (1983) 'The early development of schemas of self, of other, and of "self with other"', in J. D. Lichtenberg and S. Kaplan (eds) *Reflections on Self Psychology*, Hillsdale, NJ: Analytic Press, pp. 49–84.

—— (1985) *The Interpersonal World of the Infant*, New York: Basic Books.

—— (1989) 'The representation of relational patterns: developmental considerations', in A. Sameroff and R. Emde (eds) *Relationship Disturbances in Early Childhood*, New York: Basic Books, pp. 52–69.

Stolorow, R. and Atwood, G. (1992) *Contexts of Being*, Hillsdale, NJ: Analytic Press.

Sullivan, H. S. (1953) *The Interpersonal Theory of Psychiatry*, New York: Norton.

Thomas, E. A. C. and Martin, J. (1976) 'Analyses of parent-infant interaction', *Psychological Review* 83: 141–55.

Trevarthen, C. (1979) 'Communication and cooperation in early infancy', in M. Bullowa (ed.) *Before Speech*, New York: Cambridge University Press, pp. 321–47.

Tronick, E. (1980) 'The primacy of social skills in infancy', in D. Sawin, R. Hawkins, L. Walker, and J. Penticuff (eds) *Exceptional Infant*, vol. 4, New York: Brunner Mazel, pp. 144–58.

—— (1982) 'Affectivity and sharing', in E. Tronick (ed.) *Social Interchange in Infancy*, Baltimore, MD: University Park Press, pp. 1–8.

—— (1989) 'Emotions and emotional communication in infants', *American Psychologist* 44: 112–19.

—— Als, H. Adamson, L., Wise, S. and Brazelton, T. B. (1978) 'The infant's response to entrapment between contradictory messages in face-to-face interaction', *American Academy of Child Psychiatry* 17: 1–13.

—— and Brazelton, T. B. (1980) 'Monadic phases: a structural descriptive analysis of infant-mother face-to-face interaction', *Merrill Palmer Quarterly* 26: 3–24.

Vygotsky, L. S. (1978) *Mind in Society: the development of higher psychological processes*, Cambridge, MA: Harvard University Press.

Warner, R. (1987) 'Rhythmic organization of social interaction and observer ratings of positive affect and involvement', *Journal of Nonverbal Behavior* 11: 57–74.

Watson, J. (1985) 'Contingency perception in early social development', in T. Field and N. Fox (eds) *Social Perception in Infants*, Norwood, NJ: Ablex, pp. 157–76.

Weiss, P. (1973) *The Science of Life*, Mt. Kisco, NY: Futura.

Welkowitz, J. and Kuc, M. (1973) 'Interrelationships among warmth, genuineness, empathy and temporal speech pattern in interpersonal attraction', *Journal of Consulting and Clinical Psychology* 41: 472–3.

Wilson, A. and Malatesta, C. (1989) 'Affect and the compulsion to repeat: Freud's repetition compulsion revisited', *Psychoanalysis and Contemporary Thought* 12: 243–90.

Zeanah, C., Anders, T., Seifer, R. and Stern, D. (1990) 'Implications of research on infant development for psychodynamic theory and practice', *Journal of the American Academy of Child Psychiatry* 28: 657–68.

Zelnick, L. and Buchholz, E. (1990) 'The concept of mental representations in light of recent infant research', *Psychoanalytic Psychology* 7: 29–58.

AFTERWORD

I studied with Sid Blatt in 1971 and 1972, during my clinical psychology internship at the Connecticut Mental Health Center, a training site at the Yale University School of Medicine. We had a special match in our interests in Piaget, Werner, and the integration of developmental theory with clinical issues. Sid has been a mentor, colleague, friend, and inspiration to me for over three decades. I am honored to contribute this Festschrift for him.

Beatrice Beebe

Chapter 3

Representations in middle childhood
A dialogical perspective

Beatriz Priel

It is an honor and a pleasure to contribute to this volume dedicated to Sidney J. Blatt, one of the true pioneers of the empirical investigation of personality development and psychopathology within psychoanalytic theory. The study of personality development has inevitably led Blatt and colleagues (Behrends and Blatt 1985; Blatt, Auerbach and Levy 1997; Blatt, Brenneis, Schimek and Glick 1976; Blatt and Lerner 1983) to a concern with how patterns of relatedness with caregivers affect the individual's own capacities for interpersonal relationships and how these are further transformed into self-regulating capacities and behavior. These issues have been studied also from attachment (Bowlby 1973; Bretherton and Munholland 1999) and social cognition (Baldwin 1992; Damon and Hart 1988) perspectives. Investigations using object relations and social cognition frameworks have been focused mainly on adolescence and adulthood while attachment research centered initially on infancy and early childhood. Little is known about the transformations of patterns of relatedness into self-regulating capacities during middle childhood. This striking gap is consistent with the lack, until very recently, of studies of personality among school-aged children (Shiner 1998). This chapter's aim is to describe the application among school-aged children of Blatt and colleagues' empirical approach to the study of the transformations of early interpersonal relationships into personality structures. In the first part of the chapter, I present this theoretical approach, underscoring the dialogical perspective that has guided this line of research. Then I discuss the research pertaining to these ideas.

Within psychoanalytic theory, object relations approaches assume that children internalize basic aspects of early caretaking interactions by developing stable ways of representing these experiences (Beebe and Lachmann 1988; Blatt *et al.* 1997; Blatt *et al.* 1976; Sandler and Rosenblatt 1962; Stern 1985; Westen 1991; Westen *et al.* 1991). These internalized experiences of self with other serve as a basis for the construction of complex representational structures – object representations – that include conscious and unconscious schemas of self and other that work as templates through which experiences that affect behavior, feelings, and cognition are filtered.

Object representations are seen as complex organizing principles and as a network of concepts, affects, and images (Sandler 1994; Sandler and Rosenblatt 1962; Stern 1985). They are motivational structures that guide perception and affect processes of meaning attribution, as well as the organization of past experience and the construal of future prospects (Behrends and Blatt 1985; Greenberg and Mitchell 1983). Attachment and social cognition theories have developed similar conceptualizations of self-with-other representational structures that are called internal working models (Bowlby 1969; Main, Kaplan and Cassidy 1985) and schemas or scripts (Baldwin 1992), respectively. These representational structures of self and other are assumed to organize children's expectations and social behavior (Baldwin 1992; Bretherton 1991) and to regulate emotion and affect (Sroufe 1997). Representations of relationships are not seen as accurate reflections of real events, that is, as re-presentations of reality, but as patterns of mental activation (Fonagy 2001) or as pathways of procedural systems of relational knowing (Lyons-Ruth 1998) that might include defensive distortions (Bretherton and Munholland 1999).

Sandler characterized object representations as including two main realms: (a) a phenomenal or experiential realm (i.e., the subjective, here-and-now representation of the self and the object); and (b) a nonexperiential schema (i.e., an organization of knowledge, or a set of rules). According to Sandler and Rosenblatt (1962: 128), "Every wish involves a self-representation, an object representation, and a representation of the interaction between these." Emde (1994) expanded this idea and specified, following Luborsky and Crits-Christoph (1989), three components of the self–other interaction patterns that characterize the representational world: the wish of the self, the expected response of the other, and the response of the self. Thus, the idea of response, expected from the other or intended by the self, seems basic to the structuring of representations of relationships. The inherent responsivity that characterizes representations of relationships suggests a fundamental dialogical structure: meanings are created between partners as an emergent phenomenon.

This dialogical structure was already underscored in Spitz's (1965) observation of mother–infant mutual responsiveness to interactive cues. Spitz defined dialogue as the basic structure of mother–infant relationships and as a major tool, an instrument, of intrapsychic regulation; he suggested that reciprocal responsivity and anticipation are the very basis of preverbal and verbal interpersonal interchanges from the beginning of life. Moreover, he considered dialogical reciprocity so basic that he almost equated it with the concept of object relations (Spitz 1965). The dialogical structure of object relations provides the basis for intersubjective representations of relationships, as further developed in Beebe and Lachmann's (1988: 327) assumption that "what is represented is an emergent dyadic phenomenon, interaction structures, which cannot be described on the basis of either partner alone." Moreover, the expectation of patterns of responsiveness seems so fundamental for processes of growth and development that, in health, it is "taken for granted" from the very beginning (Rommetveit 1985: 189). Stern's observations of infant interactions with depressed mothers (1994) offer dramatic examples of a rupture of this taken-for-granted responsivity, a rupture leading to the installment of imitation instead of evolving intersubjectivity.

Using a different theoretical perspective, Vygotsky (1978, 1981) and Bakhtin (see Holquist 1990; Priel 1999) also explored the dialogical under-pinnings of the internal representations of self and other. According to Vygotsky, all higher mental functions have their origins in individual interpersonal relationships that have undergone processes of internaliza-tion:

> Any function in the child's cultural development appears twice, or on two planes. First it appears on the social plane and then on the psychological plane. First it appears between people as an interpsy-chological category, and then within the child as an intrapsychological category . . . . We may consider this position as a law in the full sense of the word, but it goes without saying that internalization transforms the process itself and changes its structure and functions.
>
> (Vygotsky 1981: 163)

Vygotsky considered internalization to be the main process by which the interpersonal transfers into the intrapsychic plane. It is important to note that, already in the quoted passage, this author, like attachment, social cognition, and object relations theorists, did not consider intrapsychic function to be a replica of its interpsychological-interpersonal precursor. Vygotsky's unique contribution, however, is his emphasis on the role of mediating symbolic or presymbolic tools, such as signs, expressions, or language, in the development of mental representations. His main con-tention is that what the child internalizes is the mediational means, the signs or words that emerge as the adult regulates the infant's and child's behavior.

A dialogical perspective highlights exchanges or relationships between coexisting, as well as between old and new object representations as fundamental for the understanding of the effects of those representations on behavior, emotion, and thought. From this perspective, the understand-ing of a specific object representation should take into account concomitant representations that may affect it in diverse ways, on the one hand as enriching agents or on the other as activating a defensive gap. This stance is congruent with the emphasis on the history of relationships as a major factor in contemporary transactional approaches to child development (Sameroff 1995), as well as with research on the negative effects of discrepant representations of caregivers (Fonagy 1996). Following this line of thought, the empirical research presented below assumes that object representations are affected not only by maturational factors and real interpersonal relationships but by coexistent object representations as well.

The empirical study of object representations

The empirical study of object representations has led to the design of methods based on responses to projective techniques, memories, dreams, and self-report inventories, all of which are intended to assess mental representations (Bell, Billington and Becker 1986; Blatt *et al.* 1997; Blatt and Lerner 1983; Krohn and Mayman 1974; Urist 1980; Westen 1991). A crucial evolution in the conceptualization and assessment of mental representations followed the development by Blatt and colleagues of the Object Relations Inventory (ORI), a projective technique for the assessment of qualitative and structural dimensions of object representations. This assessment technique is based on open narratives by individuals about parents or significant others (Blatt *et al.* 1979; Blatt *et al.* 1992; Diamond *et al.* 1991). Later, complementary procedures were developed for the assessment of representations of self (Blatt, Bers and Schaffer 1993).

The ORI is a procedure that encourages a natural narrative strategy through which the interviewee's personal idiom is conveyed. The narratives so gathered provide an experience-near account of a significant other that is very different from the responses that reflect representations of relationships through specific, imaginary, interpersonal situations suggested by the researcher (e.g., Shields, Ryan and Cicchetti 2001) or from reactions to projective techniques, such as the Rorschach, that involve unstructured and sometimes unusual stimuli (Blatt *et al.* 1976). The ORI narratives are subsequently analyzed and scored in relation to both their conscious contents and the unconscious organizational and regulatory principles involved. This scoring procedure is strongly anchored in cognitive and psychoanalytic conceptualizations of mental functioning and development (Blatt *et al.* 1992).

A major aspect of the ORI coding technique is the differentiation made between qualitative and structural aspects of mental representations, a procedure that has also been followed by other researchers of child development (see Shields *et al.* 2001). The distinction between qualitative and structural dimensions of object representations encompasses the two main areas of meaning attributed to self and other representations by Sandler (1994); whereas the structural aspects reflect the representation's organizing principles, the coding of qualitative categories assesses the phenomenological realm. The content scores refer to the presence in the narrative of explicit expressions of affection, ambitiousness, benevolence, warmth, constructive involvement, intellectuality, strength, punitiveness, criticism, nurturance and success attributed to the object and the degree to which the object is a positive versus a negative ideal. The Conceptual Level score constitutes a major structural and developmental dimension that is rated at one of five possible levels:

1   At the sensorimotor-preoperational level, the parent is experienced primarily in terms of need gratification.
2   At the concrete-perceptual level, the parent is described as separate from specific experiences of gratification and is recognized as a generalized entity in concrete, literal and demographic terms.
3   The qualities and attributes of representations at the external-iconic level are based on specific manifest properties, such as personality traits, behaviors, and interests of the parent.
4   At the internal-iconic level, representations reflect mainly an appreciation of more abstract and internal properties, like feelings and thoughts.
5   At the conceptual-representational level, the parent is represented as fully integrated and with enduring characteristics and a sense of history.

In what follows, empirical explorations of parental representations among school-aged children, as revealed by the ORI procedure, will be presented. After the basic investigation of continuities and changes of parental representations during the preschool and school years, I will present studies that focus on similarities and differences between representations of mother and father. Finally, the effects of representations of absent and new significant caregivers, as well as the relationships among these different representations, and their implications for child behavior and adjustment will be discussed.

Object representations in the preschool and school years

Over the years, Blatt and coworkers (Blatt and Behrends 1987; Blatt and Blass 1990; Blatt and Shichman 1983) proposed a developmental model of object representations that integrates object relational and cognitive-developmental conceptual frameworks. The development of object representations is assumed to progress through stages that are analogous to the stages of the development of representations of the inanimate world. The evaluation of the structural dimensions of object representations, mainly of their conceptual level, is assumed to reveal children's maturity level according to five epigenetic stages: sensorimotor, concrete perceptual, external iconic, internal iconic, and conceptual. On the other hand, the qualitative dimensions (benevolence, affective expressiveness, punitiveness, judgmental attitudes, etc.) are expected to correlate with the individual's experiential context and remain rather constant through time.

In a study intended to map the effects of age on the dimensions of object representations among 100 preschoolers (ages 5–6 years) and 106 school-aged children (ages 9–10), Priel, Myodovnick and Rivlin-Beniaminy (1995) reported a shift with age from an early focus on concrete and external attributes to an emphasis on internal attributes, as well as from egocentric and poorly differentiated to more integrated and complex representations. In addition, the qualitative aspects (e.g., benevolence and punitiveness) of children's representations were found to remain rather constant through time. These trends were recently found to continue into preadolescence (Priel *et al.* 2001; Waniel-Izhar, Priel and Besser 2003). More important, this pattern of age differences and similarities corroborates the developmental theory put forth by Blatt and colleagues, confirming the suggested multidimensionality of object relations in general and the different developmental timetables of these dimensions in particular (Westen *et al.* 1991).

A major question in the developmental study of object representations from a dialogical perspective concerns their relations with children's self-perceptions. A first attempt to answer this question can be found in a study of the relations between the object representations of school-aged children and their self-concepts (Avery and Ryan 1988). This study reports important associations between the degree of nurturance found in parental descriptions and school-age children's perceptions of cognitive and social capabilities. The question of the associations between parental representations and children's self-perceptions at earlier age levels is complex because of the known positively biased self-perceptions of preschoolers. A decline in this positive bias with age suggests that less positive self-perceptions are the result of adequate maturation. The study of the associations between parental representations and self-perceptions among preschool and school-aged children (Priel *et al.* 1995) has shown that the relations between children's self-perceptions and their parental representations' conceptual levels vary according to developmental principles. Among 9- or 10-year-old children, who characteristically maintain more or less realistic self-perceptions, higher Conceptual Level scores were significantly associated with higher assessments of social, physical, and cognitive competence, as well as with their sense of general self-worth. On the other hand, among preschool children, who characteristically overestimate their self-competence and social acceptance, parental representations with higher Conceptual Levels are associated with less idealized self-perceptions, as if greater sophistication of object relations was indicative of a lessening of self-inflation. This pattern of associations suggests the intimate intertwining of parental representations and children's self-concept and corroborates empirically the developmental underpinnings of assessments of the conceptual level of parental representations.

Although developmental processes were revealed mainly by the structural dimension of object representations, we hypothesized that both qualitative (e.g., benevolence and punitiveness) and structural dimensions (conceptual level) of object representations would predict more adaptive responses to separations from parents and to child-parent conflict situations. In a study conducted to elucidate these questions (Priel *et al.* 1995, study 2), we hypothesized that children reporting parental representations at a more advanced conceptual level and with more benign characteristics would be better able to integrate the positive and negative feelings evoked by separation and reunion situations, as well as by parent–child conflict. Specifically, qualitative dimensions of representations conveying the positive lived experience of the parent by the child were expected to be associated with positive outcomes of conflict. Higher Conceptual Level scores, on the other hand, were expected to be associated with greater frustration tolerance and a more reflective stance vis-à-vis an interpersonal conflict.

Eighty-four children were administered the ORI interview, and their responses to semiprojective reunion and conflict tasks were recorded (Priel *et al.* 1995). More benevolent parental representations and representations on a higher conceptual level were found to predict significantly the children's better adjustment to separation and reunion situations, as well as to parent–child conflicts. It is important to note here that these effects remained significant also after the very strong effects of age had been controlled. These findings provide some evidence to support the assumption that the studied dimensions of object representations tap active organizing principles of interpersonal relations and are not, for instance, prototypic descriptions characteristic of a specific age group (Leigh *et al.* 1992).

Basic to the concept of parental representations as organizing children's social behavior is the assumption that dimensions of parental representations will predict the quality of peer relationships. Empirical evidence of a significant association between children's representations of parents as nurturant on the one hand, and social acceptance as evaluated by peers on the other can already be found in Avery and Ryan's study (1988). Preliminary findings of a larger prospective project on the role played by parental representations in the development of children's social capabilities have recently corroborated these findings (Waniel-Izhar, Saban and Priel 2003). Using the Peer Nomination Inventory (Finnegan, Hodges and Perry 1996), we found significant associations between the content dimensions of parental representation and school children's prosocial behavior, as reported by each child's peers. Prosocial behavior refers to peer perceptions that a target child is willingly accepted by the group, that he or she is capable of sharing and giving things, and is friendly. More benevolent, involved, warm, and affectionate representations of mother and father were associated with higher prosocial behavior scores. In addition, higher scores on the punitiveness and judgmental dimensions of parental representations were associated with less prosocial behavior. These findings suggest that prosocial behavior, as perceived by peers, is significantly related with more benign parental representations.

Mother and father representations

The concordance between representations of different caregivers is an intriguing issue in the study of children's internal worlds. Although the study of the development of maternal representations provides an empirical basis for an understanding of the formation of representations over time, further elucidation of basic developmental processes requires the investigation of the formation of representations of fathers, as well as of other caregivers. Freud (1940: 188) believed that because the mother, in her nourishing and caregiving functions, is the infant's first love object, the mother–infant relation serves as "the prototype of all later love relationships, for both." This perspective suggests concordance between maternal and other caregiver representations. Similar predictions derive from Bowlby's (1958) assumption of monotropy in early childhood attachments – i.e., that children have a principal, preferred attachment figure who affects all other attachment patterns. Research on internal working models of attachment to mother and father shows extensive concordance, as well as important dissimilarities or nonconcordance between these working models (Belsky and Rovine 1987; Fox, Kimmerly and Schafer 1991; Steele, Steele and Fonagy 1996; van IJzendoorn and De Wolff 1997). Evidence in the developmental literature on the effects of the congruency and incongruency of object representations indicates that greater discrepancies between representations of main caregivers are associated with child maladjustment (Fonagy 1996). Moreover, Suess, Grossman and Sroufe (1992) found that combined information about attachment to both mother and father is the best predictor of play competence, conflict resolution, and behavior problems among preschoolers.

In a preliminary study of the relations between preschool ($n = 80$) and school-aged ($n = 96$) children's representations of mother and father, we (Priel and Myodovnik 1996) found a close correspondence between father and mother representations in all the dimensions scored. Although correlations between mother and father representations on qualitative dimensions (e.g., benevolence, punitiveness) were between .30 and .40, correlations between mother and father on structural dimensions (Conceptual Level, length, etc.) were between .70 and .75. A study just completed replicated these results in a sample of 115 children, aged 8 to 12 years (Waniel-Izhar and Priel 2003). These findings suggest a high concordance between the structure or organization level of mother and father representations; the concordance between the qualitative aspects of the representations is however only moderate. The findings also suggest that the structural aspects of mental representations reflect basic rules of organization while their qualitative dimensions convey the child's experiences with a specific caregiver. Moreover, these studies have also shown an important interaction between mother and father representations and the child's sex on the Conceptual Level variable. The Conceptual Level scores of mother representations among boys and of father representations among girls are significantly higher than in the mother–daughter and father–son pairs. These findings may indicate more differentiated representations of the parent of the opposite sex among school-aged children.

The representation of an unknown parent

Mental representations are assumed not just to reflect but also to construe reality (Sandler and Sandler 1998). Moreover, mental representations might not only reflect external reality but also convey the individual's particular interpretation of the experiences undergone and messages received. Even though this tenet once differentiated object relations from attachment theory approaches, distortions or defenses have also been recognized recently as important aspects of internal working models of attachment (Bretherton and Munholland 1999). To investigate how parental representations are constructed, we examined descriptions of both the present and absent parental figures of adopted children (Priel, Kantor and Besser 2000). The study of a sample of adoptees under closed adoption (i.e., neither the child nor the adoptive parents know who the biological parents are) provides a privileged perspective for the exploration of the characteristics of a representation formed without a real interactive anchor – the representation of the adoptee's biological mother. A major objective of this study was the investigation of the relations between representations of adoptive and birth mothers in the context of the adjustment of adopted children. It was assumed that the knowledge of being an adopted child might affect all object representations – not only the adoptee's representation of his or her birth mother but also the representation of the adoptive mother as well.

In order to investigate the effects of adoption on maternal representations, adoptees' adoptive mother representations were compared with maternal representations of nonadopted children. Both adoptees' representations of their adoptive mothers and nonadopted children's representations of their mothers are constructed on the basis of daily, reiterated, actual interactions, but within two very different mental contexts: the knowledge of being adopted in one case and the knowledge of being a biological offspring in the other. Two additional questions were explored: first, the similarities and differences that may exist between representations of the adoptive and the biological mother among adoptees; and second, the relation between the degree of discrepancy between these two maternal representations and the adjustment of adopted children.

Both attachment and object relations theories assume that the representations of parents are normally modulated by the child's actual interactions with them. This implies that, in the total absence of real interactions, representations by adopted children of their biological mothers might be expected to present more extreme characteristics, as compared with representations of the mothers (whether adoptive or nonadoptive) who actually raise the child. Clinical reports of adopted adults in treatment provide examples of extremely bad (Rosenberg and Horner 1991), as well as ideal, representations of biological parents (Deeg 1990). These representations may seem contradictory; however, both types of representations have an extreme, exaggerated quality.

The empirical study of adoptees' maternal representations revealed that their representations of both biological and adoptive mother have a lower conceptual level and are less benevolent and more punitive than are nonadoptees' maternal representations. These findings might suggest that having been given up is associated with negative and less developed representations of all caregivers. Moreover, adoptees' maternal representations, mainly those of their biological mothers, were found to be rather concrete and centered on physical characteristics only. When asked how they knew about their biological mothers' physical appearance, the adopted children replied that she must look the way they do. The adoptees' physical descriptions of the biological mother seem to have taken the self as a point of reference. The representations of an unknown parent thus reverse the usual developmental process: adoptees' biological mother representations apparently originate in the child's self-image (Priel *et al.* 2000). This finding sheds light on some of the complexities of the relations between lived experience and mental representation.

The comparison between representations of adoptive and biological mothers within our sample of adopted children revealed that, although the two have similar conceptual levels, biological mother representations are significantly less benign than are representations of adoptive mothers. This consistency of conceptual levels across representations parallels previous findings that this dimension reflects the individual's level of personality organization and is relatively constant and independent of the content of the representation (Blatt *et al.* 1992; Priel *et al.* 1995). In addition, the finding that representations of the birth mothers are significantly less benevolent and more punitive than are the representations of the adoptive mothers supports theoretical and clinical suggestions that, in a normal sample, the biological parent is conceived as containing the split off negative aspects of the adoptive parent (Rosenberg and Horner 1991). Finally, the degree of incongruence between the two maternal representations in the adoptee sample was found to be associated with the level of the children's externalizing symptoms (e.g., delinquent, aggressive, and hyperactive behavior). These findings corroborate basic assumptions about the importance of the integration between diverse object representations for normal development, as well as about an association between splitting and aggressive behavior (Fonagy 1996).

Preliminary results of a longitudinal research project (Priel and Manashko 2003) in progress center on the development of representations of a new caregiver among children who have been moved away from their families because of severe maltreatment. In agreement with existing research on maltreated children (Ornduff and Kelsey 1996), maternal representations were found to be significantly more negative and less mature than were representations of nonmaltreated children from a similar socioeconomic environment. Concomitantly, we found that representations of the new substitute caregiver among maltreated children had extremely positive characterisitics. These findings corroborate the adoption study evidence showing that, in conflictual situations, children report extreme lack of concordance between representations (Priel *et al.* 2000). The differences documented between biological and adoptive mother representations among adoptees and between mother and new caregiver representations among maltreated children seem to involve a specific defensive strategy. Prospective longitudinal research may provide a better understanding of the impact of diverse object representations in community and special children populations.

Epilogue

The research reviewed conveys a picture of object representations as multidimensional and underscores the importance of the relations between diverse object representations. The obtained results emphasize the effects of old object representations on new ones, as well as the importance for normal development of the integration of significant object representations. Moreover, empirical findings suggest the existence of a network of representations that includes past and present, as well as real and imaginary, interactions with significant others; different representations might be activated in different circumstances, and their relative importance might shift with age. This approach thus views development as the result of the transactions among a child's characteristics, existent representational patterns, past history, and his or her present interpersonal relationships, context, and life circumstances.

The study of parental representations and of absent and new significant caregivers strengthens the conceptualization of object representations not only as encoding of experience but as active factors in children's adjustment. Moreover, this research suggests that basic characteristics of an individual's object representations might significantly affect interpersonal relationships, as well as be affected by changes in actual relationships. However, much still remains to be explored about specific aspects of continuity and change of parental representations and their observable corollaries. The work presented here provides some evidence regarding the way in which the dialogue between theory and empirical research initiated by Sidney Blatt's creative approach to object representations leads to a renewed evaluation of the characteristics, role, and effects of mental representations of caregivers. Blatt's contribution opened as a field of investigation the similarities and differences among object representations, a field that may be compared to Primo Levi's (1975: 60) description of chemistry:

> We must distrust the almost-the-same, the practically identical, the approximate . . . . The differences can be small, but they can lead to radically different consequences . . . . The chemist's trade consists in good part in being aware of these differences, knowing them close up, and seeing their effects. And not only the chemist's trade.

References

Avery, R. R. and Ryan, R. M. (1988) 'Object relations and ego development: comparison and correlates in middle childhood', *Journal of Personality* 56: 547–69.

Baldwin, M. W. (1992) 'Relational schemas and the processing of social information', *Psychological Bulletin* 112: 461–84.

Beebe, B. and Lachmann, F. M. (1988) 'The contribution of mother-infant mutual influence to the origin of self and object representations', *Psychoanalytic Psychology* 5: 305–37.

Behrends, R. S. and Blatt, S. J. (1985) 'Internalization and psychological development throughout the life cycle', *Psychoanalytic Study of the Child* 40: 11–39.

Bell, M., Billington, R. and Becker, B. (1986) 'A scale for the assessment of object relations: reliability, validity, and factorial invariance', *Journal of Clinical Psychology* 42: 733–41.

Belsky, J. and Rovine, M. (1987) 'Temperament and attachment security in the strange situation: an empirical rapprochement', *Child Development* 58: 787–95.

Blatt, S. J., Auerbach, J. S. and Levy, K. N. (1997) 'Mental representations in personality development, psychopathology, and the therapeutic process', *Review of General Psychology* 1: 351–74.

—— and Behrends, R. S. (1987) 'Internalization, separation-individuation, and the nature of therapeutic action', *International Journal of Psycho-Analysis* 68: 279–97.

—— Bers, S. A., and Schaffer, C. E. (1993) *The Assessment of Self Descriptions*, unpublished research manual, Yale University, New Haven, CT.

—— and Blass, R. B. (1990) 'Attachment and separateness: a dialectic model of the products and processes of development throughout the life cycle', *Psychoanalytic Study of the Child* 45: 107–27.

—— Brenneis, C. B., Schimek, J. G. and Glick, M. (1976) 'Normal development and psychopathological impairment of the concept of the object on the Rorschach', *Journal of Abnormal Psychology* 35: 364–73.

Blatt, S. J., Chevron, E. S., Quinlan, D. M., Schaffer, C. E. and Wein, S. J. (1992) *The Assessment of Qualitative and Structural Dimensions of Object Representations*, unpublished research manual, Yale University, New Haven, CT.

—— and Lerner, H. (1983) 'Investigations in the psychoanalytic theory of object relations and object representations', in J. Masling (ed.) *Empirical Studies of Psychoanalytic Theories*, vol. 1, Hillsdale, NJ: Erlbaum, pp. 189–249.

—— and Shichman, S. (1983) 'Two primary configurations of psychopathology', *Psychoanalysis and Contemporary Thought* 6: 187–254.

—— Wein, S. J., Chevron, E. S. and Quinlan, D. M. (1979) 'Parental representations and depression in normal young adults', *Journal of Abnormal Psychology* 88: 388–97.

Bowlby, J. (1958) 'The nature of the child's tie to the mother', *International Journal of Psycho-Analysis* 39: 350–73.

—— (1969) *Attachment and Loss, vol. 1, attachment*, New York: Basic Books.

—— (1973) *Attachment and Loss, vol. 2, separation, anxiety and anger*, New York: Basic Books.

Bretherton, I. (1991) 'The roots and growing points of attachment theory', in C. M. Parkes, J. Stevenson and P. Marris (eds) *Attachment Across the Life Cycle*, New York: Routledge, pp. 9–31.

—— and Munholland, K. A. (1999) 'Internal working models in attachment relationships: a construct revisited', in J. Cassidy and P. R. Shaver (eds) *Handbook of Attachment: theory, research and clinical applications*, New York: Guilford Press, pp. 89–111.

Damon, W. and Hart, D. (1988) *Self-Understanding in Childhood and Adolescence*, New York: Cambridge University Press.

Deeg, C. F. (1990) 'Defensive functions and the adoptee's cathexis of the lost object', *Psychoanalysis and Psychotherapy* 8: 145–56.

Diamond, D., Blatt, S. J., Stayner, D. A. and Kaslow, N. (1991) *Differentiation-Relatedness of Self and Object Relations*, unpublished research manual (revised version), Yale University, New Haven, CT.

Emde, R. N. (1994) 'Developing psychoanalytic representations of experience', *Infant Mental Health Journal* 15: 42–9.

Finnegan R. A., Hodges, E. V. and Perry, D. G. (1996) 'Preoccupied and avoidant coping during middle childhood', *Child Development* 67: 1318–28.

Fonagy, P. (1996) 'The significance of the development of metacognitive control over mental representations in parenting and infant development', *Journal of Clinical Psychoanalysis* 5: 67–86.

—— (2001) *Attachment Theory and Psychoanalysis*, New York: Other Press.

Fox, N. A., Kimmerly, N. L. and Schafer, W. D. (1991) 'Attachment to mother/attachment to father: a meta-analysis', *Child Development* 61: 210–25.

Freud, S. (1940) 'An outline of psychoanalysis', in J. Strachey (ed. and trans.) *The Standard Edition of the Complete Works of Sigmund Freud*, vol. 23, London: Hogarth Press, pp. 144–208.

Greenberg, J. R. and Mitchell, S. A. (1983) *Object Relations in Psychoanalytic Theory*, Cambridge, MA: Harvard University Press.

Holquist, M. (1990) *Dialogism: Bakhtin and his world*, New York: Routledge.

Krohn, A. and Mayman, M. (1974) 'Object representations in dreams and projective tests', *Bulletin of the Menninger Clinic* 38: 445–66.

Leigh, J., Westen, D., Barens, A. and Mendel, M. (1992) 'Assessing complexity of representations of people from TAT and interview data', *Journal of Personality* 60: 809–37.

Levi, P. (1975) *The Periodic Table*, trans. R. Rosenthal, London: Abacus, 1986.

Luborsky, L. and Crits-Christoph, P. (1989) 'A relationship pattern measure: the core conflictual relationship theme', *Psychiatry* 52: 250–9.

Lyons-Ruth, K. (1998) 'Implicit relational knowing: its role in development and psychoanalytic treatment', *Infant Mental Health Journal* 19: 282–9.

Main, M., Kaplan, N. and Cassidy, J. (1985) 'Security in infancy, childhood and adulthood: a move to the level of representation', in I. Bretherton and E. Waters (eds) *Growing Points in Attachment: theory and research, Monographs of the Society for Research in Child Development* 50 (1–2, Serial No. 209), Chicago, IL: University of Chicago Press, pp. 66–104.

Ornduff, S. R. and Kelsey, R. M. (1996) 'Object relations of sexually and physically abused female subjects: a TAT analysis', *Journal of Personality Assessment* 66: 91–105.

Priel, B. (1999) 'Bakhtin and Winnicott: on dialogue, self and cure', *Psychoanalytic Dialogues* 9: 487–503.

—— Kantor, B. and Besser, A. (2000) 'Two maternal representations: a study of Israeli adopted children', *Psychoanalytic Psychology* 17: 128–45.

—— and Manashko, S. (2003) 'Representations of a substitute caregiver among maltreated school age children: the role of dissociation', manuscript in preparation.

—— and Myodovnick, E. (1996) 'Representations of mother and father', unpublished manuscript, Department of Behavioral Sciences, Ben-Gurion University of the Negev, Beer-Sheva, Israel.

—— Myodovnick, E. and Rivlin-Beniaminy, N. (1995) 'Parental representations among preschool and fourth-grade children: integrating object relational and cognitive developmental frameworks', *Journal of Personality Assessment* 65: 372–88.

—— Waniel-Izhar, A., Saksig-Bitton, I., Myodovnick, E., Weinberg, B., Mahalel, A. and Sisso, A. (2001) *Manual for the Coding of Parental Representations among 6–13 Year-Old Children*, unpublished research manual, Department of Behavioral Sciences, Ben-Gurion University of the Negev, Beer-Sheva, Israel.

Rommetveit, R. (1985) 'Language acquisition as increasing linguistic structuring of experience and symbolic behavior control', in J. V. Wertsch (ed.) *Culture, Communication, and Cognition: Vygotskian perspectives*, Cambridge, England: Cambridge University Press, pp. 162–204.

Rosenberg, E. B. and Horner, T. H. (1991) 'Birth parents romances and identity formation in adopted children', *American Journal of Orthopsychiatry* 61: 70–7.

Sameroff, A. J. (1995) 'General systems theories and developmental psychopathology', in D. Cicchetti and D. J. Cohen (eds) *Developmental Psychopathology*, New York: Wiley, 659–95.

Sandler, J. (1994) 'Fantasy, defense, and the representational world', *Infant Mental Health Journal* 15: 26–36.

—— and Rosenblatt, B. (1962) 'The concept of the representational world', *Psychoanalytic Study of the Child* 17: 128–45.

—— and Sandler, A. M. (1998) *Internal Objects Revisited*, London: Karnac.

Shields, A. M., Ryan, R. M., and Cicchetti, D. (2001) 'Narrative representations of caregivers and emotional dysregulation as predictors of maltreated children's rejection by peers', *Developmental Psychology* 37: 321–37.

Shiner, R. L. (1998) 'How shall we speak of children's personality in middle childhood?: a preliminary taxonomy', *Psychological Bulletin* 124: 308–32.

Spitz, R. A. (1965) 'The evolution of dialogue', in M. Schur (ed.) *Drives, Affects, Behavior*, vol. 2, New York: International Universities Press, pp. 170–92.

Sroufe, L. A. (1997) 'Psychopathology as an outcome of development', *Development and Psychopathology* 9: 251–68.

Steele, H., Steele, M. and Fonagy, P. (1996) 'Associations among attachment classifications of mothers, fathers, and their infants', *Child Development* 67: 541–55.

Stern, D. (1985) *The Interpersonal World of the Infant*, New York: Basic Books.

—— (1994) 'One way to build a clinically relevant baby', *Infant Mental Health Journal* 15: 9–25.

Suess, G. J., Grossman, K. E. and Sroufe, L. A. (1992) 'Effects of infant attachment to mother and father on quality of adaptation to preschool: from dyadic to individual organization of self', *International Journal of Behavior Development* 15: 43–65.

Urist, J. (1980) 'Object relations', in R. W. Woody (ed.) *Encyclopedia of Clinical Assessment*, vol. 2, San Francisco, CA: Jossey-Bass pp. 821–33.

van IJzendoorn, M. H., and De Wolff, M. S. (1997) 'In search of the absent father – meta analysis of infant-father attachment: a rejoinder to our discussants', *Child Development* 68: 604–9.

Vygotsky, L. S. (1978) *Mind and Society: the development of higher psychological processes*, eds M. Cole, V. John-Steiner, S. Scribner, and E. Souberman, Cambridge, MA: Harvard University Press.

—— (1981) 'The genesis of higher mental functions', in J. V. Wertsch (ed. and trans.) *The Concept of Activity in Soviet Psychology*, Armonk, NY: Sharpe pp. 144–88.

Waniel-Izhar, A. and Priel, B. (2003) 'Effects of school-aged children's representations of mother and father', manuscript in preparation.

—— —— and Besser, A. (2003) 'The role of internal representations of self and mother', manuscript submitted for publication.

—— Saban, E. and Priel, A. (2003) 'Parental representations and pro-social behavior among school age children', unpublished manuscript.

Westen, D. (1991) 'Social cognition and object relations', *Psychological Bulletin* 109: 429–55.

—— Klepser, J., Ruffins, S. A., Silverman, M., Lifton, N. and Boekamp, J. (1991) 'Object relations in childhood and adolescence: the development of working representations', *Journal of Consulting and Clinical Psychology* 59: 400–9.

Chapter 4

On spatialization

Personal and theoretical thoughts

Norbert Freedman

Psychic space is a compelling concept, but like love, it is a many splendored thing. "Give me land, lots of land . . . . Don't fence me in," so the song goes (Porter 1944). In these words and in this familiar tune we can hear an affirmation of humanity's profound longing for experiences of expansion, together with recognition of boundedness.

This yearning and this recognition enter myriad aspects of human discourse and of course psychoanalytic discourse as well. Almost every major analytic position relies on a notion of space. Grotstein (1978) has summarized this reliance on expansion and on boundedness in Freud's writings, Klein's (1930) ideas of introjection and projection are familiar to all, Viderman (1979) speaks of psychoanalytic space, Ogden (1986) contrasts analytic space with dream space, and most recently Bromberg (1998) has spoken of "standing in the spaces." Each of these positions refers to humanity's craving once more for expansion and boundedness. Here I shall attempt to place such notions of space as they can be understood within a context of more empirically grounded studies of analytic discourse.

Perspectives on psychic space

Psychic space has come to my attention from three vantage points: First, it is part of our representational world. Whether a thought, an image, a percept is rendered in two, three, or multidimensional space, it presents and re-presents the content proffered with vividness, color, or shading. I suggest that in this representational perspective the space portrayed has much to do with psychic structure. Next, psychic space also appears in its generative form. Space can be created, shaped, and implemented. Here space can anticipate content, and for that matter, it creates room so that content may take residence. Here space also refers to transitional phenomena and implies the potential for representations to develop. Space now becomes a dynamic force in its own right. Third, space is an actuality. We all are surrounded by an atmosphere, live in a country, a city, a building. This issue, space as an objective physical actuality impinging on our inner representation of space or even generating it, leads us to what I shall call the epistemological issue. In human interchanges, all three of these aspects are present at any given moment, although with varying saliency. But they form a Gestalt and refer to what I shall call the process of spatialization. Spatialization is the theme of this contribution.

Let us launch our discussion with one of Sidney Blatt's earlier contributions. During the 1970s, Blatt recognized the crucial importance of spatial representations. This was shown by his dramatic finding in a study (Blatt and Ritzler 1974) on mental structure in suicidal patients, not simply those with suicidal ideation but those who actually succeeded in committing suicide. These patients' use of transparencies in their Rorschach responses signified the loss of three-dimensional representations. Blatt and Ritzler viewed the transparency as an abortive attempt to create volume as well as depth. In their study on the manifest content of dreams, Roth and Blatt (1974) found that the emphasis on specific spatial representations like boundaries, verticality, directionality, volume, and three-dimensional integration pointed to aspects not only of pathology but also of distinct levels of personality integration. Blatt's vision of the significance of spatial representation builds upon a long line of seminal studies in psychoanalysis that I wish to summarize briefly.

The representational perspective of space is well exemplified in the work of Lewin (1973). He wrote of the dream as a screen, a two-dimensional ground of sorts onto which the figures of self and object are projected. Schilder's (1935) notion of the body image refers to the presence of a three-dimensional portrayal of the body ego, and it is this spatially elaborated representation that constitutes one's body self. Federn (1952) wrote about flexible and rigid ego boundaries, a notion that involves a conception of space in the realm of reality testing. Most recently, Anzieu (1990) has put forth the notion of skin ego, a psychic envelope both imaginary and actual, that embraces all the functions we usually designate as ego. All of these ideas assert that there is a mode of spatial representation that exists side by side, or is coordinated with, mental content but that is not reducible to this content. Through the emphasis on boundedness, each of these lines of thought contributes toward a definition of a quite stable aspect of personality and mental structure.

The Blatts also play a role in my second perspective on spatialization because the focus has to do with the creative function of space. I said the Blatts advisedly, for I refer to the joint work of Sidney Blatt and Ethel Blatt (Blatt and Blatt, 1984), which deals with the role of space in art. The Blatts offer us a new vision of the history of art forms, from Paleolithic Art, through Greco-Roman Art, to the more recent periods of impressionism, Cubism, and Modernism. Constituting the historical framework are the Piagetian modes in the development of the perception of space, with each period offering a distinct configuration. Their work is a wedding of the art historian and the cognitive scientist. But Blatt, as a scientist, recognizes that "throughout civilization the construction of concepts of space has been central to understanding human nature. Thus, there must be a common structure to the artist's creation of spatial forms and the scientist's conceptualization of space" (Blatt and Blatt 1984: 22). This recognition is central to the second aspect of space in psychoanalysis – its generative function.

Such space-creating activity, be it in art or in psychoanalysis, is inevitably implemented by the actions of the body self. It is through the sensing body self – present from the earliest moments of infancy through visual, auditory, olfactory, and synesthetic sensing and, most importantly, through motor actions – that a sense of inner space emerges and, at critical moments of the life cycle, becomes reconfirmed. This sense of an inner space is thus not only experienced but also created, and it is this creation of psychic space that is one of the threshold moments of what we have termed spatialization. When such space-creating acts appear in adult discourse, they might simply accompany verbal representation, or they may be anticipatory. They may signal the not yet verbalized or even the unthought known (Bollas 1987). They point to a transitional state that offers the opportunity for the shaping of yet unformulated thought. It is the state to which Winnicott (1971) has given the evocative name of potential space. Here space is clearly not just representational, and with the me and the not-me still to be shaped, its possibilities are manifold, its actualities still diffuse. This is spatialization proper.

For my inevitable third perspective on spatialization, I will turn to Blatt's (1995) recent contribution, which is an application of his earlier work. In his study of the Vincent Foster suicide, Blatt shows us how the collapse of inner psychic space ultimately led to the act of self-destruction. And yet, all this could not have happened without a certain set of actualities: Whitewater, Travelgate, and the incredible pressures and counterpressures of the 1994 White House. Yes, the realities of life exerted an irrevocable impact upon a very stable representational mental structure.

The actuality of a patient's treatment situation has an interesting forerunner in the history of psychoanalysis. I refer to Erikson's (1962) reinterpretation of the Dora case, in which he notes that Dora's construction and representations of Herr and Frau K. must be viewed in the unusual actuality of the patient's treatment situation – arranged as it was by Dora's father. The issue has recently come to fore not as an empirical issue but as one concerning the knowledge base of psychoanalysis. Cavell (1998) most recently stressed the necessity for recognizing an actual shared reality as a common frame that renders a dialogue feasible.

Space is a term so much used in popular culture; it seems intuitively persuasive, and as we have just seen, it has a persistent, ubiquitous presence in psychoanalytic writings. More complex is our notion of spatialization.

However, before turning to some of the empirical evidence in its support, I will tell and discuss a biographical clinical story in order to capture the spirit with which the notion of spatialization is being used here.

A biographical episode

My interest and involvement with the issue of psychic space is of very personal origin, and I thought it only appropriate to share this with the reader. For after all, it is not uncommon that the ideas we write about, the events we select for focal observations, the very themes of what we search for and research, are rooted in our own private lives.

I am a blind psychoanalyst. I have been totally blind for about five years and partially so for decades. In the transition from seeing to not seeing, I have been much concerned to sustain an effective quality of interaction and communication, of sensing, symbolizing, visualizing, and interpreting in clinical practice. In daily interactions with friends, colleagues, or patients in dyadic settings, my handicap has been of little consequence. I know the other is there, in front of me. I have little difficulty absorbing meanings – receiving, imagining, fantasizing or symbolizing – and transforming thoughts into shared language. The person opposite me – through voice, body movement, and, as you will see in a moment, olfactory cues – is alive and present. But this is possible only because of my own sense of space, and I mean my perception of physical space or of the overall physicality of the situation – the room, the distance from chair to chair, or chair to couch, the patient's entrance through the door and the sounds of his or her reclining, even the rate of breathing. The sense of physical space is also confirmed and reconfirmed by my own body movements – leaning forward or reclining. There is such a thing as optimal distance, with too far being withdrawal and too close – and I can feel it in my face – being intrusive. When distance is not optimal, I experience interference in my thinking and imagining. I then find it within myself to regulate this sense of space through my own bodily actions. Here optimal conditions of space can lead to optimal conditions of listening.

However, my mental functioning becomes severely disrupted when the spatial configuration of the environment is altered. If for some reason a usually dyadic setting switches to multiple participants, if chairs or tables are moved about, if I do not know where the voices are coming from, then I feel encroached upon, and so are my thoughts. Although I might have felt expansive at one moment, suddenly now I and my thoughts have shrunk. There appears to be a correspondence between the experience of the physical arrangement and the clarity of mental functioning. I also feel disorganized when I can no longer use my body to enhance my awareness of space. When I am in a strange place where I do not know the distances among the walls, furniture, and people, I often use the extension of the carpet as a referent.

When I lose track of the external space, I can go into psychotic-like despair, and what was clarity at one moment becomes kaleidoscopic confusion and chaos at the next. Experiences of both boundedness and expansion have disappeared. All this describes the necessity for a more or less stable frame within which I situate myself. This external frame is matched by an internal sense – a space within – that is a crucial aspect of the cohesiveness and integrity of self.

But then there is also the space between, that is, between myself and my patient. This space is much more sensitively regulated in the intimacy of analytic interaction. The space between us resides not only in my bodily motions and the patient's presence and voice quality but in the modulation of other sensory modalities as well, notably the sense of smell. I have observed over the years that the sheer quantity and intensity of fragrance use by my patients, especially the women, is much greater than is typical, I am told, in the clinical practice of my sighted colleagues. For a person accustomed to being looked at, admired, or adored, which in our culture is especially true of women, the use of perfume is a most persuasive gesture saying, "Notice me, experience me, even though you do not see me." The volume of perfume used seems to be a direct indicator of the affect of the day. I tell my patients that I can visualize what I sense or hear, but I also recognize that their experience of not being seen is a handicap that must be acknowledged for both of us.

So far I have spoken of the space within and the space between, but the story goes further. Here is an episode I encountered in my practice. It started during the 10 minute break between patients.

During the preceding session, I had received a message on my answering machine from a colleague requesting some material for a paper on which we were collaborating and that I had recorded on an audiocassette. I expected the cassette to be on the chair next to my desk, but to no avail. My secretary had moved the tape. I searched for the chair and first could not find it. Then when I did, I discovered the cassette was not on it. I felt a sense of panic, found myself pacing the floor, searching the bookshelves frantically until I located the cassette in an apparently hidden place. Several minutes had elapsed. Even though the crisis may seem to have passed, it was only now that the full brunt of affect emerged – the frustration, despair, rage at my secretary, hatred of my dependency on the external frame, and a sense of chaos. I sat down, found myself stroking my forehead and my neck, soothing cheeks and lips, and fingering my fingers. I calmed down, was able to listen to the content on the tape, and recalled the material. My reflective functions had returned. I was ready to receive my patient. I seemed to have created a space within myself.

As my patient entered, I was greeted by a wave of heavy perfume. She tended to be a perfume user generally, but I had come to learn that, for her, this amount of fragrance was a signal that she was quite depressed. It was a sign saying, "Notice me. I am here." A space had been created between us, so that her subjectivity immediately entered into my consciousness, and she knew it.

She lay down on the couch, and immediately and unwittingly, I found myself leaning forward. I wanted to receive her affect in all its dimensions. As I leaned forward, the actual space between us narrowed. I heard her despair and also relived the despair I had felt just a few moments earlier when I could not find the tape, the cassette, the words I needed to get back to my colleague. The boundaries between my patient's despair and mine fused. I felt that her subjectivity and mine had become one. As I sensed signals of confusion, I found it necessary to pull back, and I literally reclined in my chair.

It is one of the great advantages of the analytic frame that in moments of crisis we can create distance for ourselves and for our patients. By leaning back and by remaining silent, we can create physical and temporal space, and that is what I did. Then I heard her associations – a recent humiliation at work, an allusion to mother, a memory, and a questioning of me. I listened to her, reconstructing these themes, and then I offered an interpretation. I was able to both use and set aside my earlier turmoil – it was a symbolizing countertransference I was experiencing as I recognized those associations that belonged to her and those that belonged to me. I felt we had shifted from that which was immediately given to the imaginary and maybe even to the symbolic – all within a span of less than 50 minutes.

As I reflect upon this episode, I realize that my patient and I had traversed certain spatial configurations that may well be present in all clinical encounters. The first is inherent to my effort to situate myself in physical space – exploring the surface of my desk, touching bookshelves and the arrangement of my chairs, acts that reflect the affirmation of belief in the actuality of the space out there.

Next, I sought to overcome my transitory state of panic and despair by various forms of self-soothing; touching the boundaries of my skin, I seemed to have created a sense of inner body-self space that extended from the core of my body to the surface of my skin. I negotiated a transition from chaos and despair to the recognition of what I felt. I created a subjective or perhaps transitional epistemology through which I learned about my inner state.

As my patient entered the room, greeting me with a wave of perfume, she certainly demarcated a space between us. She offered me the opportunity to take in the sensation, reflect upon it, connecting it to what I knew about her clinical state. I created an object relational space, for now, through the agency of reflective functioning, I experienced her psychic presence. It was a shared intersubjective experience and, with it, an object relational epistemology.

While I sat in my chair behind her, leaning forward and then reclining again, I remembered my earlier state of panic. I relived the frustration and the state of transition once more reappeared. Momentarily I did not know where my feelings ended and where hers emerged. This situation had all the attributes of what has been termed potential space. It was a space marked by penetration and interpenetration, with diffuse boundaries. To follow the well-trodden path laid out by Winnicott (1971), we might call this realm a transitional epistemology, an uncertain mode of knowing.

In my reclining and opening up further physical distance, I found myself reflecting upon my patient's story – her emotions, her fantasies, her history, her relationship to me. I was thus traversing space within her, within me, and between us, and setting aside my tension of half an hour earlier, I created my own symbolizing space. Now we worked in tandem, two symbolizers interacting with one another. The genesis of this symbolizing attainment accrued incrementally within the confines of a single hour.

The sense of space, then, is not a simple entity. It contains various dimensions or attributes: inner body-self space, object relational space, transitional space, symbolizing space, all unfolding within the perception of an actual framework of physical space – the room, the chair, and two persons meeting. These spatial attributes are often registered in the non-verbal mode, and when they become present, they mark the presence of analytic work and, with it, a good hour. Symbolizing space may be the aimed-for achievement, but it is not attained without the prior encounter with inner (i.e., body-self space), relational space, and potential space.

The concept of spatialization in psychoanalytic dicourse: empirical studies

I formulated the foregoing reflections about myself in the context of my clinical practice some years ago. Clearly there are self-observations embedded within the context of my ongoing clinical and theoretical research. These observations describe a range of attributes of psycho-analytic space, depicted in terms of the many nuances of sensorimotor interaction that come to play in the transference-countertransference matrix. But the observations also include the ingredients of the basic perspectives of "spatialization" with which I started this essay and that has been the subject matter of empirical research that my colleagues and I have conducted. Within the personal episode, we can see the clear delineation of the representational perspectives of space, the generative perspectives of spatialization, and the actuality of space. These are all issues touched upon in recent and earlier empirical work, and I would now like to summarize some highlights. In this discussion, we will reverse the order, starting with actuality, continuing with the generative aspects of spatialization, and ending with its implications for the process of symbol formation.

The actuality of physical space and the actuality of the frame

The analytic situation, in its essence, represents an attempt to rely upon the close interplay between physical actuality and psychic life. There is the physical surround, the relative proximity or distance between the participants, and the expectation to associate and for the mind to roam. The analytic situation exemplifies the view that it is the frame that helps shape psychic life. Paradoxically, we can even note an affirmation of this view through the much-discussed "breaking of the frame," for the recognition of the impact of breaking entails a recognition of the efficacy and importance of that which is broken. It is the juxtaposition of the homogeneity of the physical surround with the expectation to generate shared meanings that creates a tension, and this tension moves the patient toward the spatialization of the inner world.

The thesis that it is the external context that can shape the mind in the direction of spatialization and, with it, the symbolizing process has led me to consider observations far removed from the analytic situation: cross-cultural studies. There it can be shown that the physical surround, the frame if you wish, can create an inner state of exploration and containment that leads to highly specific modes of reflective thought. Studies conducted during the 1940s and 1950s demonstrated the relationship between the physical habitat and crucial aspects of mental functioning (Witkin 1977). To summarize a very complex literature, there was convincing evidence that qualities of mind appeared to be shaped by the demand conditions imposed by the ecological surround (including forms of child-rearing practices). Cultural groups revealed sharp differences in modes of thinking, the articulation of the body schema, and the language organization revealed in mythology. The homogeneous surround seemed to favor psychological differentiation; the variegated surround appeared to foster dedifferentiation. One might say that these groups differed in symbolizing function and symbolizing space.

Cavell (1998) has brought home the importance of the objective space for psychoanalytic discourse through her notion of triangulation. She develops the thesis that two minds can get to know one another only through the presence of a third force: an objective world beyond that of analyst and patient. Unless one can be objective about this tertiary sphere, we are reduced to a one-person psychology. For adequate discourse, one must recognize the things we do and the room that we both inhabit. The relative separateness between analyst and patient is the result of the fact that there is an objective world that makes it possible to attain a perspective beyond one's own. In this sense, the meeting of the subjective and the inter-subjective relies on this third objective world.

These reflections, which began with a personal reverie, have suggested the direction of this inquiry: Psychic space is created by actions – by interactions – and always takes place within the framework of a physical actuality. Together, these ideas bring us to the view I am suggesting here, that the room in which we see our patients is our playground, a staging area with four walls, a ceiling, a floor, a chair, a couch, two people, and an area in between them. It is this actual arena in which transference and countertransference are born and born anew.

The generative aspects of spatialization implemented through motor action

Now, I would like to consider just how the process of spatialization can be a dynamic, motivating force in its own right. The creation of psychic space appears particularly evident when we consider the actions of the body self in the attainment of subsequent symbolic forms.

In the personal episode, I noted that every instance in the representation of space was embedded in a matrix of sensory and motor activity. Thus the experience of space was made vivid through enactment. What was described as potential space was manifest not just by words spoken but by continuous forms of sensory enervation. I observed that self-reflective space was manifest not just by verbal representations, memories or phantasies, but by various body motions and gestures defining the distance between me and my patient. It was all marked by definable actions: opening the door, turning toward the patient, reclining in the chair, and then moving forward. Then, an entire ritual of self – touching, leaning forward, and gesturing (although the patient could not see me) surrounding my interpretation. It was this enactive aspect that had led me to speak not just of a process of representation but specifically of spatialization. It is a motivated space-creating activity that gives vividness to the manifold moments of inner life.

These formulations are based not just on reminiscences of past sessions but also on a body of research data. In a recent paper, Berzofsky et al. (2001) reported on a small group of schizophrenic patients receiving dynamic psychotherapy who also agreed to the videotaping of the initial session. It was noted that patterns of bodily actions during the initial interchange were indicative of subsequent clinical course and the ability to symbolize experiences in spoken language. Three patterns of response were noted. There were the *symbolizers*, those patients able to communicate their thoughts in verbal symbolic form. Their bodily motions (head nods, hand movements, and foot kicks) were characteristically in synchrony with the phonemic rhythm of spoken language. These patients showed considerable gain in the course of treatment. There was a profile of *desymbolizers*, who portrayed a stance of frozen immobility and failed to show clinical improvement. Then there was the profile of *emergent symbolizers*. These were the patients unable to communicate their thoughts initially, but who did so later in treatment. These patients also presented a characteristic posture and gesture of address. And here we could say that bodily actions were anticipatory; they took place before patients were able to put their thoughts into verbal symbolic form.

The emergent symbolizers are of greatest clinical interest. These patients, and there were only four, showed minimal symbolization in their spoken language at the beginning of treatment, and it was only later, by the tenth or twelfth session, that various verbal symbolic forms emerged. What is noteworthy is that, at the very beginning of treatment, they showed signs of those very nonverbal signifiers that point to the potential for connectedness and to the ability to put thoughts into words. We would say they engaged in space-creating activity that subsequently evolved into an evocative dialogue. It was an instance of the generative aspect of spatialization.

Spatialization and symbol formation

With the recognition of the actuality of space as it is inherent in the frame – with the further appreciation of the propensity to create space in any dialogic interchange – we further ask just in what way do these forces from without and within contribute to the process of mental representations generally and to symbol formation in particular. What I am suggesting is that there is not just psychic space but rather specific patterns or dimensions of psychic space. These have a definable impact on the inner representational world.

These thoughts lead us to return to the opening theme of this chapter. The earlier view that the representation of space plays a role in all symbol formation is to be taken for granted, and this assertion has found its support in a long line of analytic inquiry. Now I wish to take one step further. Namely, the very act of symbol formation – that is, the creation of a symbolic form – demands the experience of space. It is a constitutive aspect of a mental process, independent of any particular content. This point of view (Cassirer 1923; Langer 1942; Werner and Kaplan 1963) has resulted in the notion of symbolic form as a determining tendency, wherein form, including space, shapes thought and thought shapes form.

It would appear on the surface that many of the forms I am about to delineate have been foreshadowed in the biographical episode. However, there is one major shift. Although it is undoubtedly true that the form that a symbol takes is unthinkable without some notion of symbolizing space, there are specific configurations of psychic space, and each appears in part a determinant of the symbolic. In the autobiographical sketch, I noted a series of spatial forms – body-self space, object relational space, etc. – all of which seemed to precede symbolizing space proper. Now I am suggesting a different perspective. I suggest that distinct qualities in the representation of space are coordinated with particular forms of symbolizing space. The attainment of the symbolic is not a dichotomous event, not an either-or phenomenon, as you might see it in French psychoanalysis or Kleinian theory. Rather we are guided by the hypothesis of incremental symbolization, wherein every act of symbolization implies an act of spatialization.

In our more recent work on the symbolization of the analytic process, we have distinguished four symbolic forms in the analytic work, and each has its own particular form of spatialization (Freedman *et al.* 2001; Freedman and Russell in press). Thus we have noted a form of *incipient symbolization* that is manifest by the naming of emotions. In the course of a clinical interchange, affect naming is a staging ground for further symbolic meaning. Although linguistically, affect naming is of course a symbolic process, clinically it functions as a transitional phenomenon, a launching pad for further meaning. Moreover, the ability to put emotional promptings into words is also accompanied, even strengthened, by rhythmic motor acts or bodily self-stimulation. During the episode reported, I experienced various modes of self-soothing that helped me sort out the sphere of that which belonged to me and that which belonged to the sphere of the not me. Both the naming of emotions (to myself) and the modes of sensorimotor actions suggest a state close to potential space.

A second form, that of *discursive symbolization*, to use a term borrowed from Susanne Langer (1942), has also been identified. Discursive symbolization comprises its own configuration of spatial attributes. In the evolving story, the patient constructs narratives within various temporal dimensions from past through present to future. The story may also be shaped by different modes of "reality," ranging from pretend mode to more elaborate fantasy depictions. It is a kind of fantasy space. The patient is also able to attribute to his or her representations of others a sense of psychic reality – a kind of object relational space. When I opened the door to receive my patient, I was hit by a wave of perfume. I surely encountered a sense of psychic reality. It was a moment of intimate distance as I quickly translated the fragrance sensed into memories of earlier sessions. I sensed her depressive state and imagined what was about to occur. In these examples of temporal space, fantasy space, or object relational space, the reader will undoubtedly note the overlap with the work on reflective functioning described by Fonagy and Target (1996) and also by Auerbach and Blatt (2002). Hence, in brief, discursive symbolization can also be regarded as a form of reflective space.

Now we must recognize that psychoanalysis entails more than the naming of affect and reflecting upon self and object. In the literature, it is usually reserved for that process wherein dynamic experiences previously inaccessible to consciousness now emerge in spoken language; appropriated they become the source of new meaning. This is *dynamic symbolization*, and it emerges in particular constellations of spoken language. It is a multidimensional construction as it reverberates in the images of the patient, the images of the listener, and the interaction of the two. Indeed it is a triangular process that can well result in a shift of defensive organization and the owning of new meaning. In the episode, as I reclined and listened to a scene from my patient's biography, an internal dialogue followed, a sudden uh huh, and I offered an interpretation that she was able to accept. It was a special moment of intersubjectivity that led to a special moment in treatment. A dynamic symbolizing space had been created.

The fourth form that we have identified is *desymbolization*, and within the frame of the current discussion, it should also be termed despatialization. It is a state marked by the negative symbol and the imperative, "I do not want to know." In reading the text of a session, we can note instances of psychic equivalence, concreteness, and an insistence on one meaning and one meaning only, with a foreclosure of affect and the use of disavowal as primary defense. Symbolizing space is throttled, and in a clinical context, impasse may ensue. Desymbolization also appeared briefly in the episode recalled. In the early moments of the sequence, I felt overcome by a barrage of sensations, helplessness, rage, or simply "not wanting to know." Only after various forms of self-touching and soothing did I allow myself to recover. I sensed the force of the negative. Was it an attack on linking (Bion 1959)? Certainly, symbolic linking was throttled. There was no space to roam.

These spatial configurations are inextricably interwoven with symbolic forms. Each serves a particular psychic function, and they all inevitably unfold in the course of a therapeutic hour, be it potential space, reflective space, dynamic space, or the collapse of space. The saliency of one or another of these spatial patterns tells much about the course of treatment. They may be indicators of difficult or regressive sessions, as opposed to working sessions, and may even be indicative of overall treatment response. Each of these spatial configurations and their concomitant functions also signify the important tasks of treatment, be it the naming of affect, reflecting upon self or object representations, or appropriating unconscious promptings so that they can be included in verbal communication. Their intimate connection to symbolic forms suggests something intrinsic to clinical change. What we are emphasizing is not just a process of implicit relational knowing but also, and crucially so, incremental symbolic knowing.

Conclusions

Personal recollections, together with empirical observations and conceptual reflections, persuade me that the notion of *psychic space*, as it appears in psychoanalytic discourse, should be considered from multiple distinct vantage points and as part of the representational process of self and others, where it is inextricably bound up with symbol formation. Then the experience of space is also initiated, implemented, shaped, and created, and this occurs inevitably through the motor system. I have termed this process spatialization, and its source is the enactive impulse. However, both the representation of space and its enactment through spatialization are further shaped by space as an objective actuality. The three parameters, occurring jointly and in interaction with each other, provide a framework for a comprehensive account of psychic life.

References

Anzieu, D. (ed.) (1990) *Psychic Envelopes*, London: Karnac Books.

Auerbach, J. S. and Blatt, S. J. (2002) 'The concept of mind: a developmental analysis', in R. Lasky (ed.) *Symbolization and Desymbolization*, New York: Other Press, pp. 75–117.

Berzofsky, M., Davis, M., Lavender, J. and Freedman, N. (2001) 'Non-verbal facilitators of symbolizing space', *Psychoanalysis and Psychotherapy* 18: 145–70.

Bion, W. R. (1959) 'Attacks on linking', *International Journal of Psycho-Analysis* 40: 308–15.

Blatt, S. J. (1995) 'The destructiveness of perfectionism: implications for treatment of depression', *American Psychologist* 50: 1003–20.

—— and Blatt, E. (1984) *Continuity and Change in Art: the development of modes of representation*, Hillsdale, NJ: Erlbaum.

—— and Ritzler, B. (1974) 'Suicide and the representation of transparency and cross-sections on the Rorschach', *Journal of Consulting and Clinical Psychology* 42: 280–7.

Bollas, C. (1987) *The Shadow of the Object*, New York: Columbia University Press.

Bromberg, P. (1998) *Standing in the Spaces*, Hillsdale, NJ: Analytic Press.

Cassirer, E. (1923) *The Philosophy of Symbolic Forms, Vol. 1 Language*, R. Mannheim (trans.), New Haven, CT: Yale University Press, 1953.

Cavell, M. (1998) 'Triangulation, one's own mind and objectivity', *International Journal of Psycho-Analysis* 79: 449–67.

Erikson, E. (1962) 'Reality and actuality: an address', *Journal of the American Psychoanaytic Association* 10: 454–61.

Federn, P. (1952) *Ego Psychology and the Psychoses*, New York: Basic Books.

Fonagy, P. and Target, M. (1996) 'Playing with reality: 1. theory of mind and the normal development of psychic reality', *International Journal of Psycho-Analysis* 77: 217–33.

Freedman, N. and Lavender, J. (in press) 'On desymbolization: the concept and observations on anorexia and bulimia', *Psychoanalysis and Contemporary Thought*.

—— and Russell, J. (in press) 'Symbolization of the analytic discourse', *Psychoanalysis and Contemporary Thought*.

—— Kagan, D., Russell, J., Schaffer, C. E. and Webster, J. (2001) *Scales of Incremental Symbolization Manuals 1–4*, unpublished manuscripts, Research Division, Institute for Psychoanalytic Training and Research, New York, NY.

Grotstein, J. (1978) 'Inner space: its dimensions and its coordinates', *International Journal of Psychoanalysis* 59: 55–61.

Klein, M. (1930) 'The importance of symbol formation in the development of the ego', in J. Mitchell (ed.) *The Selected Melanie Klein*, New York: Free Press, 1987, pp. 95–114.

Langer, S. (1942) *Philosophy in a New Key*, Cambridge, MA: Harvard University Press.

Lewin, B. (1973) *Selected Writings of Bertram D. Lewin*, New York: Psychoanalytic Quarterly.

Ogden, T. (1986) *The Matrix of the Mind: object relations and the psychoanalytic dialogue*, New York: Aronson.

Porter, C. (1944) 'Don't fence me in' (performed by Roy Rogers), in J. L. Warner (Exec. Producer) and D. Daves (Director/Writer) *Hollywood Canteen* (Motion Picture), United States: Warner Brothers.

Roth, D. and Blatt, S. J. (1974) 'Spatial representations and psychopathology', *Journal of the American Psychoanalytic Association* 22: 854–72.

Schilder, P. (1935) 'Psycho-analysis of space', *International Journal of Psycho-Analysis* 16: 274–95.

Viderman, S. (1979) 'The Analytic Space: meaning and problems', *Psychoanalytic Quarterly* 48: 257–93.

Werner, H. and Kaplan, B. (1963) *Symbol Formation*, New York: Wiley.

Williams, G. (1997) *Internal Landscapes and Foreign Bodies: eating disorders and other pathologies*, New York: Routledge.

Winnicott, D. W. (1971) *Playing and Reality*, New York: Routledge.

Witkin, H. (1977) 'Cognitive styles in personal and cultural adaptation', in *Heinz Werner Lecture Series*, vol. 2, Worcester, MA: Clark University Press, pp. 30–42.

Part II

Psychopathology

Chapter 5

Dependency, self-criticism, and maladjustment

David C. Zuroff, Darcy Santor, and Myriam Mongrain

Sidney Blatt's theorizing has ranged over the entire landscape of clinical psychology, from personality assessment to psychopathology to treatment. Of special importance is the seminal article by Blatt and Shichman (1983), the first comprehensive formulation of psychopathology as distortions of the normal developmental processes of relatedness and self-definition. This theoretical framework was elaborated in later works, including Blatt (1990), Blatt and Homann (1992), Blatt and Zuroff (1992), and Blatt, Auerbach and Levy (1997). Blatt's views, which derive from psychoanalysis, cognitive developmental theory, and attachment theory, have been responsible for over 25 years of innovative research on psychopathology, especially depression. Without attempting to summarize the entirety of Blatt's theory, we will highlight four key attributes of the theory that differentiate it from other contemporary frameworks.

First, the theory portrays maladjustment as arising from distortions or exaggerations of the normal processes of personality development; psychopathological conditions are not qualitatively distinct from normality. Various "disorders" are seen not as discrete entities but rather as differing in developmental level and focus on one or the other of the two major developmental pathways, relatedness and self-definition. Consequently, the theory permits us to understand the problems in living of people carrying a wide range of diagnostic labels – as well as those of people without diagnostic labels – in a common theoretical framework.

Second, the theory reflects a developmental orientation, with relatedness and self-definition defining trajectories across the entire life span (Blatt and Homann 1992). Although Blatt views early experiences as highly important, and personality as relatively stable, personality development is a continuing process. The theory encourages us to examine the antecedents of dependency and self-criticism, as well as factors that can mitigate maladaptive personality. Blatt's developmental perspective also implies that the manifestations of dependency and self-criticism may differ across the life span. For example, the problems in living of the self-critical adolescent are likely to differ in many ways from those of the self-critical middle-aged parent.

Third, Blatt's descriptions of the interpersonal styles associated with dependency and self-criticism are extraordinarily rich. Because these interpersonal styles are viewed as rooted in development and intimately linked to motivational and cognitive characteristics, Blatt's theory has greater explanatory power than purely interpersonal models of depression, which are unable to account for individual differences in interpersonal environments and processes. The interpersonal component of the theory is also a significant strength, especially when Blatt's ideas are compared to purely cognitive theories, which neglect the dynamic interplay among social cognition, social behaviors, and objective features of the individual's social environment.

Fourth, the theory does more than postulate that dependency and self-criticism are risk factors. It provides explanations of vulnerability in terms of underlying motivational orientations and cognitive structures (mental representations). The theory is elegantly integrated because the developmental model dovetails with the motivational, cognitive, and interpersonal components. Early life experiences are powerful determinants of preoccupations with maintaining relatedness or preserving self-worth, mental representations of self and others, and interpersonal relations.

Our approach to conducting research based on Blatt's theory has been directed by a metatheoretical commitment to dynamic interactionism (Magnusson and Endler 1977). Interactionism rejects a rigid dichotomy between person and situation and, applied to the specific context of vulnerability research, provides a framework for integrating intrapsychic (cognitive, motivational, and affective) and interpersonal vulnerability processes. As described by Zuroff (1992) and elaborated by Santor (2003), the framework includes: (a) a diathesis-stress component; (b) an interpersonal component based on Coyne's (1976) model; and (c) hypothesized linkages between the two components that are derived from the person-situation interaction literature (See Figure 5.1). The diathesis-stress component assumes that mental representations associated with dependency and self-criticism give rise to inordinately intense negative affect when stressful events are encountered. The interpersonal component assumes that dysphoria can be caused and maintained by disturbed relationships and that relationships can be disturbed by prolonged states of dysphoria. Disturbed relationships can also reduce social support, and level of support can have either direct effects on depression or moderating effects on stress.

Three additional paths represent dynamic interactions between dependency and self-criticism and the social environment. The paths from dependency and self-criticism to disturbed relationships indicate that there are systematic differences, generally of an adverse nature, in the interpersonal environments of vulnerable individuals. These differences arise because both dependency and self-criticism influence who one selects to be part of one's social network, how one perceives and remembers social

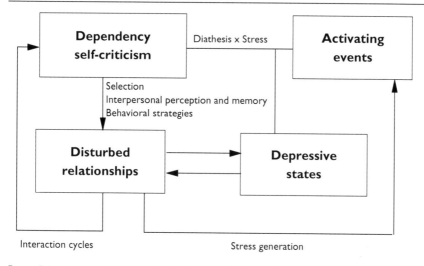

Figure 5.1   A dynamic interactionist framework for studying dependency and self-criticism

interactions, and which social behavioral strategies one employs (Santor 2003). The paths from disturbed relationships to both dependency and self-criticism indicate that living in disturbed relationships can maintain or intensify underlying vulnerabilities. The stress-generation path from disturbed relationships to activating events indicates that disturbed relationships can lead to negative events like the dissolution of relationships, loss of promotions, and family quarrels. Thus, dependency and self-criticism lead to depression through multiple pathways. In addition to diathesis-stress interactions, there are indirect paths via heightened exposure to activating events and reductions in social support.

In the remainder of this chapter, we review research stimulated by Blatt's theory. Our focus will be on studies using the Depressive Experiences Questionnaire (DEQ; Blatt, D'Afflitti and Quinlan 1976) to measure dependency and self-criticism. We begin by identifying the cognitive and motivational underpinnings of dependency and self-criticism. We then consider the developmental origins and life span implications of the two variables. Next, we review interpersonal correlates. Finally, we examine dependency and self-criticism as vulnerabilities to depressive states, although they have also been linked to anxiety disorders, personality disorders, eating disorders, substance abuse, and internalizing and externalizing problems in children.

Motivational orientations

The dependent person is overly preoccupied with obtaining nurturance and love and with preserving harmony at the expense of the development of an independent identity (Blatt 1990). In research studies, highly dependent individuals were found to have a greater number of interpersonal goals involving affiliation and intimacy and fewer achievement and individualistic goals (Mongrain and Zuroff 1995). Similarly, when implicit needs were measured, dependency was related to higher levels of intimacy motivation and to fewer agentic traits and behaviors (Saragovi *et al.* 2002). Dependent individuals engage in overly cooperative behaviors (Santor, Pringle and Israeli 2000) and act in ways that benefit friends at their own expense (Santor and Zuroff 1998). They praise disagreeing friends and rate less competent friends as superior (Santor and Zuroff 1997). They often fail to assert their competence in order to keep the peace. In summary, dependent individuals' needs for nurturance and affection come at the expense of their own individuation.

Self-criticism involves a preoccupation with establishing and maintaining a positive sense of self at the expense of relational investments (Blatt 1990). Individuals with high scores on self-criticism have been found to endorse a greater number of achievement goals and to exhibit concerns with meeting standards of excellence and doing tasks well (Mongrain and Zuroff 1995). Consistent with a preoccupation with making favorable impressions and obtaining external approval, they also demonstrate a higher number of self-presentation strivings (Mongrain and Zuroff 1995). Furthermore, with their relative lack of interest in affiliative and warm exchanges with others, self-critical persons report fewer interpersonal strivings (Mongrain and Zuroff 1995) and fewer communal traits (Saragovi *et al.* 2002). Self-critical individuals act uncooperatively in their romantic relationships (Santor *et al.* 2000); they enhance social status at a friend's expense (Santor and Zuroff 1998); and they retaliate when friends disagree with them (Santor and Zuroff 1997). These results suggest a competitive need to prove their worth, even to the detriment of interpersonal harmony.

Dependent and self-critical motivational orientations are reflected in the selection of romantic partners (Zuroff and de Lorimier 1989). Dependent women identified their ideal boyfriend as higher on needs for intimacy, whereas self-critical women prefer partners who are less nurturant but more masculine, autonomous, and aggressive. Partner preferences are one mechanism by which dependency and self-criticism influence individuals' social environments.

Cognition: content and process

Cognitive content

Mental representations are postulated to be powerfully influenced by parent–child relationships, with distinct themes expected to emerge for dependent and self-critical individuals (Blatt 1974; Blatt et al. 1979). Mongrain (1998) investigated interpersonal schemas, finding that highly dependent individuals expect to be treated more favorably by parents when they inhibit their own hostility and display friendly submissiveness. Other research has found dependency to be related to more positive, warmer representations of mothers (Sadeh, Rubin and Berman 1993). Conversely, several studies have found self-criticism to be related to negative parental representations (e.g., Brewin et al. 1992; McCranie and Bass 1984; Mongrain 1998; Rosenfarb et al. 1994; Sadeh et al. 1993). Self-critical persons expect both mother and father to be more impatient, disappointed, and critical of them, no matter what they do (Mongrain 1998). These generalized, negative perceptions may have some objective basis because parents of self-critical daughters report being less loving and more controlling (Amitay, Mongrain and Fazaa 2004). Self-critical persons' negative mental representations are not restricted to their parents; Zuroff and Duncan (1999) found that self-criticism also predicted negative relational schemas in romantic relationships.

Attachment styles provide another window through which mental representations of self and others can be examined. Zuroff and Fitzpatrick (1995) found dependency to be related to a preoccupied attachment style, which involves a negative model of self but a positive model of other. Dependent individuals fear abandonment and the loss of partners. Self-critical individuals report a fearful attachment style, characterized by negative representations of self and others. They are afraid of being rejected, are not comfortable with closeness, and do not feel they can rely on their partners (Zuroff and Fitzpatrick 1995). Their negative models of self and others leave them distrustful and avoidant of intimacy in order to protect themselves against anticipated rejection and criticism.

Perceived social support is increasingly interpreted as reflecting internal working models of attachment relationships. The negative mental representations associated with self-criticism would be expected to lead to low perceived social support, and research has consistently supported that prediction (Mongrain 1998; Moskowitz and Zuroff 1991; Dunkley, Zuroff and Blankstein 2003; Priel and Besser 2000; Priel and Shahar 2000). Low perceived social support mediated the relationship between self-criticism and depression in young adults (Dunkley et al. 2003; Priel and Shahar 2000) and in postpartum depression among first-time mothers (Priel and Besser 2000). In contrast, dependency had protective effects on postpartum depression because of perceptions of a more supportive environment (Priel and Besser 2000). These differing perceptions of social support may reflect objective differences in the respective environments of dependent and self-critical persons. However, current evidence suggests that self-criticism is strongly negatively related to perceived, but not to actual, support provided by peers (Mongrain 1998).

Cognitive processes

Cognitive distortions associated with dependency and self-criticism have also been documented. According to Blatt and Shichman (1983), the dependent configuration involves defenses that preserve the impression of harmony in relationships. Dependent women distorted their perceptions of their boyfriends during a conflict resolution task in a positive way, perceiving their boyfriends as more loving than did external raters (Mongrain *et al.* 1998). In a competitive task with a friend, dependent individuals recalled fewer disagreements than actually occurred (Santor and Zuroff 1998). The dependent person may cognitively distort perceptions in order to minimize the discomfort associated with interpersonal conflict.

Conversely, self-criticism has been associated with negative biases in self-perceptions. For example, self-critical women saw themselves as less effective and more submissive when trying to resolve conflicts with their boyfriends than did external raters (Mongrain *et al.* 1998). Self-critical adolescents rated themselves as weaker and more inadequate than did their camp counselors (Fichman, Koestner and Zuroff 1996). These negative biases may reflect schematic processing driven by negative mental representations, rather than defensive processes.

Life span development

Blatt's developmental theory (e.g., Blatt and Homann 1992) has three major implications: (a) negative parent–child interactions are crucial determinants of dependency and self-criticism; (b) dependency and self-criticism should show high levels of stability over the life span, although favorable and unfavorable experiences in significant relationships can lead to change; and (c) dependency and self-criticism can have varying correlates at different life stages.

Parent–child interaction

The majority of research on parent–child interaction has relied on retrospective, self-report methods (Blatt *et al.* 1979; Brewin *et al.* 1992; Frank *et al.* 1997; McCranie and Bass 1984; Rosenfarb *et al.* 1994). Although the limitations of such studies are evident, they have consistently found that dependency and self-criticism correlate with either parental overcontrol or parental rejection or both. Differences between the effects of mothers and fathers on boys and girls are sometimes noted, but more studies are needed before definitive conclusions can be reached.

Two studies have related parents' reports of their parenting behavior to children's reports of self-criticism. Amitay *et al.* (2004) found that self-critical mothers and fathers described themselves as more controlling and less loving towards their college-aged daughters, and these reports predicted daughters' levels of self-criticism. Thompson and Zuroff (1999) found that maternal dissatisfaction with early adolescent daughters predicted maternal coldness, which in turn predicted daughters' self-criticism. Koestner, Zuroff and Powers (1991) reported the only longitudinal study in this area, finding that maternal reports of parenting at age 5 predicted children's reports of self-criticism at age 12. Maternal rejection and restrictiveness were related to girls' self-criticism; paternal rejection and restrictiveness were related to boys' self-criticism.

Stability of dependency and self-criticism

Dependency and self-criticism have been found to be stable in young adults over periods of a few months (Zuroff et al. 1983) to a year (Zuroff, Igreja and Mongrain 1990). Only one study has examined long-term stability; Koestner et al. (1991) found that self-criticism was highly stable from age 12 to age 31 in girls but not in boys. More research is needed to determine the extent to which dependency and self-criticism are stable personality factors and to identify factors that foster stability or that favor change. Some findings suggest that the relationship between vulnerability and depression can be bidirectional, with experiences of depression leading to increases in self-criticism (Shahar et al. 2004b; Zuroff et al. 1990).

Dependency and self-criticism across the life span

Although the majority of research on dependency and self-criticism has focused on young adults, research has also examined the adolescent period. Dependency and self-criticism are related to the development of social competence and to the quality of relationships in adolescents (Fichman et al. 1994; Kuperminc, Blatt and Leadbeater 1997; Kuperminc, Leadbeater and Blatt 2001; Luthar and Blatt 1993). Evidence for increased risk associated with personality-congruent life events and vulnerability factors has been found in adolescents for dependency (Leadbeater, Blatt and Quinlan 1995). Short-term prospective studies examining developmentally specific stressors like attending summer camp have also shown that dependency and self-criticism predict specific and distinct outcomes (Fichman, Koestner and Zuroff 1996, 1997). Other research has shown that self-criticism predicts increases in both internalizing and externalizing problems (Leadbeater et al. 1999; Blatt et al. 1993), whereas long-term prospective studies have found self-criticism at age 12 to be inversely related to social adjustment during high school, as well as to academic achievement and occupational advancement (Zuroff et al. 1994).

Child-rearing and, more broadly, generativity are key developmental challenges for midlife adults. Evidence has accumulated that dependency and self-criticism have negative effects on the capacity for nurturing the next generation. Dependent mothers report higher separation anxiety with their infants (Hock and Lutz 1998) and may be more likely to thwart their children's attempts at individuation and autonomy. In laboratory studies, Thompson and Zuroff (1998, 1999) found that dependent mothers responded negatively to autonomy and competence in their early adolescent children while self-critical mothers were critical and controlling, regardless of their children's behaviors. Amitay et al. (2004) found that self-critical parents were more controlling and punitive towards daughters. Ackerman and Zuroff (1996) found that self-criticism was negatively related to generativity in midlife adults. The negative consequences of self-criticism extend to old age, where Santor and Zuroff (1994) found a negative relation between self-criticism and accepting the past, conceptualized as a facet of ego integrity.

Interpersonal implications

The mental representations of dependent people are complex. Dependent people view significant others as vital for their well-being yet lack confidence that others will provide the craved for love and support, especially if the dependent person is angry or assertive. Consequently, one would expect dependency to predict a mixed pattern of positive and negative interpersonal correlates. Dependent individuals describe themselves as more agreeable (Mongrain 1993), more intimate (Zuroff et al. 1995), more loving (Zuroff and de Lorimier 1989; Mongrain et al. 1998), and having greater social support (Priel and Shahar 2000), but not necessarily as more satisfied with their interactions or relationships (Zuroff and de Lorimier 1989; Zuroff et al. 1995). Dependent persons have also been observed to be less angry (Mongrain 1998) but more loving and submissive with their roommates (Mongrain, Lubbers and Struthers 2004) and more demanding of emotional support (Mongrain 1998). The relationships of dependent individuals may also begin on a positive note but become less satisfactory as the other person withdraws in the face of their demands (Hokanson and Butler 1992). Dependency is associated with self-reported interpersonal problems of being submissive and easily exploited by others (Alden and Bieling 1996; Fichman et al. 1994; Whisman and Friedman 1998), a pattern also observed in laboratory studies of female college-student friends (Santor and Zuroff 1997, 1998) and romantic couples (Mongrain et al. 1998; Vettese and Mongrain 2000; Santor et al. 2000). The mixture of positive and negative features in the interpersonal lives of dependent people may be reflected in Shahar and Priel's (2003) finding that dependent adolescents report more positive and more negative life events.

The pervasive, negative mental representations associated with self-criticism are expected to affect interpersonal behavior adversely. Self-criticism has been associated with less self-disclosure (Zuroff and Fitzpatrick 1995), reluctance to use social resources to deal with negative affect (Fichman *et al.* 1999), less willingness to share valuable resources (Santor and Zuroff 1998), less interpersonal warmth (Zuroff, Moskowitz and Coté 1999; Vettese and Mongrain 2000), more hostility (Mongrain *et al.* 1998; Santor and Zuroff 1997; Santor *et al.* 2000; Santor and Yazbek 2002; Zuroff and Duncan 1999), and interpersonal problems involving being overly cold and distant (Alden and Bieling 1996; Fichman *et al.* 1994; Whisman and Friedman 1998). The case histories of self-critical patients are marked by social isolation and feelings of having failed socially (Blatt *et al.* 1982). Their malevolent representations of others interfere with both their social networks (Shahar *et al.* 2004a) and their relationships with their therapists (Zuroff *et al.* 2000). Given these findings, it is not surprising that self-critical persons are dissatisfied in a wide range of relationships, including those with romantic partners, peers, parents, and their own children (Zuroff and Fitzpatrick 1995; Fichman *et al.* 1994; Zuroff *et al.* 1994; Thompson and Zuroff 1999). Problematic relationships are likely contributors to the high levels of hassles, negative life events, and chronic life difficulties that are associated with self-criticism (Mongrain and Zuroff 1994; Moskowitz and Zuroff 1991; Dunkley *et al.* 2003; Priel and Shahar 2000; Shahar and Priel 2003).

The interpersonal behaviors and relationship patterns associated with dependency and self-criticism are likely to give rise to interaction cycles that maintain or even exacerbate the personality styles. For example, in their striving for lofty standards and lack of attention to their relationships, self-critical individuals may cut themselves off from social support and prevent any corrective feedback about their negative beliefs about themselves and others. By placating others and undermining their own competence, dependent individuals may reinforce their sense of helplessness and neediness. Further, without adequate revisions of their representational world, dependent and self-critical persons are more likely to transmit their proclivities to the next generation.

Vulnerability to depressive states

Research examining dependency and self-criticism as vulnerability factors has grown dramatically in the past 25 years in terms of both the complexity of the models investigated (Blatt 1974; Zuroff and Mongrain 1987; Zuroff 1992; Santor 2003) and the manner in which vulnerability factors have been formulated and operationalized (Blatt *et al.* 1976; Hammen *et al.* 1985; Blatt *et al.* 1995; Santor, Zuroff and Fielding 1997). Evaluating the degree of support for dependency and self-criticism as vulnerability factors depends on both the nature of the vulnerability model being examined (Santor 2003) and the types of outcome being considered. One group of vulnerability studies has examined dependency and self-criticism as factors concurrently associated with symptoms, functioning, and personality traits. Event-sampling and daily diary studies have found that dependency is linked to high negative affect and that self-criticism is linked to high negative affect and low positive affect (Mongrain and Zuroff 1995; Zuroff *et al.* 1995; Zuroff *et al.* 1999; Dunkley *et al.* 2003). In addition, studies have shown that dependency and self-criticism are associated with the severity of depressed states (Zuroff *et al.* 1990), as well as with the duration and frequency of mood disturbances (Santor and Patterson 2004). Dependency and self-criticism have also been linked to theoretically consistent patterns of symptoms (Blatt *et al.* 1982) in patients and to dependent and self-critical qualities of depressed mood in students (Zuroff and Mongrain 1987; Mongrain and Zuroff 1989).

Other cross-sectional findings suggest some of the mechanisms underlying vulnerability. The dynamic interactionist framework suggests that dependency and self-criticism predict exposure to negative interpersonal and achievement life events (Dunkley *et al.* 2003; Mongrain and Zuroff 1994; Priel and Shahar 2000; Shahar and Priel 2003). As stated earlier, self-criticism is also related to impairments in perceived social support (Mongrain 1998; Dunkley *et al.* 2003) and patients' social networks (Shahar *et al.* 2004a). Additionally, dependency and self-criticism predict different maladaptive strategies for coping with stress (Dunkley *et al.* 2003) and managing negative mood (Fichman *et al.* 1999).

A second group of studies has examined dependency and self-criticism as factors moderating the impact of activating events on mood. Blatt's theory is compatible with both specificity (congruence) models emphasizing the matching of vulnerability factor and life-event domain and nonspecificity models emphasizing the assimilation of diverse life events to the predominant schemas associated with each vulnerability (Zuroff and Mongrain 1987). A large literature has developed that examines mood in prospective (Zuroff *et al.* 1990; Leadbeater *et al.* 1999), experience sampling (Dunkley *et al.* 2003; Fichman *et al.* 1999), quasi-experimental (Fichman *et al.* 1997), experimental (Blaney 2000; Gruen *et al.* 1997; Santor and Zuroff 2002; Zuroff and Mongrain 1987), and clinical studies (Segal *et al.* 1992). The weight of evidence suggests that dependency is associated with a specific vulnerability to events that threaten relatedness whereas self-criticism is associated with a broader vulnerability to threats to both relatedness and self-esteem.

Finally, a few studies have examined dependency and self-criticism as factors influencing the course of mood disorders. Self-criticism predicts poorer outcome in the short-term treatment of depression (Blatt *et al.* 1995; Blatt *et al.* 1998; Rector *et al.* 2000). Self-criticism also predicts greater vulnerability to experiencing depressive symptoms in response to stress experienced after termination (Zuroff and Blatt 2002). Segal *et al.* (1992)

found that self-critical depressed patients were more likely to relapse following achievement-related adversity, although dependent patients were found to be more vulnerable to interpersonal stressors only in the months immediately preceding relapse. This relationship was less clear cut.

Conclusion

Critics of Blatt's work (Coyne and Whiffen 1995) have argued that his personality-centered approach is a "negative heuristic" that would impede progress in the field. We believe that the exact opposite is the case. Blatt's theory has been richly heuristic, generating many novel findings and stimulating new lines of inquiry. Furthermore, his influence is deeply ingrained in several other contemporary literatures, including those addressing sociotropy and autonomy (Beck 1983), perfectionism (Flett and Hewitt 2002), and dependency (Bornstein 1993). Many psychologists decry the atheoretical framework of the current diagnostic system in psychiatry (e.g., American Psychiatric Association 1994), but Blatt's work provides the most comprehensive available alternative to conceptualizations of psychopathology as a set of biologically-based disease entities. We expect that his theoretical framework will continue to energize, direct, and inspire research for many more decades.

References

Ackerman, S. A. and Zuroff, D. C. (1996) unpublished raw data, McGill University, Montreal, Quebec, Canada.

Alden, L. E. and Bieling, P. J. (1996) 'Interpersonal convergence of personality constructs in dynamic and cognitive models of depression', *Journal of Research in Personality* 30: 60–75.

American Psychiatric Association (1994) *Diagnostic and Statistical Manual of Mental Disorders*, 4th edn, Washington, DC: American Psychiatric Press.

Amitay, O. A., Mongrain, M. and Fazaa, N. (2004) 'Love and Control: self-criticism from parents to daughters and consequences for relationship partners', manuscript submitted for publication, York University, Toronto, Ontario, Canada.

Beck, A. T. (1983) 'Cognitive therapy of depression: new perspectives', in P. J. Clayton and J. E. Barrett (eds) *Treatment of Depression: old controversies and new approaches*, New York: Raven Press, pp. 265–90.

Blaney, P. H. (2000) 'Stress and depression: a personality/situation interaction approach', in S. L. Johnson, A. M. Hayes, T. Field, P. McCabe and N. Schneiderman (eds) *Stress, Coping, and Depression*, Mahwah, NJ: Erlbaum, pp. 89–116.

Blatt, S. J. (1974) 'Levels of object representation in anaclitic and introjective depression', *Psychoanalytic Study of the Child* 29: 107–57.

—— (1990) 'Interpersonal relatedness and self-definition: two personality configurations and their implications for psychopathology and psychotherapy', in J. L. Singer (ed.) *Repression and Dissociation: implications for personality theory, psychopathology, and health*, Chicago: University of Chicago Press, pp. 299–336.

Blatt, S. J., Auerbach, J. S. and Levy, K. N. (1997) 'Mental representations in personality development, psychopathology, and the therapeutic process', *Review of General Psychology* 1: 351–74.

—— D'Afflitti, J. P. and Quinlan, D. M. (1976) 'Experiences of depression in normal young adults', *Journal of Abnormal Psychology* 85: 383–89.

—— Hart, B., Quinlan, D. M., Leadbeater, B. and Auerbach, J. (1993) 'Interpersonal and self-critical dysphoria and behavioral problems in adolescents', *Journal of Youth and Adolescence* 22: 253–69.

—— and Homann, E. (1992) 'Parent-child interaction in the etiology of dependent and self-critical depression', *Clinical Psychology Review* 12: 47–91.

—— Quinlan, D. M., Chevron, E. S., McDonald, C. and Zuroff, D. C. (1982) 'Dependency and self-criticism: psychological dimensions of depression', *Journal of Consulting and Clinical Psychology* 50: 113–24.

—— Quinlan, D. M., Pilkonis, P. A. and Shea, T. (1995) 'Impact of perfectionism and need for approval on the brief treatment of depression', *Journal of Consulting and Clinical Psychology* 63: 1–7.

—— and Shichman, S. (1983) 'Two primary configurations of psychopathology', *Psychoanalysis and Contemporary Thought* 6: 187–254.

—— Wein, S. J., Chevron, E. and Quinlan, D. M. (1979) 'Parental representations and depression in normal young adults', *Journal of Abnormal Psychology* 88: 388–97.

—— Zohar, A. H., Quinlan, D. M., Zuroff, D. C. and Mongrain, M. (1995) 'Subscales within the dependency factor of the Depressive Experiences Questionnaire', *Journal of Personality Assessment* 64: 319–39.

—— and Zuroff, D. C. (1992) 'Interpersonal relatedness and self-definition: two prototypes for depression', *Clinical Psychology Review* 12: 527–62.

—— Zuroff, D. C., Bondi, C. M., Sanislow, C. A. and Pilkonis, P. (1998) 'When and how perfectionism impedes the brief treatment of depression: further analyses of the NIMH TDCRP', *Journal of Consulting and Clinical Psychology* 66: 423–8.

Bornstein, R. F. (1993) *The Dependent Personality*, New York: Guilford Press.

Brewin, C. R., Firth-Cozens, J., Furnham, A. and McManus, C. (1992) 'Self-Criticism in adulthood and recalled childhood experience', *Journal of Abnormal Psychology* 101: 561–6.

Coyne, J. C. (1976) 'Toward an interactional description of depression', *Psychiatry* 39: 28–40.

—— and Whiffen, V. E. (1995) 'Issues in personality as diathesis for depression: the case of sociotropy-dependency and autonomy-self-criticism', *Psychological Bulletin* 118: 358–78.

Dunkley, D. M., Zuroff, D. C. and Blankstein, K. R. (2003) 'Self-critical perfectionism and daily affect: dispositional and situational influences on stress and coping', *Journal of Personality and Social Psychology* 84: 234–252.

Fichman, L., Koestner, R. and Zuroff, D. C. (1994) 'Depressive styles in adolescence: assessment, relation to social functioning, and developmental trends', *Journal of Youth and Adolescence* 23: 315–30.

—— —— and —— (1996) 'Dependency, Self-Criticism, and perceptions of inferiority at summer camp: I'm even worse than you think', *Journal of Youth and Adolescence* 25: 113–26.

Fichman, L., Koestner, R. and Zuroff, D. C. (1997) 'Dependency and distress at summer camp', *Journal of Youth and Adolescence* 26: 217–32.

—— —— —— and Gordon, L. (1999) 'Depressive styles and the regulation of negative affect: a daily experience study', *Cognitive Therapy and Research* 23: 483–95.

Flett, G. L. and Hewitt, P. L. (eds) (2002) *Perfectionism: theory, research, and treatment*, Washington, DC: American Psychological Association.

Frank, S. J., Poorman, M. O., Van Egeren, L. A. and Field, D. T. (1997) 'Perceived relationships with parents among adolescent inpatients with depressive preoccupations and depressed mood', *Journal of Clinical Child Psychology* 26: 205–15.

Gruen, R. J., Silva, R., Ehrlich, J., Schweitzer, J. W. and Friedhoff, A. J. (1997) 'Vulnerability to stress: self-criticism and stress-induced changes in biochemistry', *Journal of Personality* 65: 33–47.

Hammen, C., Marks, T., Mayol, A. and DeMayo, R. (1985) 'Depressive self-schemas, life stress, and vulnerability to depression', *Journal of Abnormal Psychology* 94: 308–19.

Hock, E. and Lutz, W. J. (1998) 'Psychological meaning of separation anxiety in mothers and fathers', *Journal of Family Psychology* 12: 41–55.

Hokanson, J. E. and Butler, A. C. (1992) 'Cluster analysis of depressed college students' social behaviors', *Journal of Personality and Social Psychology* 62: 273–80.

Koestner, R., Zuroff, D. C. and Powers, T. A. (1991) 'Family origins of adolescent self-criticism and its continuity into adulthood', *Journal of Abnormal Psychology* 100: 191–7.

Kuperminc, G. P., Blatt, S. J. and Leadbeater, B. J. (1997) 'Relatedness, self-definition, and early adolescent adjustment', *Cognitive Therapy and Research* 21: 301–20.

—— Leadbeater, B. J. and Blatt, S. J. (2001) 'School social climate and individual differences in vulnerability to psychopathology among middle school students', *Journal of School Psychology* 39: 141–59.

Leadbeater, B. J., Blatt, S. J. and Quinlan, D. M. (1995) 'Gender-linked vulnerabilities to depressive symptoms, stress, and problem behaviors in adolescents', *Journal of Research on Adolescence* 5: 1–29.

—— Kuperminc, G. P., Blatt, S. J. and Hertzog, C. (1999) 'A multivariate model of gender differences in adolescents' internalizing and externalizing problems', *Developmental Psychology* 35: 1268–82.

Luthar, S. S. and Blatt, S. J. (1993) 'Dependent and self-critical depressive experiences among inner-city adolescents', *Journal of Personality* 61: 365–86.

Magnusson, D. and Endler, N. S. (1977) 'Interactional psychology: present status and future prospects', in D. Magnusson and N. S. Endler (eds) *Personality at the Crossroads: current issues in interactional psychology*, Hillsdale, NJ: Lawrence Erlbaum, pp. 3–36.

McCranie, E. W. and Bass, J. D. (1984) 'Childhood family antecedents of dependency and self-criticism: implications for depression', *Journal of Abnormal Psychology* 93: 3–8.

Mongrain, M. (1993) 'Dependency and Self-Criticism located within the five-factor model of personality', *Personality and Individual Differences* 15: 455–62.

—— (1998) 'Parental representations and support-seeking behaviors related to Dependency and Self-Criticism', *Journal of Personality* 66: 151–73.

—— Lubbers, R. and Struthers, W. (2004) 'The power of love: Mediation of rejection in roommate relationships of dependents and self-critics', *Personality and Social Psychology Bulletin* 30: 94–105. York University, Toronto, Ontario, Canada.

—— Vettese, L. C., Shuster, B. and Kendal, N. (1998) 'Perceptual biases, affect, and behavior in the relationships of dependents and self-critics', *Journal of Personality and Social Psychology* 75: 230–41.

—— and Zuroff, D. C. (1989) 'Cognitive vulnerability to depressed affect in dependent and self-critical college women', *Journal of Personality Disorders* 3: 240–51.

—— and —— (1994) 'Ambivalence over emotional expression and negative life events: mediators of depressive symptoms in dependent and self-critical individuals', *Personality and Individual Differences* 16: 447–58.

—— and —— (1995) 'Motivational and affective correlates of dependency and self-criticism', *Personality and Individual Differences* 18: 347–54.

Moskowitz, D. S. and Zuroff, D. C. (1991) 'Contributions of personality and environmental factors to positive and negative affect in an adult community sample', poster presented at the meeting of the Canadian Psychological Association, Calgary, Alberta, Canada.

Priel, B. and Besser, A. (2000) 'Dependency and self-criticism among first-time mothers: the roles of global and specific support', *Journal of Social and Clinical Psychology* 19: 437–50.

—— and Shahar, G. (2000) 'Dependency, self-criticism, social context and distress: comparing moderating and mediating models', *Personality and Individual Differences* 28: 515–25.

Rector, N. A., Bagby, R. M., Segal, Z. V., Joffe, R. T. and Levitt, A. (2000) 'Self-criticism and dependency in depressed patients treated with cognitive therapy or pharmacotherapy', *Cognitive Therapy and Research* 24: 571–84.

Rosenfarb, I. S., Becker, J., Khan, A. and Mintz, J. (1994) 'Dependency, Self-Criticism, and perceptions of socialization experiences', *Journal of Abnormal Psychology* 103: 669–75.

Sadeh, A., Rubin, S. S. and Berman, E. (1993) 'Parental and relationship representations and experiences of depression in college students', *Journal of Personality Assessment* 60: 192–204.

Santor, D. A. (2003) 'Proximal effects of Dependency and Self-Criticism: conceptual and methodological challenges for depressive vulnerability research', *Cognitive Behaviour Therapy* 32: 49–67.

—— and Patterson, R. L. (2004) 'Frequency and duration of mood fluctuations: effects of dependency, self-criticism, and negative events', unpublished manuscript, Dalhousie University, Halifax, Nova Scotia, Canada.

—— Pringle, J. D. and Israeli, A. L. (2000) 'Enhancing and disrupting cooperative behavior in couples: effects of dependency and self-criticism following favorable and unfavorable performance feedback', *Cognitive Therapy and Research* 24: 379–97.

Santor, D. A. and Yazbek, A. (2002) 'Soliciting unfavorable social comparisons: effects of self-criticism', manuscript submitted for publication, Dalhousie University, Halifax, Nova Scotia, Canada.

—— and Zuroff, D. C. (1997) 'Interpersonal responses to threats to status and interpersonal relatedness: effects of dependency and self-criticism', *British Journal of Clinical Psychology* 36, 521–42.

—— and —— (1994) unpublished raw data, McGill University, Montreal, Quebec, Canada.

—— and —— (1998) 'Controlling shared resources: effects of dependency, self-criticism, and threats to self-worth', *Personality and Individual Differences* 24: 237–52.

—— and —— (2002) unpublished raw data, Dalhousie University, Halifax, Nova Scotia, Canada.

—— —— and Fielding, A. (1997) 'Analysis and revision of the Depressive Experiences Questionnaire: examining scale performance as a function of scale length', *Journal of Personality Assessment* 69: 145–63.

Saragovi, C., Aube, J., Koestner, R. and Zuroff, D. (2002) 'Traits, motives, and depressive styles as reflections of agency and communion', *Personality and Social Psychology Bulletin* 28: 427–41.

Segal, Z. V., Shaw, B. F., Vella, D. D. and Katz, R. (1992) 'Cognitive and life stress predictors of relapse in remitted unipolar depressed patients: test of the congruency hypothesis', *Journal of Abnormal Psychology* 101: 26–36.

Shahar, G., Blatt, S. J., Zuroff, D. C., Krupnick, J. L. and Sotsky, S. M. (2004a) 'Perfectionism impedes social relations and response to brief treatment for depression', *Journal of Social and Clinical Psychology* 23: 140–154.

—— —— Kuperminc, G. P. and Leadbeater, B. J. (2004b) 'Reciprocal relations between depressive symptoms and Self-Criticism (but not Dependency) among early adolescent girls (but not boys)', *Cognitive Therapy and Research* 28: 85–103.

—— and Priel, B. (2003) 'Active vulnerability, adolescent distress, and the mediating/suppressing role of life events', *Personality and Individual Differences* 35: 199–218.

Thompson, R. and Zuroff, D. C. (1998) 'Dependent and self-critical mothers' responses to adolescent autonomy and competence', *Personality and Individual Differences* 24: 311–24.

—— and —— (1999) 'Dependency, self-criticism, and mothers' responses to adolescent sons' autonomy and competence', *Journal of Youth and Adolescence* 28: 365–84.

Vettese, L. C. and Mongrain, M. (2000) 'Communication about the self and partner in the relationships of dependents and self-critics', *Cognitive Therapy and Research* 24: 609–26.

Whisman, M. A. and Friedman, M. A. (1998) 'Interpersonal problem behaviors associated with dysfunctional attitudes', *Cognitive Therapy and Research* 22: 149–60.

Zuroff, D. C. (1992) 'New directions for cognitive models of depression', *Psychological Inquiry* 3: 274–7.

—— and Blatt, S. J. (2002) 'Vicissitudes of life after the short-term treatment of depression: Roles of stress, social support, and personality', *Journal of Social and Clinical Psychology* 21: 473–496.

Zuroff, D. C., Blatt, S. J., Sotsky, S. M., Krupnick, J. L., Martin, D. J., Sanislow III, C. A. and Simmens, S. (2000) 'Relation of therapeutic alliance and perfectionism to outcome in brief outpatient treatment of depression', *Journal of Consulting and Clinical Psychology* 68: 114–24.

—— Moskowitz, D. S., Wielgus, M. S., Powers, T. A. and Franko, D. L. (1983) 'Construct validation of the Dependency and Self-Criticism scales of the Depressive Experiences Questionnaire', *Journal of Research in Personality* 17: 226–41.

—— and de Lorimier, S. (1989) 'Ideal and actual romantic partners of women varying in Dependency and Self-Criticism', *Journal of Personality* 57: 826–46.

—— and Duncan, N. (1999) 'Self-criticism and conflict resolution in romantic couples', *Canadian Journal of Behavioural Science* 31: 137–49.

—— and Fitzpatrick, D. A. (1995) 'Depressive personality styles: implications for adult attachment', *Personality and Individual Differences* 18: 253–65.

—— Igreja, I., and Mongrain, M. (1990) 'Dysfunctional attitudes, dependency, and self-criticism as predictors of depressive mood states: a 12–month longitudinal study', *Cognitive Therapy and Research* 14: 315–26.

—— Koestner, R., and Powers, T. A. (1994) 'Self-criticism at age 12: a longitudinal study of adjustment', *Cognitive Therapy and Research* 18: 367–85.

—— and Mongrain, M. (1987) 'Dependency and self-criticism: vulnerability factors for depressive affective states', *Journal of Abnormal Psychology* 96: 14–22.

—— Moskowitz, D. S. and Coté, S. (1999) 'Dependency, self-criticism, interpersonal behaviour and affect: evolutionary perspectives', *British Journal of Clinical Psychology* 38: 231–50.

—— Stotland, S., Sweetman, E., Craig, J. A. and Koestner, R. (1995) 'Dependency, self-criticism and social interactions', *British Journal of Clinical Psychology* 34: 543–53.

Chapter 6

Characterizing cognitive vulnerability in depression

Nasreen Khatri and Zindel V. Segal

The syndrome of depression has the dubious distinction of being one of the most prevalent forms of emotional disorder in the world (Murray and Lopez 1996). The lifetime risk for developing an episode of major depressive disorder is approximately 10 per cent for men and 20 per cent for women (McGrath *et al.* 1990; Sturt, Kumakura and Der 1984). Nearly 80 per cent of people who experience a single episode of depression will experience at least one more episode during their lifetime (Judd 1997). As well, the experience of each additional episode increases the chances of having a subsequent episode (Judd *et al.* 1998). The ubiquity and chronic nature of this syndrome has spurred the development of several effective psychological treatments (Beckham 1990). However, with evidence that recurrent bouts of depression become more likely with subsequent episodes, with up to 20 per cent of individuals becoming chronically depressed after two episodes, there is a growing need for treatments that address not just the resolution of the current episode of depression but the ongoing vulnerability patients face of suffering a relapse or recurrence (Keller *et al.* 1983; Segal and Dobson 1992).

To better inform efforts at developing treatments, researchers have drawn on accounts of depression vulnerability that point to particular risk factors that could be profitably targeted for intervention. Sidney Blatt's (1974) contributions to this literature have been seminal. They have served as a template for investigations of depression vulnerability not only within psychodynamic models but, and this is testimony to their influence, by other theoretical orientations as well. For example, in placing cognitive representation and affect regulation at the center of his theory of depression risk, Blatt's model built a conceptual bridge to cognitive accounts of depression, in which similar constructs are featured. Over time, this has led to more robust and theoretically compelling models of depression vulnerability that in turn have spawned numerous empirical tests of their validity (Segal and Dobson 1992). Much of this work is reviewed in this chapter. That such a synthetic mode of interaction occurred at a time when competition, rather than cooperation, characterized the relationship between psychodynamic and cognitive-behavioral schools of therapy illustrates a second contribution that Blatt's work has made, namely, the ability to reach across approaches for meaningful points of contact (Segal and Blatt 1993).

Blatt's psychoanalytic theory of depression: the anaclitic and introjective subtypes

Blatt's (1974; Blatt, Auerbach and Levy 1997) psychoanalytic theory of depression focuses primarily on the extent and quality of interpersonal relatedness and the nature of object representation. The secondary focus of Blatt's formulation is early childhood experiences and unconscious conflicts. From a psychoanalytic standpoint, depression emerges as a result of the disruption of one of two fundamental developmental processes, either the development of stable, nurturing, reciprocal interpersonal relationships or the development of a viable, differentiated, and well-defined sense of self. The former type of depression is termed *anaclitic*, and the latter type is termed *introjective*. Viewed in a larger context, the anaclitic–introjective dialectic echoes the universal human tension between autonomy and intimacy, or as the phrase attributed to Freud states, the two primary life tasks of love and work. Both the socially dependent, anaclitic and the hyperautonomous, perfectionistic introjective personality styles constitute a vulnerability to depression.

Blatt (1992: 172) theorizes that anaclitic psychopathology is a result of "depriving, rejecting, inconsistent, unpredictable or overindulgent parenting." These early experiences lead individuals to overemphasize the importance of social connectedness and to develop a sense of extreme sensitivity to interpersonal loss and rejection. Aloneness is experienced as intolerable and aversive. To secure the love of a nurturing other, individuals prone to anaclitic depression will go to great lengths to initiate and maintain relationships with other people. In these relationships, the anaclitic individual is excessively dependent on the other person for gratification and a sense of self-worth. Possible triggers of depression for individuals with an anaclitic style would be rejection, loss of a relationship, or any conflict that threatens the harmony of the relationship. Core conflicts that appear in anaclitic depression center around issues of protection, love, and sexuality, with attendant fears that these needs will not be met because of abandonment. The defenses most often employed to stave off painful feelings of abandonment and loneliness are avoidance through denial and repression. According to Blatt (1998), anaclitic depression occurs most often in women. Blatt has described this both in societal and psychoanalytic terms. As regards social conditioning, girls and women are encouraged to place a strong emphasis on interpersonal relatedness and nurturance. In psychoanalytic terms, women need to switch from a primary relationship with mother to other, more appropriate objects of affection (Blatt and Shichman 1983).

In contrast, Blatt (1992: 172) theorizes that introjective depression occurs as a result of parenting that is "controlling, intrusive, overly critical and punitive." These childhood experiences lead the individual to struggle to develop an excessively autonomous personality style. Intimacy is experienced as threatening and overwhelming. Thus, the focus of individuals with an introjective style is the constant striving for self-definition through achievement, self-sufficiency, and a controlled, intellectual inner life. Possible triggers for introjective depression may be a real or imagined failure to reach a goal or a feeling of loss of control, power, or independence. The conflicts that appear in introjective depression center on controlling emotions, especially anger and aggression. The defense mechanisms related to coping with emotions are counteractive and include intellectualization, overcompensation, and projection. Introjective depression occurs most often in men, who are challenged by society to gain self-definition and for whom the psychoanalytic task is to turn away from the primary identification with mother toward identification with objects of self-definition and autonomy (Blatt and Shichman 1983).

In sum, Blatt argues anaclitic depression occurs in some individuals with a history of neglect and deprivation within their relationships with primary caregivers. These individuals develop a sense of themselves as vulnerable and in need of protection and nurturance. Their difficulties center around securing and maintaining interpersonal relationships that will shield them from the possibility of loneliness and abandonment. Their defensive structure is avoidant and involves denial and repression. Alternatively, Blatt proposes introjective depression occurs in individuals who experienced harsh, controlling, and demanding parenting as children. These individuals internalize a punitive, self-critical, and perfectionistic stance and strive to achieve an exaggerated sense of self-definition through solitary pursuits and activities, many of which involve work, power, and control. The anaclitic individual focuses on interpersonal relationships to the exclusion of achieving sufficient self-definition that conceivably could remove the need for such social dependence. The introjective person strives to attain a painful level of independence at the cost of developing intimacy that may ease the constant need to achieve abstract goals. In this way, the anaclitic and the introjective personality each create an affective vulnerability to depression.

Beck's cognitive model of depression

Beck's (1967, 1976) cognitive model of depression emphasizes the central role of negative cognitions in the onset and maintenance of depressive disorders. Depressive symptoms are understood as manifestations of three aspects of negative cognition – the negative cognitive triad, cognitive distortions, and schemas. The negative triad is a pattern of negative judgments made about oneself, others, and the future. In the negative triad, the self is perceived as flawed, others are judged as not meeting one's needs or even harmful, and the future is viewed with a sense of helplessness and hopelessness. Cognitive distortions are negatively biased ways of perceiving experiences that occur because of inaccuracies in information processing and misinterpretations of events. These inaccuracies and misinterpretations lead individuals to arrive at conclusions about experiences that fulfill their negative predictions about them (Segal 1988). Examples of negative distortions include *black-and-white thinking*, in which people and events are judged to be either completely good or bad, *catastrophizing*, in which an individual tends to expect the absolute worst-case scenario for any situation, and *disregarding positive evidence*, in which a person may focus on the one negative aspect of an experience (e.g., of a work evaluation), although 95 per cent of the feedback was positive (Beck 1983).

The basis of the negative triad and cognitive distortions is the schema. According to Beck (1976), a schema is a relatively stable cognitive structure that supports errors and distortions in thinking. A schema is a theoretical representation of the base of self-knowledge; it is hypothesized in depressed individuals to be mostly negative in content. The term *schema* was originally used in cognitive psychology to refer to a construct in which previous knowledge exerts an influence on memory and perception of new information (Bartlett 1932). We will combine the view of the schema as a knowledge base with that of the schema as an implicit memory system in our discussion of vulnerability to depression.

In terms of psychopathology, Beck (1967) states that a negative cognitive schema may constitute a vulnerability or cognitive marker for depression. Essentially, the depression-prone person may be unaware of a propensity for negative thinking that nonetheless increases the risk for developing a depressive disorder. Moreover, this vulnerability may remain inactive or latent until the individual encounters a stressor with an emotional tone and valence that is reminiscent of the negative early life experiences that contributed to the development of the negative schema. Clearly, although many individuals experience adverse events in childhood, not all go on to develop negative cognitive schemas that make them vulnerable to depression. According to Beck, one difference between individuals who become depressed and those who do not is the level of dysfunctional attitudes they have about experiences in their lives.

Dysfunctional attitudes refer to extremely rigid and strongly held ideas about the meaning of any given situation – for example, "If everybody does not love and accept me, then I am worthless" (Weissman 1979). Research findings indicate that there is a correlation between dysfunctional attitudes and depression (Segal and Shaw 1986). Finally, once the latent schema is activated, a cascade of negative thoughts may appear without conscious intention. These negative cognitions are referred to as *automatic thoughts*. Automatic thoughts are the final cognitive output of schema-based distortions about the self, others, and the future and are activated by stressful experiences that are emotionally congruent with painful early experiences. They attack the vulnerable schema and result in the assertion of dysfunctional attitudes. An example of this scenario may unfold as follows. An individual who experienced neglect from primary caregivers as a child may develop a schema that centers on thoughts and attitudes of being unlovable. In adulthood, following the rejection by a romantic partner, the individual may experience an activation of the latent schema "I'm unlovable," and dysfunctional attitudes may actively emerge: "If so-and-so doesn't love me, then I'm worthless." With the schema now fully activated, the individual experiences depressive symptoms that are maintained moment to moment by automatic thoughts in which other interpersonal experiences are interpreted as punitive and rejecting. The generalized negative thinking may result in negative automatic thoughts, such as "Why was she late for my appointment, she must be avoiding me" and "She didn't return my call because I'm not worth it," in unrelated social situations.

Cognitive subtypes of depression: sociotropy and autonomy

According to Beck's (1983) theory, *sociotropy* and *autonomy* are two personality styles that are predisposing to depression. Sociotropy (interpersonal dependency) is a "person's investment in positive interchange with others" (Beck 1983: 272). Sociotropic individuals tend to have a strong need for approval and belonging and simultaneously fear social rejection. This personality style has been demonstrated to be positively correlated with depression, vulnerability, and psychopathology more generally (Bieling, Beck and Brown 2000). The highly sociotropic individual seeks social connectedness as a confirmation of self-worth and actualization. The loss or disruption of a relationship with a valued other is experienced as intolerable. The interpersonal loss is taken as evidence of a core defect, an innate flaw that precludes one from securing a stable, loving relationship. The sociotropic individual's relationships are characterized by dependence and a need to be nurtured by others. There is an underlying sense of vulnerability, unlovability, and lack of emotional agency.

In comparison with sociotropy, autonomy is "the person's investment in preserving and increasing his/her independence, mobility and personal rights" (Beck 1983: 272). Autonomous individuals prize goal attainment and fear loss of control or failure. They are focused on meeting their own high standards, are not particularly concerned with others' views of them unless these views involve comparisons of status-related factors like wealth or career success, and like to pursue their goals without being encumbered by others. They may appear to have an exaggerated sense of independence, and they avoid intimate relationships as they attempt to control all variables in their environment. The autonomous individual's chief vulnerability appears to be in the excessive criticism of self and others and the perfectionism that lead to isolation, lack of social support, and disinclination to seek help when appropriate. Objective or perceived failures to achieve or meet perceived goals lead to depression. For autonomous individuals, there appears to be an underlying sense of inadequacy, fear of losing control, and humiliation.

Convergence of psychoanalytic and cognitive approaches to depression

Both Blatt (1974, 1998) and Beck (1967, 1976; Beck et al. 1979) have posited views of vulnerability to depression that include several descriptive commonalities. First, both believe that vulnerability can be separated into two distinct types of personality style and functioning. Blatt (1974; Blatt et al. 1997) posited the anaclitic–introjective distinction in personality. Although the introjective individual avoids intimacy and is focused upon self-definition through high levels of independence, self-sufficiency, and affective control, the anaclitic person is centered on securing intimacy at the exclusion of developing a viable self-definition. Similarly, Beck (1983) has introduced the autonomy–sociotropy dimension, in which autonomous individuals prize freedom, control, and achievement and avoid intimacy and in which sociotropic individuals value social acceptance and approval and fear social rejection. Clearly the two theorists converge on the basic structure and polarity of their personality typologies. Second, both Beck (1983) and Blatt developed scales for measuring these underlying personality dimensions. Blatt, D'Afflitti and Quinlan (1976, 1979) developed the Depressive Experiences Questionnaire (DEQ), which contains scales for dependency and self-criticism. Beck and colleagues have developed both the Dysfunctional Attitudes Scale (DAS; Weissman and Beck 1978; Cane et al. 1986) and the Sociotropy–Autonomy Scale (SAS; Beck et al. 1983). Third, although possibly emphasized more in Blatt's earlier work, both theorists make mention of the gender-based nature of the personality styles. That is, autonomous and introjective individuals tend to be men, and anaclitic and sociotropic individuals tend to be women (Blatt and Shichman 1983; Beck 1983).

Nevertheless, there are also several important points of divergence between Blatt's and Beck's conceptualizations, especially at the level of gender-based etiology of subtypes, content of schemas, state-trait aspects of the schemas, and treatment indications that flow from the different formulations. First, whereas Beck has a purely cognitive formulation that emphasizes mainly present and future-focused vulnerability to depression, Blatt (1992: 184) takes a wider view that encompasses "characteristic instinctual preoccupations, unconscious conflicts, cognitive organization, defenses and personal experiences throughout the life cycle." Thus Blatt's view is that the vulnerability to depression emerges in early life, concurrent with the development of gender identity and often in interaction with it. Unlike Blatt, Beck does not specify the exact conditions and temporal specificity that lead to depressogenic cognitive schemas.

Second, the content of schemas is another source of divergence between the theorists. Beck (1983) maintains that the cognitive schema comprises a constellation of distortions, dysfunctional attitudes, and automatic thoughts that lead the individual to interpret life experiences in an overly negative manner. Blatt and Maroudas (1992) state that there are many aspects to the schemas, including conflicts, cognitive organization, and defenses; in other words they describe a cognitive–affective schema. One of the difficulties with a cognitive–affective schema is that it is parsimonious in description but is not so easily given to empirical examination as is a cognitive formulation. It is important to remember that Beck's views of schemas were influenced by the social cognition literature, in which mental representations of events led to emotional experience. The role of emotions in the cognitive theory of depression can best be viewed as one type of response to the activation of a cognitive schema, whereas, for Blatt, the emotions may act as the antecedents, precipitants, and products of the depressive schema.

Third, there is some debate about the state-trait nature of depressive subtypes. Initially, Blatt had stated that once the vulnerability to either the anaclitic or the introjective subtype is established in early adulthood, there is no switching back and forth between subtypes of depression (Blatt and Bers 1992; Blatt and Maroudas 1992). However, Beck asserts that the different vulnerabilities may be activated at different times by different stressors (Beck 1983). This statement was supported by data that demonstrated that cognitive distortions thought to cause depression were not stable and measurable in a remitted state (e.g., reviewed in Hammen 1997; Ingram et al. 1998). More recent work has indicated that a state-trait vulnerability model may be a more accurate reflection of the stability of schemas. Specifically, recent findings indicate that some measures, such as the DAS, remain relatively constant between episodes but that measures of automatic negative cognition appear to remain less constant when depression is in a remitted state (Zuroff et al. 1999).

Last, treatment indications emerging from the two theories diverge markedly. The standard cognitive-behavioral treatment for depression is 16 to 20 sessions of present-focused psychotherapy based on behavioral activation techniques, cognitive monitoring, and reduction of automatic reactivity to negative thoughts and attitudes. Between sessions, patients are asked to test out their interpretations and beliefs through the use of behavioral experiments and thought records. During the session, the therapist employs Socratic questioning of patients to guide them to a less reactive and more evidence-based construal of their experience. In contrast, the psychoanalytic approach to the treatment of depression is long-term psychotherapy, in which the focus of treatment includes the exploration of early childhood events, past and current conflicts, and defenses.

Evidence for psychoanalytic and cognitive subtypes of depression

The evidence for Blatt's and Beck's personality-based subtypes of depression emerges from three areas: the validation of subtype assessment measures, findings related to subtype-congruent vulnerabilities (i.e., the matching hypothesis), and differential responses to treatment aimed at alleviating depressive symptoms based on subtypes.

Thus, first, as mentioned previously, Blatt and Beck have respectively developed measures of anaclitic–introjective and sociotropic–autonomous personality styles. These are the DEQ from Blatt's research group and the DAS and the SAS from Beck's. These instruments have been validated by several independent researchers, with factor analysis supporting the two-factor structure of these proposed personality styles.

Second, as hypothesized, if an individual is identified as having a certain type of vulnerability to depression, for example the introjective–autonomous type, then one would expect to observe schema-congruent stressors as the most likely candidates to precipitate an episode of the disorder. For example, the models predict that, if a person scoring extremely high on autonomous features like self-criticism and perfectionism encounters a career setback, that individual is more likely to become depressed than if encountering the loss of a personal relationship. This matching hypothesis has been supported empirically in both the cognitive and psychoanalytic realms. Substantial support has accrued for the hypothesis that life stressors congruent with personality style are more likely to precipitate depression (Blatt and Zuroff 1992; Nietzel and Harris 1990; Segal and Dobson 1992; Zuroff and Mongrain 1987).

Third, the evidence in support of these subtypes that comes from treatment specificity is, at best, indirect. Studies have found that patients with higher cognitive functioning tend to benefit more in cognitive behavior therapy, whereas patients with higher social functioning tend to benefit more in interpersonal therapy, a form of psychodynamic therapy that explores personal relationships and their role in the onset and maintenance of depression (Blatt and Felsen 1993; Blatt et al. 1996).

Conclusion: evidence for the schema model of depression

With respect to empirical investigation of the proposition, shared by Blatt and Beck, that vulnerability to depression results from disordered cognitive–affective schemas, several relevant studies have been performed. In general, these have relied on semantic priming and construct activation as a means by which putative vulnerability representations can be accessed in order to examine their effects on information processing in vulnerable yet asymptomatic (remitted) individuals. A common design involves a laboratory-based mood challenge procedure to induce transient dysphoric mood in groups at high and low risk for relapse. Consistent with prediction, formerly depressed patients generally evidence a more depressogenic processing style (or mood-linked cognitive reactivity) while they are feeling sad but are no different from controls when euthymic (see Ingram *et al.* 1998 for a review). Furthermore, Segal *et al.* (1999) reported that the degree to which mood-linked cognitive reactivity increased in the face of a mood challenge significantly predicted the likelihood of reappearance of a depressive episode up to 30 months later.

These are among the first clinical data to suggest that changes in cognitive processing arising from the experience of dysphoria can predict future symptom return. They suggest that some aspects of depressive self-representation may emerge if properly primed or elicited. Furthermore the content of such representations seems to be in line with clinical accounts of negative, self-deprecatory views of the self (Beck 1967; Blatt 1974). With respect to treatment development, prophylactic approaches designed to reduce this reactivity might involve attempts to deautomatize these processes, perhaps through the teaching of metacognitive skills that serve to render this type of mood-linked processing more accessible to effortful reflection (Blatt and Bers 1993; Segal and Blatt 1993). Future work will need to address itself to these remaining challenges.

References

American Psychiatric Association (1994) *Diagnostic and Statistical Manual of Mental Disorders* (4th ed.), Washington, DC: American Psychiatric Press.

Bartlett, F. C. (1932) *Remembering*, London: Cambridge University Press.

Beck, A. T. (1967) *Depression: clinical, experimental and theoretical aspects*, New York: Harper and Row.

—— (1976) *Cognitive Therapy and the Emotional Disorders*, New York: International Universities Press.

—— (1983) 'Cognitive therapy of depression: new perspectives', in P. J. Clayton and J. E. Barnett (eds) *Treatment of Depression: old controversies and new approaches*, New York: Raven Press, pp. 265–290.

—— Epstein, N., Harrison, R. P. and Emery, G. (1983) 'Development of the

Sociotropy-Autonomy Scale: a measure of personality factors in psychopathology', unpublished manuscript', University of Pennsylvania, Philadelphia, PA.

—— Rush, A. J. Shaw, B. F. and Emery, G. (1979) *Cognitive Therapy of Depression*, New York: Guilford Press.

—— Steer, R. A. and Brown, G. K. (1996) *Beck Depression Inventory Manual* (2nd edn), San Antonio: Psychological Corporation.

Beckham, E. E. (1990) 'Psychotherapy of depression research at crossroads: direction for the 1990s', *Clinical Psychological Review* 10: 207–28

Bieling, P. J., Beck, A. T. and Brown, G. K. (2000) 'The Sociotropy-Autonomy Scale: structure and implications', *Cognitive Therapy and Research* 24: 763–80.

Blatt, S. J. (1974) 'Levels of object representation in anaclitic and introjective depression', *Psychoanalytic Study of the Child* 24: 107–57.

—— (1990) 'Interpersonal relatedness and self-definition: two personality configurations and their implication for psychopathology and psychotherapy', in J. L. Singer (ed.) *Repression and Dissociation: implications for personality theory, psychopathology and health*, Chicago: University of Chicago Press, pp. 299–335.

—— (1991) 'A cognitive morphology of depression', *Journal of Nervous and Mental Disease* 179: 449–58.

—— (1992) 'The differential effect of psychotherapy and psychoanalysis with anaclitic and introjective patients: the Menninger Psychotherapy Research Project revisited', *Journal of the American Psychoanalytic Association* 40: 691–724.

—— (1998) 'Contributions of psychoanalysis to the understanding and treatment of depression', *Journal of the American Psychoanalytic Association* 1: 723–52.

—— Auerbach, J. S. and Levy, K. N. (1997) 'Mental representations in personality development, psychopathology, and the therapeutic process', *Review of General Psychology* 1: 351–74.

—— and Bers, S. A. (1993) 'The sense of self in depression: a psychodynamic perspective', in Z. V. Segal and S. J. Blatt (eds) *The Self in Distress: cognitive and psychodynamic perspectives*, New York: Guilford, pp. 171–210.

—— D'Afflitti, J. P. and Quinlan, D. M. (1976) 'Depressive Experiences Questionnaire', unpublished manuscript, Yale University, New Haven, CT.

—— and Felsen, I. (1993) 'Different kinds of folks may need different kinds of strokes: the effect of patients' characteristics on therapeutic process and outcome', *Psychotherapy Research* 3: 245–59.

—— and Maroudas, C. (1992) 'Convergence of psychoanalytic and cognitive behavioral theories of depression', *Psychoanalytic Psychology* 9: 157–90.

—— Quinlan D. M., Zuroff D. C. and Pilkonis P. A. (1996) 'Interpersonal factors in brief treatment of depression: further analyses of the National Institute of Mental Health Treatment of Depression Collaborative Research Program', *Journal of Consulting and Clinical Psychology* 64: 162–71.

—— and Shichman, S. (1983) 'Two primary configurations of psychopathology', *Psychoanalysis and Contemporary Thought* 6: 187–254.

—— Wein, S. J., Chevron, E. S. and Quinlan, D. M. (1979) 'Parental representations and depression in normal young adults', *Journal of Abnormal Psychology* 88, 388–97.

—— and Zuroff, D. C. (1992) 'Interpersonal relatedness and self-definition: two prototypes for depression', *Clinical Psychology Review* 121: 527–62.

Cane, D. B., Olinger, L. J., Gotlib, I. H. and Kuiper, N. A. (1986) 'Factor structure of the Dysfunctional Attitudes Scale in a student population', *Journal of Clinical Psychology* 42: 307–9.

Elkin, I., Shea, M. T., Watkins, J. T., Imber, S. D., Sotsky, S. M., Collins, J. F., Glass, D. R., Pilkonis, P. A., Leber, W. R., Dockerty, J. P., Fiester, S. J. and Parloff, M. B. (1989) 'NIMH treatment of depression collaborative research program: general effectiveness of treatments', *Archives of General Psychiatry* 46: 310–16.

Frank, E., Anderson, B., Reynolds III, C. F., Ritenour, A. and Kupfer, D. J. (1994) 'Life events and the research diagnostic criteria endogenous subtype: a confirmation of the distinction using the Bedford College methods,' *Archives of General Psychiatry* 51: 519–24.

Gilligan, C. (1982) *In a Different Voice*, Cambridge, MA: Harvard University Press.

Gotlib, I. H. (1983) 'Perception and recall of interpersonal feedback: negative bias in depression', *Cognitive Therapy and Research* 5: 399–412.

—— and Cane, C. B. (1987) 'Construct accessibility and clinical depression: a longitudinal investigation', *Journal of Abnormal Psychology* 96: 199–204.

Hammen, C. (1997) *Depression*, London: Psychology Press.

—— (2000) 'Vulnerability to depression in adulthood', in R. E. Ingram and J. M. Price (eds) *Vulnerability to Psychopathology: risk across the lifespan*, New York: Guilford, pp. 226–67.

—— Ellicott, A., Gitlin, M. and Jamison, K. R. (1989) 'Sociotropy/autonomy and vulnerability to specific life events in patients with unipolar depression and bipolar disorders', *Journal of Abnormal Psychology* 98: 154–60.

Ingram, R. E., Miranda, J. and Segal, Z. V. (1998) *Cognitive Vulnerability to Depression*, New York: Guilford Press.

Judd, L. L. (1997) 'The clinical course of unipolar major depressive disorders', *Archives of General Psychiatry* 54: 989–91.

—— Akiskal, H. S., Maser, J. D., Zeller, P. J., Endicott, J., Coryell, W., Paulus, M. P., Kunovac, J. L., Leon, A. C., Mueller, T. I., Rice, J. A. and Keller, M. B. (1998) 'A prospective 12–year study of the subsyndromal and syndromal depressive symptoms in unipolar major depressive disorders', *Archives of General Psychiatry* 55: 694–700.

Keller, M. B., Lavori P. W., Lewis, C. E. and Klerman, G. L. (1983) 'Predictors of relapse in major depressive disorder', *Journal of the American Medical Association* 250: 3299–304.

Lewinsohn, P. M., Steinmetz, J. L., Larson, D. W. and Franklion, J. (1981) 'Depression related cognitions: antecedent or consequence?', *Journal of Abnormal Psychology* 90: 213–19.

McGrath, E., Keita, G. P., Strickland, B. R. and Russo, N. F. (eds) (1990) *Women and Depression: risk factors and treatment issues: final report of the American Psychological Association's National Task Force on Women and Depression*, Washington, DC: American Psychological Association.

Miranda, J. (1992) 'Dysfunctional thinking is activated by stressful life events', *Cognitive Therapy and Research* 16: 473–83.

—— and Persons, J. B. (1988) 'Dysfunctional attitudes are mood-state dependent', *Journal of Abnormal Psychology* 9: 776–9.

—— Persons, J. B. and Byers, C. N. (1990) 'Endorsement of dysfunctional beliefs depends on current mood state', *Journal of Abnormal Psychology* 99: 237–41.

Moore, R. G. and Blackburn, I. M. (1994) 'The relationship of sociotropy and autonomy to symptoms, cognition and personality in depressed patients', *Journal of Affective Disorders* 32: 239–45.

—— and —— (1996) 'The stability of sociotropy and autonomy in depressed patients undergoing treatment', *Cognitive Therapy and Research* 20: 69–80.

Murray, C. J. and Lopez, A. D. (eds) (1996) *The Global Burden of Disease: a comprehensive assessment of mortality and disability from diseases, injuries, and risk factors in 1990 and projected to 2020*, Cambridge, MA: Harvard University Press.

Nietzel, M. T. and Harris, M. J. (1990) 'Relationship of dependency and achievement/autonomy to depression', *Clinical Psychology Review* 10: 279–97.

Persons, J. B. and Miranda, J. (1992) 'Cognitive theories of vulnerability to depression: reconciling negative evidence', *Cognitive Therapy and Research* 16: 485–502.

Radloff, L. S. (1975) 'Sex differences in depression: the effects of occupation and marital status', *Sex Roles* 1: 249–65.

Roberts, J. E. and Kassel, J. D. (1996) 'Mood state congruence in cognitive vulnerability to depression: the roles of positive and negative affect', *Cognitive Therapy and Research* 20: 1–12.

Robins, C. J. and Luten, A. G. (1991) 'Sociotropy and autonomy: differential patterns of clinical presentation in unipolar depression', *Journal of Abnormal Psychology* 100: 74–7.

Roediger, H. L. and McDermott, K. B. (1992) 'Depression and implicit memory: commentary', *Journal of Abnormal Psychology* 101: 587–91.

Russo, N. F. and Sobel, S. B. (1981) 'Sex differences in the utilization of mental health facilities', *Professional Psychology* 12: 7–19.

Safran, J. D., Vallis, T. M., Segal, Z. V. and Shaw, B. F. (1986) 'Assessment of core cognitive processes in cognitive therapy', *Cognitive Therapy and Research* 10: 509–26.

Segal, Z. V. (1988) 'Appraisal of the self-schema construct in cognitive models of depression', *Psychological Bulletin* 103: 147–62.

—— and Blatt, S. J. (1993) *The Self in Emotional Distress: cognitive and psychodynamic perspectives*, New York: Guilford Press.

—— and Dobson, K. S. (1992) 'Cognitive models of depression: report from a consensus development conference', *Psychological Inquiry* 3: 219–24.

—— Gemar, M. C. and Williams, S. (1999) 'Differential cognitive response to a mood challenge following successful cognitive therapy or pharmacotherapy for unipolar depression', *Journal of Abnormal Psychology* 108: 3–10.

—— and Ingram, R. E. (1994) 'Mood priming and construct activation in tests of cognitive vulnerability to unipolar depression', *Clinical Psychology Review* 14: 663–95.

—— and Muran, J. C. (1993a) 'A cognitive perspective on self-representation in depression', in Z. V. Segal and S. J. Blatt (eds) *The Self in Emotional Distress: cognitive and psychodynamic perspectives*, New York: Guilford Press, pp. 131–63.

—— and —— (1993b) 'The sense of self in depression: a psychodynamic perspective: commentary', in Z. V. Segal and S. J. Blatt (eds) *The Self in Emotional Distress: cognitive and psychodynamic perspectives*, New York: Guilford Press, pp. 211–17.

Segal, Z. V. and Shaw, B. F. (1986) 'Cognition in depression: a reappraisal of Coyne and Gotlib's critique', *Cognitive Therapy and Research* 10: 671–93.
—— Truchon, C., Gemar, M., Guirguis, M. and Horowitz, L. M. (1995) 'A priming methodology for studying self-representation in major depressive disorder', *Journal of Abnormal Psychology* 104: 205–13.
Sturt, E., Kumakura, N. and Der, G. (1984) 'How depressing life is: life morbidity risk for depressive disorder in the general population', *Journal of Affective Disorders* 7: 104–22.
Stroop, J. R. (1935) 'Studies of interference in serial verbal reactions', *Journal of Experimental Psychology* 18: 643–62.
Teasdale, J. D. and Dent, J. (1987) 'Cognitive vulnerability to depression', *Cognition and Emotion* 2: 247–74.
Weissman, A. N. (1979) 'The Dysfunctional Attitude Scale: a validation study' (Doctoral dissertation, University of Pennsylvania, 1978), *Dissertation Abstracts International* 40: 1389–90B.
—— and Beck, A. T. (1978) 'Development and validation of the Dysfunctional Attitudes Scale: a preliminary investigation', paper presented at the annual meeting of the American Educational Research Association, Toronto, Canada.
Zuroff, D. C., Blatt, S. J., Sanislow, C. A., III, Bondi, C. M. and Pilkonis, P. A. (1999) 'Vulnerability to depression: reexamining state dependence and relative stability', *Journal of Abnormal Psychology* 108: 76–9.
—— and Mongrain, M. (1987) 'Dependency and self-criticism: vulnerability factors for depressive affective states', *Journal of Abnormal Psychology* 96: 14–22.

Chapter 7

The development of schizophrenia
A psychosocial and biological approach[1]

Stephen Fleck

Concerning schizophrenia, Adolph Meyer (1950–52) stated over 90 years ago: "We are justified in directing our attention to factors we see at work in the life histories of our patients instead of resorting to mystifying theoretical assumptions." Many of these mystifying assumptions are still with us, although some may be less mystifying thanks to the advances in neurobiological research during the last several decades. These produced findings that are relevant "factors" as they distinguish neurotransmitter functions and aberrations in some schizophrenic patients as compared with other patients. But even so, the role of these transmitter differences, most notably in the dopamine-dependent network, as well as their etiological significance, remain "mysterious."

Likewise, investigating the personal histories and the social matrix surrounding patients early in life, usually the family, has revealed significant deviations in the background of schizophrenic patients compared with other patients or non-ill persons, but the specificity of these findings is also unclear (Alanen 1958; Doane *et al.* 1986; Leff and Vaughan 1985; Lidz and Fleck 1985; Wynne 1968). Although Meyer did not separate social life events from psychological and biological developments (hence "Psychobiology"), I believe it is in order to consider the development of schizophrenia a tridimensional course of events – social life events as studied meticulously by Holmes and Rahe (1967) and others (Dohrenwend *et al.* 1978; Malla *et al.* 1990), personal events, especially psychobiological and emotional trauma (Fromm-Reichmann 1948; Sullivan 1962), and biological events or vicissitudes, not necessarily inborn (Halbreich *et al.* 1988; Kandel *et al.* 1983; Sachar *et al.* 1963).

In the last quarter century, there have been a number of attempts to reconcile, if not integrate, biological and psychosocial phenomena, e.g., the investigations of post-traumatic syndromes (Kolb 1987; Kolb and Multipassi 1982; Pitman *et al.* 1987; van der Kolk *et al.* 1985), Reiser's monograph *Mind, Brain and Body* (1984), and with regard to schizophrenia in particular, essays by Ciompi (1988a), Extein and Bowers (1979), Haracz (1985) and Scheflen (1981). There have also been relevant animal studies

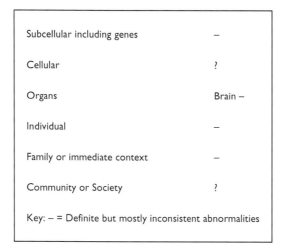

Subcellular including genes	–
Cellular	?
Organs	Brain –
Individual	–
Family or immediate context	–
Community or Society	?
Key: – = Definite but mostly inconsistent abnormalities	

Figure 7.1   The systems hierarchy

exploring the establishment of memory, e.g., those by Kandel *et al.* (1983) and by Goldman-Rakic (1982). Therefore it seems useful to consider this illness from a systems perspective with disturbances on several levels, eschewing, as is appropriate in systems theory, any single causal chain in favor of cybernetic mechanisms.

In terms of system hierarchies we can at this time consider the levels shown in Figure 7.1 implicated as malfunctioning or disorganized, although none of these aberrations is a sole or sine-qua-non factor as far as we can determine now (Buchsbaum 1990; Ciompi 1988a; Garza-Trevino *et al.* 1990; Lidz and Fleck 1985; Mesulam 1990; Reiss, Plomin and Hetherington 1991; Wynne 1968). All we can suggest is that if most or all of the systems levels shown are intact, beginning with the genes, schizophrenia would not occur (Weinberger 1987).

In considering development in the various system parameters, I want to emphasize the conditioning paradigm and Kandel's work (1979) as a way to understand some normal and abnormal facets of early brain developments as well as of memory and feelings, i.e., personality development and organization. Long ago, French (1933) and Kubie (1934) simultaneously, although independently, presented some plausible parallels between Pavlovian conditioning and psychoanalytic therapy. French emphasized that Pavlov's "differentiation" occurs in response to "conflict" and also pointed out that if the conflict becomes too intense, reactions either become generalized or stop altogether. Obviously, catatonia and some passive "negative-symptoms" schizophrenics come to mind.

Kubie believed that inhibition in the Pavlovian sense is essential to focusing and the conditioned reflex formation, and that inhibition can be lifted only if there is lack of reinforcement (as in the analytic situation where the analyst's passivity and silence facilitate disinhibition). I cite these observations not for historical reasons but because I continue to believe as do Kandel and his coworkers (1983) that learning and the establishment of memory depend on appropriate stimuli, reinforcement and inhibition of irrelevant stimuli even though, as I pointed out long ago, learning and memory acquisition are more complex phenomena than Pavlov's original conditioning paradigm (Fleck 1953). Kandel's investigation with the snail Aplysia confirms this complexity as he has shown how different synaptic channels are involved in short-term and long-term memory, respectively (Kandel *et al.* 1983). The latter concerns and interests us of course in considering psychotherapy and other treatments from a developmental perspective.

Besides Kandel's studies, elucidating primitive learning and memory establishment in a simple organism or nervous system, we have also learned that higher brain functions do not evolve via discrete pathways and enduring localization but involve modular organization and integration (Mountcastle 1979). Sherrington (1907) seemed to fathom this when he pointed to the hierarchical organization of the central nervous system, although more latter-day investigations point to a "heterarchical" evolvement and organization of higher brain functions and of mentality (Grigsby and Schneider 1991). These recent formulations of subcortical and cortical organization are based on many quite diverse investigations, such as Luria's work with frontally-lobectomized dogs (1972); Mountcastle's investigations of module functions (1979); findings of "secondary repertoires" related to failure to disconnect – I would say inhibit – modules or functional systems age-appropriately, thus resulting in interfering projections (Carlsson and Carlsson 1990; Cowan 1973; Feinberg 1982; Huttenlocher *et al.* 1982; Kimberle and Donahue 1991). Leckman and coworkers (1981) hypothesized that dopamine centers mature late in adolescence, and they related poor premorbid functioning to delays in that system's maturation – presumably a failure to inactivate the excessive number or dopaminergic axons or modules of childhood.

This is one possible model for the presumed failure to achieve age-appropriate inhibitions or disconnections of modular cortical systems in the service of establishing focused, meaningful, purposeful and adaptive cerebral integration. The extensive investigations of neurotransmitter systems in recent decades have often been flawed by overinterpretation, claims that the key to understanding schizophrenia is in the dopamine system or some deficit in pituitary-adrenal integration, or in some polypeptide aberration, etc. Recently the serotonin complex has also been revived as playing an etiological role (Garza-Trevino *et al.* 1990). Declarations that neurochemical findings tell us the cause of schizophrenia seem premature and often disregard the continued plasticity of the central nervous system in adulthood, as well as the dependency of these evolving systems early in life, maybe even intrauterine life, on stimulation (or lack of it), i.e., dependency on the extracorporeal environment (Emde 1982, 1990; Leckman *et al.* 1980; Ruthrich, Matthies and Ott, 1982).

The aforementioned plasticity of the brain has been emphasized by a number of investigators (Haracz 1985; Kimberle and Donahue 1991) beginning with the findings of Rosenzweig *et al.* (1972) that increased stimulation in young animals results in increased cortical cell mass. Thus, findings of reduced cortical mass in the brains of some schizophrenics (Andreasen *et al.* 1982), especially in those with so-called negative symptoms, might be viewed as atrophy or attrition of disuse or developmental failure, but need not be irreversible, as recovery after traumatic tissue injury demonstrates (Cotman and Nadler 1978; Flaum, Arndt and Andreasen 1990; Goldman-Rakic 1982; Kirkpatrick and Buchanan 1990; Lynch, Deadwyler and Cotman 1973). Considering brain plasticity and the capacity for change or reorganization at any age is in line with practically all recent investigations of brain structure, brain functioning and brain chemistry (Feinberg 1982; Gazzaniga 1985; Haracz 1985; Huttenlocher *et al.* 1982; Raisman and Field 1973; Ruthrich *et al.* 1982; Sawaguchi and Goldman-Rakic 1991; Weinberger 1987). To quote one eminent investigator: Goldman-Rakic stated in 1979 "The structure and pattern of neuroconnections are genetically determined, but can be altered by various influences from the outside world, including unbalanced sensory experience – in other words, immature connections require functional validation" (cited in Reiser 1984: 121).

It is apparent that dopamine plays a role in both the establishment and functioning of the neural substrate of higher mental activity like memory but its exact role or that of the dopamine-dependent modules remain unclear (Bowers 1980; Heritch 1990; Wood and Flowers 1990). Moreover, one form of learning or memory has hardly been investigated biologically; that is imprinting which may play a specific role in bonding and attachment behavior (Bowlby 1984; Horn 1985).

Besides contradictory findings concerning the dopamine system and other chemical or endocrine factors studied, radiological findings also have been variable (Andreasen *et al.* 1982; Flaum *et al.* 1990). Most methods are cross-sectional rather than sequential or longitudinal. We need to find out what happens to dilated ventricles or dopamine excess or pituitary-adrenal axis variations over time and especially what, if any, changes might accompany therapeutic progress (Carlsson and Carlsson 1990; Leckman *et al.* 1980; Pettegrew *et al.* 1991; Sachar *et al.* 1963; Sturgeon *et al.* 1981). We have now no definite biological marker for schizophrenia, not in the chemical realm, not in eye-movement aberrations nor in PET or SPECT studies (Mesulam 1990; Notradonato *et al.* 1989; Szymanski, Kane and Lieberman 1991).

From a systems viewpoint it does not matter which is the cart and which is the horse, because linear similes are wrong anyway; genetic, chemical or metabolic conditions may be the horse at some times and psychosocial events may "lead" at other times (Chapman, Hinkle and Wolff 1960; Reiser 1984; Reiss et al. 1991; Ruthrich et al. 1982). Such a view is reinforced by the recent findings that post-traumatic syndromes in veterans are accompanied by lasting neurochemical changes, e.g., disregulation of noradrenalin and the locus ceruleus (Aghajanian 1982) and changes in various transmitters coincident with cognitive and behavioral deficits produced by inescapable stress. Acute stress and panic in veterans with PTSD can be brought about by external stress or noise reminiscent of combat sounds, by psychological stimuli like sudden recall or dreams, as well as by changes in the chemical substrate responding ideopathologically to some random stress (Butler et al. 1990; Dobbs and Wilson 1960; Kardiner 1941; Kolb 1987; Krystal et al. 1989; Lidz 1946; Orr 1990; Pitman et al. 1987). The Corsons (1990) have demonstrated lasting changes in presumably constitutionally violent dogs, induced first with drugs but sustained later without medication. This work suggests that genetic factors can be overcome or compensated for postnatally – or aggravated by adverse inputs or experiences. Traumatic life events are not limited to veterans. Psychiatric case histories are replete with abuse in both physical and psychological spheres. The communication studies of Singer, Wynne and Toohey (1979) and Alanen's earlier study of mother–patient interactions (1958), and our own investigation of the families of schizophrenic patients (Lidz and Fleck 1985) all have pointed retrospectively to aberrations and deviations in the early social environment of schizophrenic patients. Bizarre rearing practices are not necessarily abusive but are perplexing and frightening, besides failing to prepare a child properly for extrafamilial interactions. Similar adverse psychosocial inputs have been noted in other conditions, and (with the possible exception of communication deviancy) these findings cannot be claimed to be specific for the development of schizophrenia any more than this is necessary for the neuronal and synaptic differences discovered so far. Moreover, there remains the diagnostic uncertainty of schizophrenia or the schizophrenias (Pettegrew et al. 1991).

However, the three parameters studied necessarily by very different methods should not necessarily be seen as contradictory or mutually exclusive. Obviously, throughout childhood, personality patterns and characteristics which have interactional utility and validity must be established via learning from others who must be trustworthy, consistent and caring. MacLean (1985) has pointed out the essentiality of trust and reliance on maternal signals in the "coevolution of the brain and family." Equally obvious is the fact that personality development and psychological organization must entail "coevolution" of neurophysiological organization, and family (social) interactions. Personality development or changes do not stop at "maturity" as seems to have been assumed earlier in this century (Levinson 1978; Minuchin 1985).

"Plasticity" is not limited to the brain but is a given in the psychosocial sphere, involving besides conditioning, imprinting and inhibitions, the more complex evolutions of speech, thought and abstract ideation. Each step involves and depends on excitatory or inhibitory inputs, and is influenced by the affective climate within and around the individual. If simulation is confusing or even abusive during a person's development or later as exemplified by post-traumatic syndromes, disorganization may occur in the substrate as it does in the behavioral sphere. Beginning with the latter we now know how frequently abuse in childhood, sexual or physical, as well as psychological is a strikingly common finding in various personality disorders and psychotic conditions (Bowlby 1984; Breslau *et al.* 1991; Day 1989; Hartmann *et al.* 1984; Hawkins 1991; Kraemer 1985). In one such study, 46 per cent of hospitalized psychotic women, not all schizophrenic, gave a history of incestuous abuse when no pointed effort was made to elicit such histories (Beck and van der Kolk 1987). Similarly, I found many years ago that almost 25 per cent of consecutive state hospital admissions reported instances of incest when appropriate inquiry was made part of the routine medical history. The majority of the patients were schizophrenics but not all of them (Fleck *et al.* 1959). Yet whereas traumatic inputs are potentially pathogenic, they, like other aberrations, biologic or psychosocial do not correlate consistently with the emergence of a particular psychopathology.

Trauma aside, neurochemical changes and aberrations need not be brought into the system by the genes (Tienari *et al.* 1987), but can be viewed or understood as conditioned results of confusing, unclear if not traumatizing inputs, not to mention chemical abuse (Glass and Bowers 1970). It has been well known that some schizophrenics eventually can get and remain well without medication, once recovered, usually thanks to comprehensive psychosocial treatments over a significant period of time as demonstrated by Alanen *et al.* (1991), Ciompi (1988b), and others (Benedetti 1985; Fleck 1980; 1990; Fromm-Reichmann 1948; Lidz and Lidz 1982; Wynne 1978); in a sense such patients have relearned or experienced reconditioning with regard to reality perception and self-sense and often acquired social know-how for the first time. Their stress vulnerability may diminish and we can assume that their neurochemistry also has changed, maybe returned to non-pathological levels and equilibria, or achieved these for the first time, but this needs to be demonstrated (Bellack *et al.* 1990; Cotman and Nadler 1978; Sturgeon *et al.* 1981).

A few decades ago, I treated a young man who was admitted to the Yale Psychiatric Institute from his college with a florid psychosis. He was the only child of two estranged, not divorced but strange, parents. He was closely tied to his mother who moved 3,000 miles to the East Coast to be near him, knowing beforehand that her visiting would be limited to a few hours at most. While staying in a nearby city, she undertook some adult education courses, including one on psychology, in order to be of help to her son. During one of her visits she reported that her teacher had given them all examinations and he had praised the class for doing very well in answering the questions concerning conditional reflexes, except for one student who presented the perfect paradigm for creating an experimental neurosis. The mother rather proudly reported to her son that she was that student. Eventually, that patient recovered and has been well for over three decades without medication.

What must be stressed in the pathogenesis of traumatic situations is the inability to escape (Krystal *et al.* 1989; van der Kolk *et al.* 1985). Whether it is the cage where conditioning experiments are carried out (Fleck and Gantt 1949) or the abused child in the family, or the soldier in a combat situation – an important element in addition to confusion, uncertainty, helplessness, is the fact that there is no escape. Going back to Cannon's paradigm, neither fight nor flight is possible (Cannon 1934). In the family the child's fight (e.g. temper tantrums) is ineffectual, and the soldier in a Vietnam-like situation cannot fight because the enemy is invisible. In neither event is flight possible, or at least not a realistic option. In childhood trauma, the enemy is the psychologically abusive parent who is also invisible in a sense, because that same parent is also one's caretaker and nurturer, as Gregory Bateson once reported of a schizophrenic veteran who sent his mother a Mother's Day card which read, "To somebody who is like a mother" (personal communication).

The role of the genes remains unclear (Goldberg *et al.* 1990); they might produce weakened or vulnerable transmitter systems, or an imbalance among several, and thus may handicap the establishment of wholesome and realistic modular hierarchies and heterarchies. However, establishing the connections required for a secure sense of self and accepting or acquiring a sense of shared realities, depend on learning, on memory development as well as memory extinction at least from levels of consciousness (Feinberg 1982; Haracz 1985; Kraemer 1985; Weinberger 1987) and on the affective climate in the group, regardless of inborn defects (Emde 1982, 1990; Sturgeon *et al.* 1981). All these operations depend on post-natal psycho-social inputs (or their lack) from the organism's context. This context, of course, is primarily and usually one's family or delegated early caretakers. They are in particular critically involved in language development and acquisition, and as Luria (1973) and others have pointed out, language is the one essential factor that gives coherence to human existence and experience. Linguistic aberrations are demonstrable clinically in schizophrenics and their families, as shown most cogently by the communication studies of Singer, Wynne and Toohey (1979), and others (Doane *et al.* 1986; Hoffman, Stopak and Andreasen 1986). However, traumatic and confusing

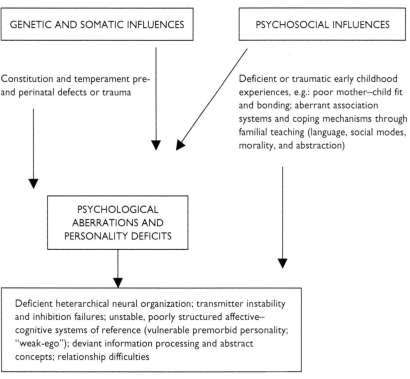

Neuro-chemical instability or aberration plus overload in form of
adulthood or age-appropriate expectations or other crisis

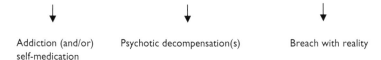

Addiction (and/or)   Psychotic decompensation(s)   Breach with reality
self-medication

COMPREHENSIVE TREATMENTS

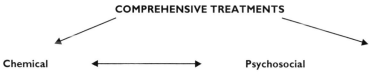

Chemical   ◄──────────►   **Psychosocial**

Possible effect and aberrant
neurotransmitters and promote
necessary inhibition:
reorganization of modules

Establish trusting/psychoeducational
relationship with patient; holding
and facilitating environment; family
therapy as indicated (focus on EE. etc.);
habilitation or rehabilitation

Figure 7.2   Development of schizophrenia
        Source: Partly modified from Ciompi (1988b).

inputs or inability to "hear" are not limited to language per se. Often in the background of schizophrenic patients one finds parental oblivion to or denial of what others say or even have indicated as their course of action. One mother who didn't want her daughter to get married tried to stop the daughter's plans by denying that there was a date set for the wedding, and by refusing to make or participate in on-going preparations for the event. Although this daughter had managed to get along with her disturbed mother and was not schizophrenic like her less fortunate sister, she suffered a psychotic depression several years later.

It has not been my intention to explore schizophrenia as such or demonstrate the neurobiological substrate of various symptoms. However, I believe schizophrenia is best conceptualized as a mixed maldevelopment of the neurologic, psychologic and social dimensions of personality, rooted in early or inborn weakness of neuromodular organization which is compromised further by aberrant and contradictory social inputs (Figure 7.2). These deviant inputs are exemplified by the language pathology observed in schizophrenics and their families, and language competence is essential for a secure self-sense as well as for social effectiveness – two major deficiencies in schizophrenics. Such a view encompasses interrelated systems highlighting the cybernetic nature of the problem in contrast to the search for a cause or causes as a linear chain of events. Consequently, therapeutic and preventive measures must also be multi-dimensional and the mix determined for each patient instead of assigning him or her to a routine program simply because it is there.

Acknowledgement

Critical comments and suggestions by Drs M. B. Bowers and B. S. Bunney are gratefully acknowledged, as is the editorial assistance of Anna Singer.

Note

1 This chapter is newly edited from 'The Development of Schizophrenia: A Psychosocial and Biological Approach', published in A. Werbart and J. Cullberg (eds) (1992) *Psychotherapy of Schizophrenia: facilitating and obstructive factors*, Oslo, Norway: Scandinavian University Press, pp. 179–92.

References

Aghajanian, G. K. (1982) 'Central noradrenergle neurosis: a locus for functional interplay between alpha-2 adrenoceptors and opiate receptors', *Journal of Clinical Psychiatry* 46: 20–4.

Alanen, Y. O. (1958) 'The mothers of schizophrenic patients', *Acta Psychiatrica et Neurologica KjoBenhavn* (Suppl. No. 124): 359.

—— Lehtinen, K., Raekkoelaeinen, V and Aaltonen, J. (1991) 'Need-adapted treatment of new schizophrenic patients: experiences and results of the Turku project', *Acta Psychiatrica Scandinavica* 83: 363–72.

Andreasen, N. C., Smith, M. R., Jacoby, G. C., Dennert, J. W. and Olsen, S. A. (1982) 'Ventricular enlargement in schizophrenia: definition and prevalence', *American Journal of Psychiatry* 139: 292–6.

Beck, J. and van der Kolk, B. A. (1987) 'Behavioral correlates of incest histories in chronically hospitalized women', *American Journal of Psychiatry* 144: 1474–6.

Bellack, A. S., Mueser, K. T., Morrison, R. L., Tierney, P. and Podell, K. (1990) 'Remediation of cognitive deficits in schizophrenia', *American Journal of Psychiatry* 147: 1650–5.

Benedetti, G. (1985) 'Möglichkeit und Grenzen der Psychotherapie bei Schizophrenen', in H. Stierlin, L. C. Wynne and M. Wirsching (eds) *Psychotherapie und Social Therapie der Schizophrenie*, Berlin and Heidelberg, Germany: Springer.

Bowers, M. B., Jr. (1980) 'Biochemical processes in schizophrenia: an update', *Schizophrenia Bulletin* 6: 393–403.

Bowlby, J. (1984) 'Violence in the family as a disorder of the attachment and caregiving systems', *American Journal of Psychoanalysis* 44: 9–27.

Breier, A., Schreiber, J. L., Dyer, J. and Pickar, D. (1991) 'National Institute of Mental Health longitudinal study of chronic schizophrenia: prognosis and predictors of outcome', *Archives of General Psychiatry* 48: 239–46.

Breslau, N., Davis, G. C., Andreski, P. and Peterson, E. (1991) 'Traumatic events and PTSD in an urban population of young adults', *Archives of General Psychiatry* 48: 216–22.

Buchsbaum, M. S. (1990) 'The frontal lobes, basal ganglia, and temporal lobes as sites for schizophrenia?', *Schizophrenia Bulletin* 16: 377–89.

Butler, R. W., Braff, D. L.. Rausch, J. L., Jenkins, M. A., Sprock, J. and Geyer, M. A. (1990) 'Physiological evidence of exaggerated startle response in a subgroup of Vietnam veterans with combat-related PTSD', *American Journal of Psychiatry* 147: 1308–12.

Cannon, W. B. (1934) *Bodily Changes in Pain, Hunger, Fear and Rage*, New York: Appleton.

Carlsson, M. and Carlsson, A. (1990) 'Schizophrenia: a subcortical neurotransmitter imbalance syndrome?', *Schizophrenia Bulletin* 16: 425–32.

Chapman, L. F., Hinkle, L. E., Jr. and Wolff, H. G. (1960) 'Human ecology, disease, and schizophrenia', *American Journal of Psychiatry* 117: 193–204.

Ciompi, L. (1988a) *Aussenwelt/Innenwelt*, Göttingen, Germany: Vandenhoeck & Ruprecht.

—— (1988b) 'Learning from outcome studies: toward a comprehensive biological-psychosocial understanding of schizophrenia', *Schizophrenia Research* 1: 373–84.

Coe, C. L., Glass, J. C. and Wiener, S. G. (1983) 'Behavioral, but not physiological adaptation, to repeated separation in mother and infant primates', *Psychoneuroendocrinology* 8: 401–9.

Corson, S. A. and Corson, E. O. (1990) 'Are there instincts of aggression and violent behavior?', *Neurosciences* 16: 15–28.

Cotman, C. W. and Nadler, J. V. (1978) 'Reactive synaptogenesis in the hippocampus', in C. W. Cotman (ed.) *Neuronal Plasticity*, New York: Raven Press, p. 227.

Cowan, W. M. (1973) 'Neuronal death as a regulative mechanism in the control of cell number in the nervous system', in D. M. Rockstein (ed.) *Development and Aging in the Nervous System*, New York: Academic Press, pp. 19–41.

Day, R. (1989) 'Schizophrenia', in G. W. Brown and T. O. Harris (eds) *Life Events and Illness*, New York: Guilford, pp. 113–37.

Doane, J. A., Goldstein, M. J., Miklowitz, D. J. and Falloon, I. R. H. (1986) 'The impact of individual and family treatment on the affective climate of families of schizophrenics', *British Journal of Psychiatry* 148: 279–87.

Dobbs, D. and Wilson W. P. (1960) 'Observations on the persistence of traumatic war neurosis', *Journal of Nervous and Mental Disease* 21: 40–6.

Dohrenwend, B. S., Krasnoff, L., Askenasy, A. R. and Dohrenwend, B. P. (1978) 'Exemplification of a method for scaling life events: the PERI life events scale', *Journal of Health and Social Behavior* 19: 205–29.

Emde, R. N. (1982) *The Development of Attachment and Affiliative Systems*, New York: Plenum Press.

—— (1990) 'Mobilizing fundamental modes of development: empathic availability and therapeutic action', *Journal of the American Psychoanalytic Association* 38: 881–913.

Extein, I. and Bowers, M. (1979) 'State and trait in psychiatric practice', *American Journal of Psychiatry* 136: 690–3.

Feinberg, I. (1982) 'Schizophrenia and late maturational brain changes in man', *Psychopharmacology Bulletin* 18(3): 29–31.

Flaum, M., Arndt, S. and Andreasen, N. C. (1990) 'The role of gender in studies of ventricle enlargement in schizophrenia: predominantly male effect', *American Journal of Psychiatry* 147: 1327–32.

Fleck, S. (1953) 'Vigilance (orienting behavior), conditional reactions, and adjustment patterns in schizophrenic and compulsive patients', *Annals of the New York Academy of Sciences* 56: 342–79.

—— (1980) 'Some observations on the nature and value of psychotherapy with schizophrenic patients', in J. S. Strauss, M. Bowers, T. W. Downey, S. Fleck, S. Jackson, and I. Levine (eds) *The Psychotherapy of Schizophrenia*, New York: Plenum, pp. 55–63.

—— (1990) 'Holding and facilitating: families and therapeutic agencies', in C. N. Stefanis *et al.* (eds) *Psychiatry: a world perspective, vol. 3*. Amsterdam: Elsevier Science Publishers.

—— Lidz, T., Cornelison, A., Schafter, S. and Terry, D. (1959) 'The intrafamilial environment of the schizophrenic patient: incestuous and homosexual problems', in J. H. Masserman (ed.) *Individual and Family Dynamics*, New York: Grune & Stratton.

—— and Gantt, W. H. (1949) 'Functional conditioning of behavior based on electrically-induced convulsions', *Federation Proceedings* 8: 1.

French, T. M. (1933) 'Interrelations between psychoanalysis and the experimental work of Pavlov', *American Journal of Psychiatry* 12: 1165–203.

Fromm-Reichmann, F. (1948) 'Notes on the development of treatment of schizophrenics by psychoanalytic psychotherapy', *Psychiatry* 11: 263–73.

Garza-Trevino, E. S., Volkan, N. D., Cancro, R. and Contreras, S. (1990) 'Neurobiology of schizophrenic syndromes', *Hospital and Community Psychiatry* 41: 971–80.

Gazzaniga, M. S. (1985) 'The Social Brain: discovering the networks of the mind, New York: Basic Books.

Glass, G. S. and Bowers, M. D., Jr. (1970) 'Chronic psychosis associated with long-term psychotomimetic drug abuse', Archives of General Psychiatry 23: 97–103.

Goldberg, T. E., Rasland, J. D., Torrey, E. F., Gold, J. M., Bigelow, L. B. and Weinberger, D. R. (1990) 'Neuropsychological assessment of monozygotic twins discordant for schizophrenia', Archives of General Psychiatry 47: 1066–72.

Goldman-Rakic, P. S. (1982) 'Neuronal development and plasticity of association cortex in primates', Neurosciences Research Program Bulletin 20: 520–32.

Grigsby, J. and Schneider, J. L. (1991) 'Neuroscience, modularity and personality theory: conceptual foundation of a model of complex human functioning', Psychiatry 54: 21–38.

Halbreich, U., Olympia, J., Glogowski, J., Carson, S., Axelrod, S. and Chin-Ming, Y. (1988) 'The importance of past psychological trauma and pathophysiological process as determinents of current biological abnormalities', Archives of General Psychiatry 45: 293–4.

Haracz, J. L. (1985) 'Neural plasticity in schizophrenia', Schizophrenia Bulletin 11: 191–229.

Hartmann, E., Milofsky, E., Vaillant, G., Oldfield, M., Falke, R. and Ducey, C. (1984) 'Vulnerability to schizophrenia: prediction of adult schizophrenia using childhood information', Archives of General Psychiatry 41: 1050–6.

Hawkins, J. (1991) 'Bowers on the river Styx', Harvard Magazine 93: 43–52.

Heritch, A. J. (1990) 'Evidence for reduced and dysregulated turnover of dopamine in schizophrenia', Schizophrenia Bulletin 16: 605–15.

Hoffman, R. E., Stopak, S. and Andreasen, N. C. (1986) 'A comparative study of manic vs. schizophrenic speech disorganizations', Archives of General Psychiatry, 43: 831–8.

Holmes, T. H. and Rahe, R. H. (1967) 'The Social Readjustment Rating Scale', Journal of Psychosomatic Research 11: 213–18.

Horn, G. (1985) 'Imprinting and the neural basis of memory', Advances in Behavioral Biology, 28: 21–9.

Huttenlocher, P. R., de Courten, C., Garcy, L. J. and Van der Loos, H. (1982) 'Synaptogenesis in human cortex – evidence for synapse elimination during normal development', Neuroscience Letters 33: 247–52.

Kandel, E. R. (1979) 'Cellular insights into behavior and learning', Harvey Lectures 73: 19–92.

—— Abrams, T., Bernier, L., Carew, T. S., Hawkins, R. D. and Schwartz, J. H. (1983) 'Classical conditioning and sensitization share aspects of the same molecular cascade in Aplysia', Cold Spring Harbor Symposium on Quantitative Biology 48(2): 821–30.

Kardiner, A. (1941) The Traumatic Neuroses of War, New York: P. Hoeber.

Kimberle, M. and Donahue, J. P. (1991) 'Reshaping the cortical motor map by unmasking latent intracortical connections', Science 251: 944–7.

Kirkpatrick, B. and Buchanan, R. W. (1990) 'The neural basis of the deficit syndrome of schizophrenia' Journal of Nervous and Mental Disorders 178: 545–55.

Knight, R. P. (1939) 'Psychotherapy in acute paranoid schizophrenia with successful outcome: a case report', Bulletin of the Menninger Clinic 1: 97–105.

Kolb, L. C. (1987) 'A neuropsychological hypothesis explaining posttraumatic stress disorders', *American Journal of Psychiatry* 144: 989–95.

—— and Multipassi, L. R. (1982) 'The conditioned emotional response: A subclass of chronic and delayed post-traumatic disorder', *Psychiatric Annals* 12: 979–87.

Kraemer, G. W. (1985) 'Effects of differences in early social experiences on primate neurobiological-behavioral development', in M. Reite and T. Field (eds) *The Psychobiology of Attachment and Separation*, Orlando, FL: Academic Press.

Krystal, J. H., Kosten, T. R., Southwick, S., Mason, J. W., Perry, B. D. and Giller, E. L. (1989) 'Neurobiological aspects of PTSD: review of clinical and pre-clinical studies', *Behavior Therapy* 20: 177–98.

Kubie, L. S. (1934), 'Relation of the conditioned reflex to psychoanalytic technic', *Archives of Neurology and Psychiatry* 53: 1137–42.

Leckman, J. F., Bowers, M. B., Jr. and Sturges, J. S. (1981) 'Relationship between estimated premorbid adjustment and CSF homovanillic acid and 5-hydroxyindoleacetic acid levels', *American Journal of Psychiatry* 138: 472–7.

—— Cohen, D. J., Shaywitz, B. A., Caparulo, B. K., Heninger, G. R. and Bowers, M. B., Jr. (1980) 'CSF monoamine metabolites in child and adult psychiatric patients: a developmental perspective', *Archives of General Psychiatry* 37: 677–81.

Leff, J. P. and Vaughan, C. E. (eds) (1985) *Expressed Emotion in Families: its significance for mental illness*, New York: Guilford.

Levinson, D. J. (1978) *The Seasons of a Man's Life*, New York: Knopf.

Lidz, T. (1946) 'Nightmares and the combat neuroses', *Psychiatry* 9: 37–49.

—— and Fleck, S. (1985) *Schizophrenia and the Family*, New York: International Universities Press.

—— and Lidz, R. W. (1982) 'Curative factors in the psychotherapy of schizophrenic patients, in S. Slipp (ed.) *Curative Factors in Dynamic Psychotherapy*, New York: McGraw-Hill.

Luria, A. R. (1973) *The Working Brain*, New York: Basic Books.

Lynch, G., Deadwyler, S. and Cotman, C. (1973) 'Postlesion axonal growth produces permanent functional connections', *Science* 180: 1364–6.

MacLean, P. D. (1985) 'Brain evolution relating to family, play, and the separation call', *Archives of General Psychiatry* 42: 417–505.

Malla, A. K., Cortese, L., Shaw, T. S. and Ginsberg, B. (1990) 'Life events and relapse in schizophrenia: a one-year prospective study', *Social Psychiatry and Psychiatric Epidemiology* 25: 221–4.

Mesulam, M. M. (1990) 'Schizophrenia and the brain', *New England Journal of Medicine* 322: 842–5.

Meyer, A. (1950–52). *The Collected Papers of Adolph Meyer*, ed. E. E. Winters, Baltimore, MD: Johns Hopkins University Press.

Minuchin, P. (1985) 'Families and individual development: provocations from the field of family therapy', *Child Development* 56: 289–302.

Mountcastle, V. P. (1979) 'An organizing principle for cerebral function: the unit module and the distributed system', in F. O. Schmitt and F. G. Wordan (eds) *The Neurosciences: fourth study program*, Boston, MA: MIT Press.

Notradonato, H., Gonzalez-Avilez, A., Van Heertum, R. L., O'Connell, R. A. and Yudd, A. P. (1989) 'The potential value of cerebral SPECT scanning in the evaluation of psychiatric illness', *Clinical Nuclear Medicine* 14: 319–22.

Orr, S. P. (1990) 'Psychophysiologic studies of post-traumatic stress disorder', in E. L. Giller (ed.) *Biologic Assessment of Post-Traumatic Stress Disorder*, Washington, DC: American Psychiatric Press.

Pettegrew, J. W., Keshavan, M. S., Panchaligam, K., Strylhor, S., Kaplan, D. B., Tretta, M. G. and Allen, M. (1991) 'Alterations in brain high energy phosphate and membrane phospholipid metabolism in first-episode, drug-naive schizophrenics: a pilot study of the dorsal prefrontal cortex by in vivo phosphorus 31 nuclear magnetic resonance spetroscopy', *Archives of General Psychiatry* 48: 563–7.

Pitman, R. K., Orr, S. P., Laforgue, D. I., DeJong, J. B. and Claiborn, J. M. (1987) 'Psychophysiology of posttraumatic stress disorder imagery in Vietnam combat veterans', *Archives of General Psychiatry* 44: 970–5.

Raisman, G. and Field, P. M. (1973) 'A quantitative investigation of the development of collateral reinnervation after partial deafferentation of the septal nuclei', *Brain Research* 50: 241–64.

Reiser, M. F. (1984) *Mind, Brain and Body*, New York: Basic Books.

Reiss, D., Plomin, R. and Hetherington, E. M. (1991) 'Genetics and psychiatry: an unheralded window on the environment', *American Journal of Psychiatry* 148: 283–91.

Robins, L. N. and Barrett, J. E. (eds) (1989) *The Validity of Psychiatric Diagnosis*, New York: Raven Press.

Rosenzweig, M. R., Bennett, E. L. and Diamond, M. C. (1972) 'Brain changes in response to experience', *Scientific American* 226(2): 22–9.

Ruthrich, H., Matthies, H. and Ott, T. (1982) 'Long-term changes in synaptic excitability of hippocampal cell populations as a result of training', in C. A. Marsan and H. Matthies, (eds) *Neuronal Plasticity and Memory Formation*, New York: Raven Press pp. 589–94.

Sachar, E. J., Mason, J., Kolmer, H. S. and Artiss, K. L. (1963) 'Psycho-endocrine aspects of acute schizophrenic reactions', *Psychosomatic Medicine* 25: 510–35.

Sawaguchi, T. and Goldman-Rakic, P. S. (1991) 'D1 dopamine receptors in prefrontal cortex: involvement in working memory', *Science* 251: 947–50.

Scheflen, A. E. (1981) *Levels of Schizophrenia*, New York: Brunner/Maazel.

Sherrington, C. (1907) *The Integrative Action of the Nervous System*, New York: Scribner.

Singer, M. T., Wynne, L. C. and Toohey, M. L. (1979) 'Communication disorders and the families of schizophrenics', in L. C. Wynne, R. L. Cromwell and S. Matthysse (eds) *The Nature of Schizophrenia*, New York: John Wiley, pp. 499–511.

Sturgeon, D., Turpin, G., Kuipers. L., Berkowitz, R. and Leff, J. P. (1981) 'Psychophysiological responses of schizophrenic patients to high and low expressed emotion relatives: a follow-up study', *British Journal of Psychiatry* 145: 62–9.

Sullivan, H. S. (1962) *Schizophrenia as a Human Process*, New York: Norton.

Szymanski, S., Kane, J. M. and Lieberman, J .A. (1991) 'A selective review of biological markers in schizophrenia', *Schizophrenia Bulletin* 17: 99–111.

Tienari, P., Sorri, A., Lahti, L., Naarala, M., Wahlberg, K. E., Moring, J., Pohjola, J. and Wynne, L. C. (1987) 'Genetic and psychosocial factors in schizophrenia: the Finnish adoptive family study', *Schizophrenia Bulletin* 13: 477–84.

Tremayne, P. and Barry, R. J. (1990), 'Applied orienting response research: some examples', *Pavlovian Journal of Biological Science* 25: 132–41.

van der Kolk, B. A., Greenberg, M. S., Boyd, H. K. and Rysal, J. (1985) 'Inescapable shock, neurotransmitters and addition to trauma: towards a psychobiology of posttraumatic stress', *Biological Psychiatry* 20: 314–25.

Weinberger, D. R. (1987) 'Implications of normal brain development for the pathogenesis of schizophrenia', *Archives of General Psychiatry* 44: 660–9.

Wood, F. B. and Flowers, D. L. (1990) 'Hypofrontal vs. hyposylvian bloodflow in schizophrenia', *Schizophrenia Bulletin* 16: 413–24.

Wynne, L. C. (1968) 'From symptoms to vulnerability and beyond: an overview', in L. C. Wynne, R. L. Cromwell and S. Matthysse (eds) *The Nature of Schizophrenia*, New York: Wiley, pp. 698–714.

AFTERWORD

Since the original publication of this paper, there has been nothing reported that would alter the essence of my formulation. Two important publications should be mentioned, although they are not in conflict with my general thesis. These are a comprehensive treatise on schizophrenia by Alanen (1997), possibly the most painstaking overview since Manfred Bleuler's (1972) *Die Schizophrenen Geistestorungen* and the study by Sidney J. Blatt and Richard Ford (1994) of treatment results in Austen Riggs patients. Neither of these studies invalidates my earlier publication reprinted here. Nor has there been any significant discovery or advance in neurobiologic research of schizophrenia in the past nine years of the "Decade of the Brain" (Carlsson 1995).

However, there has been progress regarding the psychosocial treatment and management of psychotic patients in Scandinavian countries and Great Britain. In the United States such progress has not occurred (except in a few small private hospitals like the Austen Riggs Center) because of the severe funding curtailments imposed by managed care dictates. These general fund restrictions have not only curtailed patient care, whether private or public, but also diminished psychiatric education in that, for the most part, patients are not available for adequate psychotherapy programs because of financial restrictions.

References

Alanen, Y. O. (1997) *Schizophrenia: its origins and need-adapted treatment*, trans. S. L. Leinonen, London: Karnac Books.

Blatt, S. J. and Ford, R. (1994) *Therapeutic change: an object relations approach*, New York: Plenum Press.

Bleuler, M. (1972) *Die schizophrenen Geistesstorungen im Lichte langjahriger Kranken- und Familiengeschichten*, trans. S. M. Clemens (1978) *The Schizophrenic*

Disorders: long-term patient and family studies, New Haven, CT: Yale University Press.

Carlsson, A. (1995) 'Neurocircuitries and neurotransmitter interactions in schizo-phrenia', *International Clinical Psychology* 10 (Suppl. No. 3): 25–8.

Chapter 8

Another "lens" for understanding therapeutic change

The interaction of IQ with defense mechanisms[1]

Phebe Cramer

In 1992, Sidney Blatt published a paper in the *Journal of the American Psychoanalytic Association* that profoundly changed our thinking about psychotherapy, and the efficacy of different modes of therapeutic treatment. Previously, data from the Menninger Psychotherapy Research Project had indicated that there was little difference in the therapeutic outcome of patients who had been treated with psychoanalysis, as compared with those who had been seen in supportive-expressive psychotherapy. However, Sid's reanalysis of these data, looking at them through a new lens, revealed a different understanding of the relation between type of therapy and treatment outcome. In careful reanalyses of the outcome data, Sid demonstrated that the responsiveness of patients to the two types of treatment was importantly determined by personality differences in the patients. Patients who could be identified as having an *anaclitic* personality organization – those who were primarily focused on interpersonal relatedness and who used avoidant defenses like denial – showed more positive change when provided with supportive-expressive psychotherapy. In contrast, patients who could be identified as having an *introjective* personality organization – those who were primarily focused on issues of self-definition, autonomy and self-worth and who used counteractive defenses like projection – showed greater positive change when treated by psychoanalysis. The very important discovery of this work demonstrated that the nature of the therapeutic outcome depended on the *interaction* between personality organization of the patient and treatment mode.

In this chapter, I propose to look again at therapy outcome data through a new lens – i.e., to consider another patient variable that may be important in predicting therapeutic change and to consider the interaction of this variable with others already identified as being critical. To skip ahead for a moment, I propose to examine the role that intelligence, which surely belongs among the ego functions of the patient, plays in therapeutic change. But first, I will discuss the importance of another group of ego functions – namely, the mechanisms of defense – as these have been found to relate to therapy outcome. In this section, I review and expand on what was discovered from the Riggs study of therapeutic change (Blatt and Ford 1994).

A theory of defense mechanism development

When Sid Blatt and Dick Ford were in the midst of their extensive study of psychotherapy patients treated at the Austen Riggs Center, I had finally completed the development of a method to assess defense mechanism use through the analysis of narrative material from Thematic Apperception Test (TAT) stories (Murray 1943). Further, the method had been used to substantiate the hypothesis that when children's self-esteem is threatened, or when they experience trauma, they make greater use of the defense mechanisms available to them (Cramer and Gaul 1988; Dollinger and Cramer 1990).

This method had been developed to test out a theory of defense mechanism development (Cramer 1991) across the period from early childhood through late adolescence. I had proposed that, as children mature, and particularly as their cognitive functioning becomes more complex, changes in defense use would ensue. Specifically, I hypothesized that young children would rely primarily on the cognitively simple defense of denial. However, I suggested that eventually this defense would become ineffective and would be superceded, in later childhood and adolescence, by the defense of projection. In the later adolescent period, when the issue of identity development is salient, I hypothesized that the defense of identification would become prominent. When empirical studies with children of different ages were carried out, the results confirmed the theory – namely, that defense use showed the developmental progression described (Cramer 1991).[2]

The Riggs study

Among the excellent test protocols available in the Riggs study, there were TAT stories told at the time of patient admission to the hospital and told again after 15 months of treatment. Although the defense coding method had not been applied to adult stories at that point, here was clearly an exciting opportunity to determine whether this method would be relevant for understanding patient pathology and sensitive to changes in defense mechanism use over the course of treatment.

An initial pilot study with a small group of Riggs patients suggested that there were meaningful relations between defense use and scores on various measures of symptoms of psychopathology, interpersonal relations, and investment in object relations. On this basis, we decided to go ahead with the project of coding the use of defense mechanisms in the TAT stories of 90 patients, as these occurred during the standard psychological assessment at admission and again 15 months later. The coding of these stories occurred without the coder's knowing from which point in treatment the stories came and without knowledge of the patient's diagnosis, gender, or other test results. Subsequently, defense scores from early and later in treatment were compared. Initially, in keeping with Sid's interest in the anaclitic and introjective personality, the data were also sorted in this way.

Our first report of these data (Cramer, Blatt and Ford 1988) focused on the relation between the use of defenses and psychological symptoms, interpersonal functioning, and object relations, as these were found at the time of admission. An immediate, important finding was that these relations occurred almost exclusively within the anaclitic group. For the anaclitic patients, at admission to the hospital, high use of denial was significantly associated with two of the Strauss-Harder (1981) symptom scales – Bizarre Disorganized and Bizarre Retarded.[3] Also, high use of denial and of projection were both associated with unsatisfactory interpersonal involvement, as measured by the Fairweather scale (Fairweather et al. 1960), and by poor capacity for interpersonal relatedness (Menninger Factor 1 scale; Harty et al. 1981). In contrast, high use of Identification, a more mature defense, was negatively related to evidence of psychotic symptoms (Strauss-Harder scale) and was related to positive interpersonal involvement (Fairweather scale) and to good capacity for interpersonal relatedness (Menninger scale).[4] For the anaclitic patients, the defense measures were also found to be related to Rorschach measures of disordered thinking. The primitive defense of denial was positively related to having a low $F+$ per cent (indicative of poor perceptual accuracy), a large number of pure C responses (indicative of unmodulated affect), and to indications of thought disorder, contaminations, and confabulations.

The results of this first study thus indicated that, for anaclitic patients, the level of pathology, as determined from rating scales and from Rorschach measures, was related to level of defense use. The use of low-level, primitive defenses was associated with more symptomatology, poorer interpersonal functioning, and greater thought disorder as the patient entered the hospital.

Our next investigation was concerned with questions of how patients changed in defense use after a 15-month period of treatment and how this change might be related to changes in symptoms and interpersonal functioning (Cramer and Blatt 1990, 1993). This study found a significant decrease in patients' defense use after 15 months of treatment. Moreover, this decrease was significantly correlated with a decrease in Bizarre Disorganized symptoms.

Further examination of the results through the anaclitic–introjective lens, now in combination with patient gender, revealed a very interesting pattern. Most typically, anaclitic patients are women while introjective patients are men. But this is not always the case; in this disturbed patient group, a third of the men had an anaclitic personality organization, and a third of the women were described as introjective. Cramer and Blatt (1993) designated these patients as being *gender incongruent* for personality organization and suggested that this incongruence may be a source of inner conflict. In the Riggs study, there were 14 anaclitic men and 17 introjective women (in contrast to 28 anaclitic women and 31 introjective men). Further study of these groups demonstrated how a gender-incongruent identity was related to intensified defense use. At admission to the hospital, gender-incongruent patients used defenses that were consistent with the opposite gender. That is, anaclitic men tended to use more denial (statistically more frequent among women) while introjective women used more projection (statistically more frequent among men). However, after 15 months of treatment, the gender-incongruent patients shifted from gender-incongruent to gender-congruent defenses – that is, anaclictic men used more projection and introjective women used more denial.

The meaning of this change in gender-related defenses is perhaps best understood by examining changes in the defense of identification, a defense that is closely linked to identity development (Erikson 1968). Here, we must distinguish between the normal developmental process of identification and the use of identification as a defense mechanism. As part of normal development, the growing child internalizes the attitudes, values, and personality characteristics of important others. However, under certain circumstances, such as loss of the other through death or prolonged absence, or in other circumstances that create conflict, anxiety, or loss of self-esteem, identification may be used for defensive purposes.

In the developmental process of identification, a growing boy generally will identify with significant boys and men, acquiring their masculine characteristics, whereas a girl will usually identify with girls and women and thus acquire feminine characteristics. However, in the case of the anaclitic boy or man, he has taken on defenses and other personality characteristics usually found in women, while the introjective girl or woman has taken on defenses and characteristics usually found in men. In these gender-incongruent patients, there is a tension or conflict between the nature of their personality organization and their biological sex. Under these circumstances, to maintain the conflicted identity, and to manage the attendant anxiety and protect self-esteem, identification is used as a defense. This defensive identification includes the more primitive processes of incorporation and introjection (Meissner 1974).

Cramer and Blatt (1993) expected that as the identity conflict was resolved, the use of identification would decrease, and this is what we found. For the gender-incongruent anaclitic male and introjective female patients, the use of identification significantly decreased after 15 months of treatment. Along with the change in the gender-related defenses of denial and projection, we took this finding to reflect a decrease in the patients' anxiety stemming from a conflicted initial identity. With further treatment, we might expect to find an increase in the more mature forms of the defense of identification.

This study also demonstrated that changes in defense use during treatment were related to changes in clinical symptomatology, interpersonal relations, and investment in object relationships. To summarize these results, we found that for gender-incongruent patients an *increase* in gender-congruent defenses was related to psychological improvement. Further, a *decrease* in the defense of identification among gender-incongruent patients was related to better psychological functioning. Again, the implication of the use of the defense of identification by gender-incongruent patients was highlighted. We theorized that, in these patients, strong use of identification may be indicative of psychological disturbance, or conflict, rather than an indication of psychological strength. In contrast, for gender-congruent patients, a decrease in gender-congruent defenses of denial and projection and an increase in the use of identification was related to psychological improvement. For these patients, better functioning was linked to less use of immature defenses and greater use of a more mature defense.

One further study, based on the Riggs data, compared the change in defense use of patients diagnosed as psychotic with that of patients diagnosed with a severe personality disorder (e.g., borderline personality disorder; Cramer 1999a). As compared to the personality disorder patients, psychotic patients at admission to the hospital had higher total defense scores and especially showed greater use of the primitive defense of denial. After 15 months of treatment, psychotic patients had reduced their use of all three defenses, with the largest reduction occurring for the defense of denial. In this study, patients who had been clinically rated as most improved after treatment were compared with those determined to be least improved. As expected, it was the most improved patients who showed a decrease in defense scores after treatment, primarily because of the decrease in the use of denial.

What is the status of IQ in clinical research?

It is an interesting and curious fact that the large majority of contemporary investigations of personality do not include IQ among the seriously considered factors of importance to study. If considered at all, IQ is frequently used as a control variable, matching groups so as to rule out, or make unimportant, any possible influence of IQ on the findings of the study. Yet the assessment of intelligence and the development of the IQ measure represents the earliest success by psychologists to measure complex psychological functioning, and the IQ measure continues to be the best standardized procedure among our battery of assessment procedures. Moreover, an assessment of IQ as part of the diagnostic battery is considered important by clinicians of varying theoretical positions, and the concept of IQ is more familiar to the general public than are many of our other clinical constructs. However, apart from the study of neurologically-based psychopathology, IQ is generally overlooked or given minimal mention in research studies of personality and therapeutic change.

The Riggs study provides an opportunity to look more closely at the role of IQ in therapeutic change. For each of the 90 patients, Full Scale, Verbal, and Performance IQ scores from the Wechsler Adult Intelligence Scale or Wechsler-Bellevue Scales I or II (Wechsler 1955) were available from the clinical assessment done at admission and again after 15 months of treatment. However, only two paragraphs in *Therapeutic Change* (Blatt and Ford 1994) were devoted to a discussion of findings involving IQ. The first paragraph notes that both Full Scale and Performance IQ scores increased significantly during treatment (Blatt and Ford 1994: 87). The second reference to IQ (Blatt and Ford 1994: 151) points out that there were significant correlations between changes in IQ scores and changes in clinical symptoms. Possibly because of the difficulty of interpreting this finding, or possibly because of the many other variables to be studied, no further analysis of the implications of the IQ findings were reported.

We may ask at this point what is the status of IQ in research investigations of personality and clinical change? Is IQ (should IQ be) simply a control variable? Or, might IQ be an independent variable that predicts change? Alternatively, is it better to conceptualize IQ as a dependent variable that is predicted *by* pathology change? The very interesting finding reported by Blatt and Ford (1994) that there were significant correlations between changes in IQ scores and changes in clinical symptoms is directly relevant to the important question of whether improved intellectual functioning contributes to the lessening of symptoms – i.e., is responsible for decreased pathology (IQ is an independent variable) – or instead whether the reduced pathology facilitates better intellectual functioning (IQ is a dependent variable). Correlational data do not allow us to answer that question, although more complex statistical analyses may provide a method to assess causal relations.

In any case, the finding that IQ change is related to symptom change strongly suggests that IQ should be considered along with other intrapsychic variables in the investigation of how change occurs in clinical symptoms and personality. Intelligence, as assessed by IQ measures, represents a variety of ego functions – reasoning, judgment, memory, perception – and thus might reasonably be expected to be related to change that is influenced by ego functioning. In the next section of the chapter, I consider the question of how IQ, as another component of ego functioning, may add to, or interact with, the use of defense mechanisms in predicting personality and personality change.

Defense mechanisms plus IQ predict personality change

In this section, I discuss the initial discovery, and subsequent confirmation, that defense mechanisms interact with IQ level in predicting personality maturity and favorable personality change. In the first study (Cramer 1999b), I focused on the relation between levels of ego development (Loevinger 1976) and the use of defense mechanisms. Because level of ego development is defined, in part, by the capacity to control impulses, it seemed possible that there should be a correspondence between ego level and the use of defense mechanisms. For example, at the lowest levels of ego development (termed, by Loevinger, Impulsive and Self-Protective), there is minimal conscious control of impulses, and the feared consequences of impulse expression result in what A. Freud (1936) termed *objective anxiety*. Thought processes at these early stages tend to be simplistic and organized around dichotomies (good–bad, yes–no); troubles are located outside of the self, and blame is externalized. Thus one might expect that immature defenses, such as denial and projection, would be characteristic of adults who are at these early ego developmental levels.

At the next highest levels of ego development – the Conformist and Self-Aware levels – there is a major shift in impulse control The need to control impulses is now consciously recognized. However, the source of control is seen as being external to the self. Conscious control is based on the adoption of social norms and adherence to rules. The influence of these external constraints renders the need for defense control of impulses to be less important.

At the highest levels of ego development, impulse control is internalized. The awareness of inner conflict, which may either be tolerated or defended against, develops. In the latter case, some relation between these higher ego levels and defense mechanism use should be found. However, now that the conflict is consciously recognized, mechanisms based on disavowal (e.g., denial) or externalization (e.g., projection) would not be expected to be prominent.

Overall, this conceptual linking suggests a curvilinear relation between ego level and defense use.[5] At low levels of ego development, the use of low level immature defenses would be expected. At mid-range levels of ego development, defense use should be minimal, because impulse control is taken over by social rules of conduct. At highest levels of ego development, the use of defenses may increase, depending on the tolerance of the individual for internal conflict.

Using data from the Block and Block (1980) longitudinal study of San Francisco Bay Area residents, I was able to study the relation between ego level, measured by both Loevinger's Sentence Completion Test and prototype matching of personality descriptions, and the use of defense mechanisms. (For a full description of the method, see Cramer 1999b). As a first step, I determined the correlation between ego level at age 23 and the use of denial, projection, and identification, as determined from the coding of TAT stories. The results indicated that the relations were curvilinear: people with both low and high ego levels used more defenses, and those with mid-range ego levels used fewer defenses.

For this sample of young adults, there was also available a measure of Wechsler Adult Intelligence Scale IQ. It seemed that as ego functions, IQ, defense use, and ego level might be interrelated. Indeed, IQ was significantly, and positively, correlated with ego level. However, using simple linear correlations, IQ was unrelated to defense use. Nevertheless, inspection of the data suggested that the interrelation of these variables might be more complex. Specifically, although there was no linear relation between IQ and defenses, and no linear relation between defenses and ego level, it appeared that the *interaction* between IQ and defenses was a predictor of ego level.

A series of regression analyses bore this out. When the participants were separated into higher IQ ($M = 128$) and lower IQ ($M = 107$) groups, it became clear that the use of defense mechanisms had different implications for each group when predicting ego level. For lower IQ individuals, the use of denial predicted higher ego levels. However, for individuals with higher IQs, the use of denial predicted lower ego levels. Similarly, IQ and projection interacted in predicting ego level. Again, for lower IQ individuals, the use of projection predicted higher ego level; the opposite was true for higher IQ individuals.

These findings may be understood as follows: When IQ is lower, the use of defense mechanisms may compensate for the lower IQ, allowing the individual to reach higher levels of ego development than would be possible if these compensatory mechanisms were not available. However, for higher IQ individuals, the use of age-inappropriate defenses like denial is a deterrent to ego development. When lower and higher IQ individuals are combined into a single group, this has the consequence of masking the effect of IQ, such that there appears to be no (linear) relation between defense mechanisms and ego level.

This discovery of a reciprocal, compensatory relation between defenses and IQ in predicting positive ego development prompted me to look at this phenomenon in another arena of personality. Currently, many researchers in the field of personality rely on the five-factor model (McCrae and Costa 1990) to guide studies of personality. Systematic study of the many extant personality scales designed to measure a large variety of different dispositions and traits has suggested that these various traits may be best understood as representing five underlying personality dimensions. These five dimensions have been demonstrated, through factor analysis, to best account for the numerous aspects of personality being assessed by the variously named self-report measures. The five factors have been designated as Neuroticism, Extraversion, Openness to experience, Agreeableness, and Conscientiousness. There has been some disagreement among researchers whether these personality dimensions become fixed and immutable in adulthood by age 30 or whether personality change continues throughout adulthood. To answer this question, a longitudinal study following the same individuals as they move through the adult years was needed.

The opportunity to carry out such a study came to me through collaboration with the Institute of Human Development at the University of California, Berkeley. From their longitudinal study, data were available to determine the participants' standing on each of the five factors at three different points in their adult lives. In this study (Cramer 2003), the same group of 155 men and women were followed across adulthood, from approximately age 30 to age 60. The results indicated that significant personality change occurs during adulthood, with Agreeableness, Extraversion, and Conscientiousness increasing with age, Neuroticism decreasing, and Openness initially increasing but then decreasing by age 60. More interesting, for the purposes of the present essay, is that, for all five personality traits, the interaction between IQ and defense mechanisms was found to be a significant predictor of both personality and personality change.[6] Further, the nature of that prediction was consistent across traits. For individuals with a lower IQ, strong defense use was related to a more positive personality picture. For example, lower IQ men ($M = 107$) who used projection were more Conscientious than those who did not use projection. In contrast, the use of defenses by higher IQ men ($M = 127$) was related to the opposite, more negative personality picture. For example, higher IQ men who used projection were less Conscientious than those who did not use projection. Similar results were found for women. Thus, as in the previous study, for lower IQ individuals, the use of defenses – even immature defenses – is seen as compensatory, in that the defense use is associated with positive personality traits and with reduction of less desirable traits. However, the use of these defenses by higher IQ individuals is a negative indicator for personality well-being.

Looking at therapeutic change through the lens of the interaction between IQ and defense mechanisms

In the Riggs study, change was assessed by comparing scores from the time of hospital admission with similar scores obtained after 15 months of treatment. In the present analysis, I focus on the 79 most disturbed patients (those diagnosed with psychosis or with borderline or narcissistic personality disorders). Clinical change was seen most clearly in these patients, where a statistical comparison of their functioning before and after 15 months of treatment indicated that the presence of pathological symptoms had decreased and that the quality of interpersonal functioning had improved.

The next question was how IQ might contribute to clinical change and, especially, whether defense mechanisms would interact with IQ in predicting clinical change. The earlier research, studying normal personality dispositions, had found that defenses appeared to compensate for lower IQ, such that the use of defenses by lower IQ individuals was associated with a more positive personality organization – e.g., higher ego level, greater conscientiousness, and better adjustment. For these individuals, greater defense use was associated with an increase in positive dispositions. What, then, might we expect the relation between defense use and IQ to be when considering negative dispositions – i.e., dimensions of psychopathology?

To investigate this question, a series of analyses was carried out to determine the role of defenses and IQ in predicting change in symptoms and interpersonal functioning. For each of the clinical outcome change measures, the variables of IQ, change in the three defenses (denial, projection, and identification), and the interaction of IQ with these defense changes were entered into a regression analysis to determine the strongest predictors of clinical change. Thus, for each outcome variable, it could be determined whether outcome change could be predicted by defense change, by IQ, or by the interaction between IQ and defense change. If this interaction was significant, it would indicate that defense change predicts clinical change in a different way for lower IQ ($M = 109$), as compared with higher IQ ($M = 128$), patients.[7]

In discussing the results of these several regression analyses, I consider first the independent contributions of denial, projection, identification, and IQ for predicting clinical change. As regards the relation between defense change and symptom change, the results of the regression analyses indicated that a decrease in the use of denial was associated with a decrease in Bizarre Disorganized symptoms, a decrease in projection was associated with a decrease in Impulsivity (Menninger Factor 2 scale; Harty *et al.* 1981), and a decrease in identification was associated with a decrease in Bizarre Retarded symptoms. In contrast, IQ by itself did not predict clinical change.

On the basis of these results, it would appear that defense change plays a role in clinical change but that IQ is unrelated to change. However, when the *interaction* between defense change and IQ was considered, it became apparent that this interaction predicts clinical change.

The results of the interaction analyses presented a consistent picture across the clinical symptom and interpersonal functioning variables. For lower IQ patients, a decrease in the use of defenses after 15 months of treatment predicted a decrease in symptom level and an increase in interpersonal functioning. Thus, for lower IQ patients, a decrease in the use of identification predicted a decrease in Neurotic symptoms, a decrease in the use of projection predicted a decrease in Bizarre Retarded symptoms, and a decrease in denial predicted a decrease in Impulsivity. Likewise, for lower IQ patients, a decrease in identification and in projection both predicted an improvement in interpersonal functioning (Fairweather scale).

The corollary of this finding, however, is that an increase in defense use by lower IQ patients predicted increased symptom manifestation. In turn, this suggests that, for seriously *disturbed* individuals of lower IQ, defenses function to support their pathological symptoms; in the earlier studies of *psychologically healthy* individuals with lower IQ, defenses functioned to support favorable personality characteristics. In general, then, for lower IQ individuals, defenses function to maintain or strengthen the existing personality organization – an adaptive, positive organization in psychologically healthy individuals or a pathological organization in psychologically disturbed individuals. A decrease in the use of defenses among these lower IQ individuals will result in a decrease of positive traits in healthy individuals and of pathological symptoms in disturbed individuals.

For the higher IQ patients, the reverse association between defense and symptom change was found. For these individuals, midway through their treatment, an increase in defense use predicted decreased symptoms and more adequate interpersonal functioning. This pattern suggested that defenses are functioning to control or suppress manifestations of pathology. Thus, an increase in the use of identification predicted a decrease in Neurotic symptoms and more adequate interpersonal functioning (Fairweather and Menninger Factor 1 scales). An increase in the use of projection predicted a decrease in Bizarre Retarded symptoms and improved interpersonal functioning (Fairweather scale), and an increase in denial predicted a decrease in Impulsivity.

Some tentative speculations regarding the implications of these findings for therapy

On a speculative level, there may be some issues to consider regarding the focus of therapy with patients of varying IQ levels. For seriously disturbed patients of lower IQ, defenses appear to support or contribute to their psychopathology. Thus, a reduction in defense mechanism use would be expected to decrease pathology and to increase the quality of interpersonal functioning. In this case, the analysis of defense mechanisms in therapy would be expected to be associated with positive change.

In contrast, the analysis of defenses in higher IQ individuals in a seriously disturbed patient group might be expected to lead, at least temporarily, to greater evidence of disturbance and less adequate functioning. *These patients will likely appear to get worse before they get better.* This is because, for higher IQ patients, defenses function to control pathological symptoms and modulate the expression of pathological maladaptive behavior. If defenses are reduced, so is adaptive functioning; symptom expression is also increased. Here we should keep in mind that this description represents a point in the treatment of these patients (15 months after treatment began) when they were in the process of change, but the change was not complete. With further treatment, a reduction in pathology would be expected.

Conclusion

Sidney Blatt's (1992) work demonstrated the importance of the interaction between treatment modality and the patient's personality organization for therapeutic outcome. The present chapter offers an addition to this interactional focus. It suggests that the implications of the use of defense mechanisms – and, by extension, the effect of the analysis of defense mechanisms – for therapeutic outcome will be different for patients of different levels of intelligence. Again, it is the interaction between two variables – in this case, defense and IQ – that will predict therapeutic outcome.

Final note

Sid Blatt is one of the warmest, most positive, and most supportive psychologists I know. It was his interest in my approach to assessing defense mechanisms through the analysis of TAT stories that encouraged me to continue working with this method. Because of Sid's interest, this method was used in the Riggs study, from which we published three papers and a chapter in *Therapeutic Change*. Despite initial skepticism from academic journals, Sid's optimism and steadfastness demonstrated to me how benign resistance to rejection could lead to positive outcome. It was a lesson that I carried with me as I continued to work in an area of research that did not fit neatly into either academic psychology or the community of psychoanalysis. Sid's initial buoyancy about my work helped keep me afloat; for this I am most grateful.

Notes

1 Appreciation is expressed to Richard Q. Ford for his helpful comments on this chapter.
2 These findings have also been confirmed by Porcerelli *et al.* (1998). Subsequent research (Cramer 1997), using a longitudinal design in which the same children were followed over a number of years, demonstrated the same decrease in the use of denial (between ages 6–6 and 7–3) and an increase in the use of projection (between ages 7–3 and 7–10).
3 The scales were subsequently designated as Labile Affect and Flattened Affect.
4 The various scales are fully described in Blatt and Ford (1994).
5 These ideas are developed more fully in Cramer (1999b).
6 The prediction of personality change from defenses and IQ was based on

hierarchical multiple regression analyses in which the predictors included the personality score from the previous age.

7 Statistically, this would indicate that IQ moderates the effect of defense change on outcome.

References

Blatt, S. J. (1992) 'The differential effect of psychotherapy and psychoanalysis on anaclitic and introjective patients: the Menninger Psychotherapy Research Project revisited', *Journal of the American Psychoanalytic Association* 40: 691–724.

—— and Ford, R. Q. (1994) *Therapeutic Change: an object relations perspective*, New York: Plenum Press.

Block, J. H. and Block, J. (1980) 'The role of ego-control and ego-resiliency in the organization of behavior', in W. A. Collins (ed.) *Studying Lives Through Time*, Washington, DC: American Psychological Association, pp. 9–41.

Cramer, P. (1991) *The Development of Defense Mechanisms: theory, research and assessment*, New York: Springer.

—— (1997) 'Evidence for change in children's use of defense mechanisms', *Journal of Personality* 65: 233–47.

—— (1999a) 'Future directions for the Thematic Apperception Test', *Journal of Personality Assessment* 72: 74–92.

—— (1999b) 'Ego functions and ego development: defense mechanisms and intelligence as predictors of ego level', *Journal of Personality* 67: 735–60.

—— (2003) 'Personality change in later adulthood is predicted by defense mechanism use in early adulthood', *Journal of Research in Personality* 37: 76–104.

—— Blatt, S. J. and Ford, R. Q. (1988) 'Defense mechanisms in the anaclitic and introjective personality configuration', *Journal of Consulting and Clinical Psychology* 56: 610–16.

—— and Blatt, S. J. (1990) 'Use of the TAT to measure change in defense mechanisms following intensive psychotherapy', *Journal of Personality Assessment* 54: 236–51.

—— and —— (1993) 'Change in defense mechanisms following intensive treatment, as related to personality organization and gender', in W. Ehlers, U. Hentschel, G. Smith, and J. G. Draguns (eds) *The Concept of Defense Mechanisms in Contemporary Psychology*, New York: Springer: pp. 310–20.

—— and Gaul, R. (1988) 'The effects of success and failure on children's use of defense mechanisms', *Journal of Personality* 56: 729–42.

Dollinger, S. and Cramer, P. (1990) 'Children's defensive responses and emotional upset following a disaster: a projective assessment', *Journal of Personality Assessment* 54: 116–27.

Erikson, E. (1968) *Identity: youth and crisis*, New York: Norton.

Fairweather, T., Fairweather, G. W., Simon, R., Gebhard, M. E., Weingarten, E., Holland, J. L., Sanders, R., Stone, G. B. and Reahl, J. E. (1960) 'Relative effectiveness of psychotherapeutic programs: a multicriteria comparison of four programs for three different patient groups', *Psychological Monographs* 74, 5 (Whole no. 492).

Freud, A. (1936) *The Ego and the Mechanisms of Defense*, New York: International Universities Press.

Harty, M., Cerney, M., Colson, D., Coyne, L., Frieswyk, S., Johnson, S. and Mortimer, R. (1981) 'Correlates of change and long-term outcome', *Bulletin of the Menninger Clinic* 45: 209–28.

Loevinger, J. (1976) *Ego Development*, San Francisco: Jossey-Bass.

McCrae, R. R. and Costa, P. T. (1990) *Personality in Adulthood*, New York: Guilford Press.

Meissner, W. W. (1974) 'The role of imitative social learning in identificatory processes', *Journal of the American Psychoanalytic Association* 28: 43–67.

Murray, H. A. (1943) *Thematic Apperception Test Manual*, Cambridge, MA: Harvard University Press.

Porcerelli, J. H., Thomas, S., Hibbard, S. and Cogan, R. (1998) 'Defense mechanism development in children, adolescents, and late adolescents', *Journal of Personality Assessment* 71: 411–20.

Strauss, J. S. and Harder, D. W. (1981) 'The Case Record Rating Scale: a method for rating symptom and social function data from case records', *Psychiatry Research* 4: 333–45.

Wechsler, D. (1955) *Manual for the Wechsler Adult Intelligence Scale*, New York: Psychological Corporation.

Part III

Assessment

Chapter 9

Sidney Blatt's contributions to the assessment of object representations

Barry Ritzler

The construct of object representation is the cornerstone of object relations theory. Its importance is not limited to this specific theory, but extends to all psychodynamic theories because of its origins in Freud's writings (1914) and subsequent extensions by Rapaport (1950), Schafer (1968), and others (e.g., Fairbairn 1963). Cognitive behaviorists might also find object representations to be a useful construct (Blatt and Auerbach 2000) if they were not so biased by its association with psychoanalysis.

Object relations theory developed when psychoanalysis moved from Freud's original emphasis on drive theory to a focus on interpersonal relationships essential to personality development. Its emergence was consistent with an emphasis on the concept of the object in developmental theory (e.g., Piaget 1937; Werner 1948; Werner and Kaplan 1963). In psychoanalysis, Klein (1952), Winnicott (1965), and Kohut (1971) were foremost in proposing that internalized, largely unconscious images of parental figures and the child's relationship with the parents formed the foundation for later personality development and adaptation. In particular, Mahler (Mahler, Pine and Bergman 1975) identified stages in the development of object relations and disturbances that arise from problems during the developmental process.

Object relations theory (A. Freud 1965; Fraiberg 1969; Fairbairn 1954; Guntrip 1969; Kernberg 1967) therefore emphasizes the central role of the concept of the object in ego development. Early experiences of rejection, neglect, or both are hypothesized as major contributing factors to later impairment in object relations. In severe cases, early trauma in object relations is hypothesized to result in the disruption of normal development. Such early disruptions lead to later disturbances that are characterized by cognitive distortions in the conceptualization of self and others that interfere with effective adult relationships. For example, Fairbairn (1954) cited the schizophrenic patient's disturbed preoccupation with human relationships as evidence for the validity of his object relations theory's explanation of the psychotic cognitive deficit. Searles (1965) also argued that schizophrenic patients showed little cognitive impairment when relating to the nonhuman environment, but often broke down under the high anxiety and subjective stress of interpersonal situations. Subsequently, treatment methods have developed for the modification and improvement of internal object representations that result in more effective interpersonal relationships (Greenberg and Mitchell 1983). But like any potentially useful theoretical construct, object representation requires effective assessment procedures for testing hypotheses generated by the construct. Sidney Blatt has made major contributions to the development and refinement of assessment methods for operationalizing object representations.

Early contributions

The development of Blatt's methods for assessing object representations began with a study of thought disorder and boundary disturbances on the Rorschach (Blatt and Ritzler 1974). Three manifestations of thought disorder – fabulized combinations, confabulations, and contaminations – were found to be characteristic of psychotic patients at progressively more severe levels of clinical disorganization. The authors concluded that psychoses, particularly schizophrenia, were associated with disturbances in the boundaries of internal object representations.

Following the boundary disturbance study, Blatt, Wild and Ritzler (1975) reviewed psychoanalytic and experimental research literature to conclude that schizophrenia is the result of fundamental disturbances in the early development of object representations. In this theoretical paper, the authors emphasized the importance of developing methods for accurate assessment of object representations.

Measures of object representations

After the early foundation papers, Blatt *et al.* (1976) developed the Concept of the Object Scale (COS), a coding system for assessing the articulation, differentiation, and integration of object representations projected in Rorschach responses. In their effort to develop a method for projective assessment of object representations, 37 participants were assessed in a longitudinal study at ages 11–12, 13–14, 17–18, and 30. Normal development showed a significant increase in highly articulated, well-differentiated, and integrated human responses depicting constructive, reciprocal relationships. A comparison sample of 48 adolescent and young adult psychiatric patients also was assessed. Compared to the normal participants, the patients gave human responses that were more inaccurately perceived, distorted, and partial and more engaged in unmotivated, incongruent, nonspecific, and malevolent activity. Patients also gave more accurately perceived human responses at lower levels of development and more inaccurately perceived human responses at higher levels of development. The authors discussed the role of object relations in normal, adaptive functioning, as well as in the development of complex but maladaptive behavior.

Further development of the COS

After the COS was introduced, Ritzler *et al.* (1980) conducted a replication study examining paranoia and premorbid adjustment in schizophrenic individuals. The results of the Ritzler *et al.* study were nearly identical to those of Blatt *et al.* (1976), with no major differences with regard to level of premorbid adjustment (i.e., good versus poor) or to paranoia (i.e., paranoid versus nonparanoid) among schizophrenic patients. The authors reasoned that schizophrenic individuals cannot effectively use existing ego potential for higher levels of integrated and organized behavior. Instead, the greater ego resources are absorbed in the unrealistic fantasy and symptomatic behavior that interfere with, rather than, facilitate effective adaptation.

Several other studies evaluating the validity of the COS followed the initial efforts by Blatt *et al.* (1976) and Ritzler *et al.* (1980). For instance, Spear and Lapidus (1981) used the COS to examine human representations on the Rorschach of 55 severely disturbed inpatients grouped under the diagnostic categories of obsessive/paranoid borderline personality, hysterical/impulsive borderline personality, and nonparanoid, undifferentiated schizophrenia. Consistent with the authors' predictions, the obsessive/paranoid borderline group displayed higher levels of object representations according to the COS.

Later, Blatt and Lerner (1983) selected five prototypic patients from different diagnostic categories to demonstrate the value of a systematic assessment of object representations. The authors showed that a combination of object relations theory and Rorschach methodology yielded very effective understandings of the essential distinctions among different diagnoses. For instance, they assessed the Rorschach of a woman diagnosed with an hysterical personality disorder in the following manner:

A major problem in her representational world seems to be her occasional inappropriate articulation . . . [and] difficulty assuming responsibility for her own action, as indicated by the fact that all of her responses are essentially unmotivated. She sees the world in relatively positive terms, but she seems to lack a sense of inner direction and purpose. Events simply seem to happen to her. Interactions between females are represented as cooperative and reciprocal, but interactions between a female and a male are more problematic and filled with a sense of passivity and danger.

(Blatt and Lerner 1983: 23)

For each example, Blatt and Lerner also showed how assessment of object representations was meaningful for studying change in the psychotherapeutic process.

Lerner and St. Peter (1984) compared the COS scores of outpatient neurotic and borderline patients and hospitalized borderline and schizophrenic patients. Again, consistent with predictions, the schizophrenic patients displayed lower levels of object representations on the Rorschach than did borderline patients. Differences in the expected direction were found between outpatients and hospitalized borderline patients for accurately perceived responses. However, the inpatient borderline patients unexpectedly displayed the highest levels of differentiation, articulation, and integration for inaccurate responses and produced more inaccurate responses in these categories than did the other diagnostic groups.

Finally, Fritsch and Holmstrom (1991) modified Blatt's scale by weighting the quality of each response by its form level to calculate a continuous score combining developmental maturity and accuracy that yielded a more effective correspondence with the functional level of psychotic and nonpsychotic individuals.

Assessment of the representations of significant figures

The Rorschach is limited in its potential for assessing human object representations because responses with human qualities usually occur in low to moderate frequencies. Consequently, Blatt turned from the Rorschach to another method, a scale for the assessment of the representations of parents and other significant figures that consistently yielded more information for the assessment of object representations (Blatt *et al.* 1979).

Blatt *et al.* (1979) used the assessment of open-ended descriptions of parents to predict intensity and types of depressive experiences in 121 undergraduates. Participants' descriptions of their parents were scored according to the Conceptual Level (CL) Scale, a method that categorized the descriptions into five conceptual levels (from lowest to highest level of development): (a) the sensorimotor-preoperational level, at which ". . . the parent is described primarily by his/her activities in reference to the gratification or frustration he or she provides"; (b) the concrete perceptual level, at which ". . . the parent is described as a separate entity, but the description is primarily in concrete, literal, often physical terms"; (c) external iconic level, at which ". . . the parent is described primarily on the basis of his/her functional attributes"; (d) the internal iconic level, at which ". . . the parent is described . . . in terms of internal dimensions such as values, thoughts, and feelings"; and (e) the conceptual level, at which ". . . the parent is described in a way that integrates all the prior levels" (Blatt *et al.* 1979: 390). In addition to the CL scale, Blatt *et al.* (1979) constructed 12 qualitative-thematic dimensions for rating parental descriptions, and they also rated the descriptions for length. When the 12 qualitative-thematic scores and the length of the descriptions were subjected to a principal-components factor analysis with varimax rotation, two primary factors, Nurturant and Striving, emerged. The three main rating scales that Blatt *et al.* constructed for rating parent representations (CL, Nurturant, and Striving), when taken together, compared favorably with a semantic differential procedure (Osgood, Suci and Tannenbaum 1957) for describing the parents. Both methods successfully discriminated the dimensions of depression targeted in the study, but there were significant differences between the two measures. The three dimensions of the semantic differential were predictive of traditional measures of depression, as was the Nurturant factor identified by Blatt *et al.*, but the pattern of correlations between depression and the CL scale suggested that the relationship between depression and cognitive development is complex and may not be linear.

Several studies were published that had relevance for the reliability and validity of these rating scales for significant-figure descriptions. Bornstein and O'Neill (1992) were able to distinguish between 66 adult psychiatric inpatients and 66 normal participants with regard to (a) the valence of attitudes toward parents, (b) ambivalence toward parents, and (c) conceptual level of the parental representations. Marziali and Oleniuk (1990) expanded the coding system to account for multiple levels of representations within the same individual and found differences between five borderline and five nonpatient women. Borderline participants clearly showed lower levels of object differentiation. Bornstein *et al.* (1991) analyzed the test-retest reliability of the rating scales. They found that scores on the qualitative-thematic scales were moderately stable for participants (undergraduates) living away from home and not stable for participants still living at home. However, scores for ambivalence, length of description, and conceptual level of representations were quite stable for both groups.

Following the initial Blatt *et al.* (1979) study, Blatt *et al.* (1992) developed a revised manual for the assessment of the qualitative and structural dimensions of object representations. Eventually, Quinlan *et al.* (1992) examined the reliability and validity of the revised version of the manual. Using data from 213 undergraduates, they rated 12 qualitative-thematic aspects of parental descriptions, as well as the length and degree of ambivalence. They identified four factors for this revised scale: Benevolence, Punitiveness, Ambivalence and Length. The first three factors accounted for 71 per cent of the variance. These three substantive factors were meaningfully correlated with external criteria for assessing depression: a semantic differential, a self-rating depression scale, and the Depressive Experiences Questionnaire constructed by Blatt, D'Afflitti and Quinlan (1976).

Recently, using results for 279 undergraduates, Heck and Pincus (2001) carried out a principal components analysis of the rating scales for significant-figure descriptions and found three stable factors: agency, communion, and structure. This is a radically different factor structure from that found by Quinlan *et al.* (1992). Obviously, the underlying structure of the measure is not consistently replicable and needs further study.

The Differentiation-Relatedness scale

In 1990, Diamond *et al.* developed a 10–point scale to quantitatively assess the degree of differentiation and relatedness of open-ended descriptions of self and others. The Differentiation-Relatedness (D-R) Scale defined the following 10 levels, in order of increasing articulation, stabilization of object representations, and a sense of mutual, empathic relatedness: Levels 1 and 2, lack of differentiation between self and others; Level 3, mirroring; Level 4, idealization or denigration; Level 5, fluctuation between negative and positive attributes of the same object; Levels 6 and 7, increasing acceptance of complexity and ambiguity; Level 8, empathically interrelated representations of self and other; Level 9, reciprocal and mutually facilitating interactions; and Level 10, the highest level of integrated representations in reciprocal and mutual relationships. This scale was assessed for reliability and validity in several studies following the Diamond *et al.* (1990) original presentation, i.e., Blatt *et al.* 1996; Blatt, Auerbach and Aryan 1998; and Levy, Blatt and Shaver 1998. Eventually, Blatt and Auerbach (2001) gave a comprehensive presentation of the use of significant-figure descriptions in assessing object representations. They used the method to track the psychotherapeutic change of 40 severely disturbed, treatment-resistant inpatients. They collected scores from descriptions of self, mother, father, and therapist and rated them on the D-R Scale. As treatment progressed, representations became less dominated by polarization and splitting and evolved into more consolidated object constancy. Two prototypical cases were presented. The article is an excellent source for instruction in assessment of object representations and personality assessment in general.

Thematic Apperception Test

Cramer, Blatt and Ford (1989), with a sample of 90 severely disturbed inpatients, compared object representation scores on the Rorschach with measures of defense mechanisms taken from the Thematic Apperception Test (TAT; Morgan and Murray 1935; Murray 1943). The level of defense was related to the developmental level of object representations on the Rorschach. Specifically, denial, projection, and identification represented different levels on a developmental continuum of defenses from primitive to sophisticated or from mature to immature. Encouraged by the relationships identified in this initial study, Rosenberg *et al.* (1994) used a lexically based, quantitative approach to assess object relations from the TAT with the same sample of hospitalized patients. The results showed that TAT narratives represent a valid source of information for assessing the quality of object representations.

Although Cramer and Blatt did not follow up on their promising start with using the TAT for assessment of object representations, other authors have developed TAT rating methods with demonstrated reliability and validity. For instance, Porcerelli and Dietrich (1994) introduced the Dietrich Object Relations and Object Representations Scale for the TAT, showing that it effectively differentiated between 102 psychiatric patients and 48 normal controls. Also, Westen (1991) developed the Social Cognition and Object Relations Scale (SCORS), a frequently used instrument for assessing object representations on the TAT that measures the dimensions of complexity, affect tone, capacity for emotional investment in relationships, and understanding of social causality. Since its development, the SCORS, although somewhat cumbersome in its scoring procedures, has been used for many studies of object representations.

Applications

The value of a psychological assessment method depends on the extent to which it provides meaningful data for clinical and research purposes. Blatt's methods for assessing object representations have been widely used in research on parent introjects, therapy outcome, and psychiatric diagnoses.

Parent introjects

Blatt and Homann (1992) discussed the role of parent–child relationships in the development of depression by reviewing studies of attachment patterns in infants and young children, interactions of depressed mothers with their children, and depressed adults' retrospective accounts of early experiences with their parents. The authors concluded that negative representations of parents are central to the development of depression.

Using the parental description methodology described earlier, Blatt et al. (1979) found that negative representations of parents correlated with several measures of depression. Also, they found that the more negative qualities attributed to parents and the more immature the conceptual level of parental representations, the greater the intensity and severity of depression. Later, Bornstein, Galley and Leone (1986) administered the Rorschach to 193 male undergraduates to compare a measure of orality with the CL Scale and the qualitative dimensions of parental representations. They found that the orality score was negatively correlated with descriptions of the mother as nurturing and positively correlated with descriptions of the father as nurturing. There was no significant relationship between orality and the overall conceptual level of parental representations. Because orality should be associated with students' experiences with and perceptions of their parents, the authors speculate that the lack of a significant relationship between orality and conceptual level of the parental representations may be due to the undergraduates' tendencies to describe their parents in socially desirable terms.

Also using the parent-description method, Levy, Blatt and Shaver (1998) identified relationships between attachment styles and parent representations. Securely attached participants produced descriptions with higher levels of differentiation, elaboration, benevolence, and nonpunitiveness than did participants with dismissing and ambivalent attachment styles. Participants with fearful attachment styles also had highly differentiated parental descriptions, but described their parents less benevolently and more ambivalently than did individuals with secure attachments.

In a unique study assessing undergraduates with the Blatt CL Scale, Herr and Lapidus (1998) found that opposition to nuclear armament was correlated with mature levels of parental representations. Also, empathy, based on Blatt's developmental level scores, was higher in those opposed to nuclear armament.

Therapy outcome

Blatt, Auerbach and Levy (1997) summarize the theoretical proposition that personality development, psychopathology, and the therapeutic process can be more effectively understood through the construct of object representation. Several studies using Blatt's methods for assessing object representations provide data that support this hypothesis.

In companion articles, Diamond et al. (1990) and Gruen and Blatt (1990) presented case studies that demonstrate that progress in psychotherapy parallels positive changes in representations of self and others. Diamond et al. (1990) used significant-figure descriptions and the Rorschach to assess self and object representations in four borderline women. The Rorschach was coded for separation-individuation by a method developed by Coonerty (1986) that evolved from Blatt's methods. Critical features of interpersonal relationships and interactions demonstrated problems in self–other differentiation and intersubjectivity. Shifts in the configuration of Rorschach responses, shifts that demonstrated changes in separation-individuation and intersubjectivity, occurred as treatment progressed.

In another small-sample study, Blatt et al. (1991) followed eight severely disturbed adolescents and young adults over the course of long-term, intensive treatment and found that changes in the level of clinical functioning were accompanied by changes in the conceptual level and degree of differentiation and articulation of parental representations. In a much larger study, Blatt et al. (1996) collected open-ended descriptions of self and others from 40 hospitalized adolescent and young adult patients in long-term psychotherapy. Again, clinical progress was consistent with changes in the structure, content, and articulation of object representations. More positive attitudes developed toward mother and therapist while attitudes toward father became more negative. In an even larger project, Cook, Blatt and Ford (1995) used path analysis of data derived from Rorschach measures of object relations to study 90 patients hospitalized for at least a year. The patients who benefited most from treatment were those who were able overtly to express disturbed thinking and describe destructive inter-actions while maintaining a relatively high level of object representations.

Responding to criticisms by Bein (1998) of the studies of object represen-tations and therapy outcome, Blatt *et al.* (1998) argued that, to understand the effectiveness of the object representation construct for explaining pro-gress in therapy, one must appreciate the research findings in the context of severe pathology and long-term treatment. Seriously disturbed, treatment-resistant patients present challenges to the therapist that can be effectively met by a focus on the quality and content of object representations. To assess these factors, Blatt's methods are invaluable.

Diagnosis

Studies of diagnostic groups also have demonstrated the construct validity of Blatt's methods for assessing object representations. The early studies of schizophrenia (i.e., Blatt *et al.* 1976; Ritzler *et al.* 1980) were partially replicated by Johnson and Quinlan (1993), who found that a role-playing test showed greater discrimination than the Rorschach between schizo-phrenic patients and normal controls when both procedures were scored according to the COS. Later, Auerbach and Blatt (1997) scored the object representation level of the self description of a 15-year-old schizophrenic patient to demonstrate typical problems in self–other differentiation.

Many studies have used Blatt's methods to test his theory of depression. One example is a study by Jarmas and Kazak (1992) that investigated depression in 84 adult children of alcoholics. As predicted, the majority of participants showed introjective depression, with corresponding distur-bances in object representations. In a study of 49 bulimic women, Aronson (1986) used the CL scale to compare object representation levels with bulimic symptom patterns. She found that object representation levels were predicted by five symptom variables: frequency of laxative use, use of starvation, vomiting frequency, amount of drinks per day, and inpatient residence status.

Dissertations

For a master teacher and theoretician like Sidney Blatt, there is no more fitting tribute than dissertations by graduate students using methods and ideas he developed. Although dissertations receive only faculty review, they are fairly extensive research projects that make meaningful contributions to the knowledge concerning assessment methods and theoretical constructs. Many dissertations have used Blatt's methods for assessing object representations.

Attachment style

The popular construct of attachment style (Bowlby 1969) has been the focus of several dissertations using Blatt's object representation assessment methods. Rothstein (1997), using the COS, and Posner (2000), using the CL Scale found no relationship between attachment styles and object representations. However, Levy (2000), using the CL Scale and White (2001), using the procedures for assessing object representations with written descriptions of others (Blatt et al. 1992) found positive correlations between security of attachment and level of object representation.

Therapy

Two dissertations completed by students at Columbia University assessed the object representations of self and therapist with a sample of 28 outpatient adults using the COS method for assessing parental object representations. Bender (1996) found significant relationships between degree of psychopathology, attachment and object representations during the course of therapy. Arnold (1998) found the same relationships in a nine-month follow-up assessment after an average of 46 therapy sessions and also found a relationship between levels of object representation and therapy outcome.

Women's issues

Several dissertations using Blatt's methods for assessing object representations have focused on women's issues. Rosenbaum (1998) assessed the object representations of undergraduates and determined that both men and women had relatively negative concepts of women's power. Coe (1999) used the same methodology in finding that women high in the state of loneliness had malevolent object representations of their mothers while women high in the trait of loneliness had developmentally higher object representations of their fathers. Gerber (2000) assessed self and other descriptions to discover that battered women had lower levels of representations of self, partner, and father.

Other topics

Dissertations on more exotic topics also have yielded meaningful results with Blatt's procedures. Lambert (1999) assessed the dreams of patients with schizophrenic and major depressive diagnoses and found that the schizophrenic patients reported dreams with lower levels of object representations. Kern (2000) also used the assessment of object representations in dreams to show that Chicano and Anglo undergraduates showed similar patterns of object representations, except for the finding that the dreams of Anglos showed more action. Finally, Engelmann (1995) used the COS to assess the representations of the concept of God in the written descriptions of God by religious and nonreligious Roman Catholics. As predicted, the religious participants showed significantly more differentiated God representations.

Future implications

Blatt's well-established methods for assessing object representations provide psychodynamically oriented psychologists with effective tools for personality assessment, treatment planning, and research. For instance, the continuing application and development of object relations theory are enhanced by these methods that allow internal object representations to be validly described and quantified.

Although Blatt's thesis that object representations is a construct that has potential relevance for cognitive behavior psychologists (Blatt and Auerbach 2000) has fallen on deaf ears, his methods can be applied effectively to phenomena that behaviorists often study. That is, Blatt's methods for assessing conceptual levels of internal representations of others might constitute effective means for operationally defining cognitive and emotional processes that have eluded behaviorists who have formed biases against projective assessment on the basis of scant information and experience. Perhaps more effort is needed to disseminate Blatt's methods and research outside the realm of psychoanalytically oriented publications. A step in this direction might be to include Blatt's methods in graduate level classes on empirically validated approaches to personality assessment. Certainly, the interest shown in Blatt's methods by young psychologists conducting their dissertations indicates that the assessment of object representations with Blatt's methods has a promising future.

Parent representations, the material most commonly subjected to object representations assessment, seem to provide dependable information for understanding the phenomenon. The only representation likely to have greater relevance for understanding the individual is the self-representation (Auerbach and Blatt 1996, 1997, 2001). However, because parental representations seem to have the most temporal stability (Bornstein et al. 1991), they may continue to yield the data of choice. The lack of correspondence between two separate factor analyses (i.e., that by Quinlan et al. [1992] and that by Heck and Pincus [2001]) of parental description scales suggests that this popular method requires further study. Nevertheless, it seems apparent that understanding internal representations of parents is a key to effective personality assessment.

Blatt's contributions to the assessment of object representations recently has been extended to the Rorschach Comprehensive System (Exner 1993). Following research conducted by Burns and Viglione (1996), a new variable has been added to the System that incorporates many of the features of the original COS. The Interpersonal Perception cluster of variables in the Comprehensive System has been enhanced by the addition of the Human Response Variable (HRV), a measure that results from the application of an algorithm for assessing the quality of responses with human characteristics. Nearly every element in the algorithm is an element of the COS (Exner 2000).

In developing the HRV, Burns and Viglione (1996) relied on object relations theory to guide their analyses. They proposed that the result of their work is a measure that provides a valid and reliable assessment of internal object representations. Exner (2000: 323), in keeping with the empirical, atheoretical foundations of the Comprehensive System articulates the following interpretive hypotheses for the HRV:

> Good Human Response answers correlate with interpersonal histories that are usually considered to be effective and adaptive. People who give numerous GHR answers typically are well regarded by others and their interpersonal activities tend to be reasonably free of chaos . . . . Poor Human Responses correlate highly with patterns of interpersonal behavior that are ineffective or maladaptive. Individuals who give numerous PHR answers usually have interpersonal histories that are marked by conflict and/or failure.

It is clear that Blatt's methods for assessing object representations will continue to provide psychologists with effective procedures for operationalizing theoretical constructs that are important for understanding human behavior. The dissertation studies that follow from Blatt's work are a prime example of the future potential of the object representations assessment methods. Some areas such as multicultural assessment and treatment planning need much further study, but the established reliability and validity of Blatt's methods and their modifications provide an avenue for greater understanding of this very important theoretical construct in the future.

A major result of the continuing use of Blatt's methods for assessing object representations is the development and expansion of his theoretical perspective on personality development (Blatt *et al.* 1997), psychopathology (Blatt and Levy 1998), and clinical theory (Blatt and Auerbach 2001). Recently, Blatt and colleagues have begun to link his methods for assessing object representations to the understanding of attachment (Levy *et al.* 1998) and self-reflexivity (Auerbach and Blatt 2001). Indeed, this line of research suggests that Blatt's methods for assessing object representations are effective and necessary tools for continued theory development and understanding of both the self and human relationships.

References

Arnold, B. (1998) 'A follow-up study of post-termination effects of psychotherapy on self-representation, representation of the therapist, and symptomatology', *Dissertation Abstracts International* 58(12-B): 6799.

Aronson, J. K. (1986) 'The level of object relations and severity of symptoms in the normal weight bulimic patient', *International Journal of Eating Disorders* 5: 669–81.

Auerbach, J. S. and Blatt, S. J. (1996) 'Self-representation in severe psychopathology: The role of reflexive self-awareness', *Psychoanalytic Psychology* 13: 297–341.

—— and —— (1997) 'Impairment of self-representation in schizophrenia: the roles of boundary articulation and self-reflexivity', *Bulletin of the Menninger Clinic* 46: 297–316.

—— and —— (2001) 'Self-reflexivity, intersubjectivity, and therapeutic change', *Psychoanalytic Psychology* 18: 427–50.

Bein, E. (1998) 'How well does long-term psychoanalytically oriented inpatient treatment work? A review of a study by Blatt and Ford', *Psychotherapy Research* 8: 30–41.

Bender, D. S. (1996) 'The relationship of psychopathology and attachment to patients' representations of self, parents, and therapist in the early phase of psychodynamic psychotherapy', *Dissertation Abstracts International* 57(5-B): 3400.

Blatt, S. J. and Auerbach, J. S. (2000) 'Psychoanalytic models of the mind and their contributions to personality research', *European Journal of Personality* 14: 429–47.

—— and —— (2001) 'Mental representation, severe psychopathology, and the therapeutic process', *Journal of the American Psychoanalytic Association* 49: 113–59.

—— —— and Aryan, M. (1998) 'Representational structures and the therapeutic process', in R. F. Bornstein and J. M. Masling (eds) *Empirical Studies of Psychoanalytic Theories, vol. 8: empirical studies of the therapeutic hour*, Washington, DC: American Psychological Association.

—— —— and Levy, K. N. (1997) 'Mental representations in personality development, psychopathology, and the therapeutic process', *Review of General Psychology* 1: 351–74.

—— Berman, W. H., Cook, B. P. and Ford, R. Q. (1998) 'Effectiveness of long-term, intensive, inpatient treatment for seriously disturbed young adults: A reply to Bein', *Psychotherapy Research*, 8: 42–53.

—— Brenneis, C. B., Schimek, J. G. and Glick, M. (1976) 'Normal development and psychopathological impairment of the concept of the object on the Rorschach', *Journal of Abnormal Psychology* 85: 364–73.

Blatt, S. J., Chevron, E. S. Quinlan, D. M., Schaffer, C. E. and Wein, S. J. (1992) 'The assessment of qualitative and structural dimensions of object representations', unpublished manuscript, Yale University, New Haven, Connecticut.

—— D'Afflitti, J. P. and Quinlan, D. M. (1976) 'Experiences of depression in normal young adults', *Journal of Abnormal Psychology* 85: 383–9.

—— and Homann, E. (1992) 'Parent-child interaction in the etiology of dependent and self-critical depression', *Clinical Psychology Review* 12: 47–91.

—— and Lerner, H. (1983) 'The psychological assessment of object representation', *Journal of Personality Assessment* 47: 7–28.

—— and Levy, K. N. (1998) 'A psychodynamic approach to the diagnosis of psychopathology', in J. W. Barron (ed.) *Making Diagnosis Meaningful: enhancing evaluation and treatment of psychological disorders*, Washington, DC: American Psychological Association, pp. 73–109.

—— and Ritzler, B. A. (1974) 'Thought disorder and boundary disturbances in psychosis', *Journal of Consulting and Clinical Psychology* 42: 370–81.

—— Stayner, D. A., Auerbach, J. S. and Behrends, R. S. (1996) 'Change in object and self-representations in long-term, intensive, inpatient treatment of seriously disturbed adolescents and young adults', *Psychiatry* 59: 82–107.

—— Wein, S. J., Chevron, E. S. and Quinlan, D. M. (1979) 'Parental representations and depression in normal young adults', *Journal of Abnormal Psychology* 88: 388–97.

—— Wild, C. M. and Ritzler, B. A. (1975) 'Disturbances of object representations in schizophrenia', *Psychoanalysis and Contemporary Science* 4: 235–88.

—— Wiseman, H., Prince-Gibson, E. and Gatt, C. (1991) 'Object representations and change in clinical functioning', *Psychotherapy* 28: 273–83.

Bornstein, R. F., Galley, D. J. and Leone, D. R. (1986) 'Parental representations and orality', *Journal of Personality Assessment* 50: 80–9.

—— —— —— and Kale, A. (1991) 'The temporal stability of ratings of parents: test-retest reliability and influence of parental contact', *Journal of Social Behavior and Personality* 6: 641–9.

—— and O'Neill, R. M. (1992) 'Parental perceptions and psychopathology', *Journal of Nervous and Mental Disease* 180: 475–83.

Bowlby, J. (1969) *Attachment and Loss, vol. 1: attachment*, New York: Basic Books.

Burns, B. and Viglione, D. J., Jr. (1996) 'The Rorschach Human Experience Variable, interpersonal relatedness, and object representation in nonpatients', *Psychological Assessment* 8: 92–9.

Coe, J. E. (1999) 'Developmental perspectives on women's experiences of loneliness', *Dissertation Abstracts International* 59(5-A): 3206.

Cook, B., Blatt, S. J. and Ford, R. Q. (1995) 'The prediction of therapeutic response to long-term intensive treatment of seriously disturbed young adult inpatients', *Psychotherapy Research* 5: 218–30.

Coonerty, S. (1986) 'An exploration of separation-individuation themes in the borderline personality disorder', *Journal of Personality Assessment* 50: 501–11.

Cramer, P., Blatt, S. J. and Ford, R. (1989) 'Defense mechanisms in the anaclitic and introjective personality configuration', *Journal of Consulting and Clinical Psychology* 56: 610–16.

Diamond, D., Kaslow, N., Coonerty, S. and Blatt, S. J. (1990) 'Changes in separation-individuation and intersubjectivity in long-term treatment', *Psychoanalytic Psychology* 7: 363–97.

Engelmann, T. C. (1995) 'Religious experiences: psychiatric status, religiosity and god images', *Dissertation Abstracts International* 55(11-B): 5065.

Exner, J. E., Jr. (1993) *The Rorschach: a comprehensive system: vol. 1, basic foundations*, 3rd edn, New York: Wiley.

—— (2000) *A Primer for Rorschach Interpretation*, Asheville, NC: Rorschach Workshops.

Fairbairn, W. R. D. (1954) *An Object Relations Theory of the Personality*, New York: Basic Books.

—— (1963) 'Synopsis of an object-relations theory of the personality', *International Journal of Psychoanalysis* 44: 224–5.

Fraiberg, S. (1969) 'Libidinal object constancy and mental representation', *Psychoanalytic Study of the Child* 24: 9–47.

Freud, A. (1965) *Normality and Pathology in Childhood: assessments of development*, New York: International Universities Press.

Freud, S. (1914) 'On narcissism: an introduction', trans. C. M. Baines, in *Collected Papers*, vol. 4, ed. E. Jones, New York: Basic Books, 1959, pp. 30–59.

Fritsch, R. C. and Holmstrom, R. W. (1991) 'Assessing object representations as a continuous variable: a modification of the Concept of the Object on the Rorschach scale', *Journal of Personality Assessment* 55: 319–34.

Gerber, J. D. (2000) 'Imagining the child: maternal representations of the child as a function of the quality of the mother's object relations', *Dissertation Abstracts International* 60(9-B): 4887.

Greenberg, J. R. and Mitchell, S. A. (1983) *Object Relations in Psychoanalytic Theory*, Cambridge, MA: Harvard University Press.

Gruen, R. J. and Blatt, S. J. (1990) 'Change in self- and object representation during long-term dynamically oriented treatment', *Psychoanalytic Psychology* 7: 399–422.

Guntrip, H. (1969) *Schizoid Phenomena, Object Relations and the Self*, New York: International Universities Press.

Heck, S. A. and Pincus, A. L. (2001) 'Agency and communion in the structure of parental representations', *Journal of Personality Assessment* 76: 180–4.

Herr, C. E. and Lapidus, L. B. (1998) 'Nuclear weapons attitudes in relation to dogmatism, mental representation of parents, and image of a foreign enemy', *Journal of Peace Psychology* 4: 59–68.

Jarmas, A. L. and Kazak, A. E. (1992) 'Young adult children of alcoholic fathers: depressive experiences, coping styles, and family systems', *Journal of Consulting and Clinical Psychology* 60: 244–51.

Johnson, D. R. and Quinlan, D. M. (1993) 'Can the mental representations of paranoid schizophrenics be differentiated from those of normals?', *Journal of Personality Assessment* 60: 588–601.

Kern, C. (2000) 'Object representation in dreams of Chicanos and Anglos', *Dissertation Abstracts International* 60(12-B): 6369.

Kernberg, O. (1967) 'Borderline personality organization', *Journal of the American Psychoanalytic Association* 15: 641–85.

Klein, M. (1952) *Developments in Psychoanalysis*, London: Hogarth Press.

Kohut, H. (1971) *The Analysis of the Self*, New York: International Universities Press.

Lambert, L. M. (1999) 'Lingering impressions: a comparative study of the dream life of schizophrenic and major depressive patient groups, and the use of the dream in informing the therapy', *Dissertation Abstracts International* 60(2-B): 0834.

Lerner, H. D. and St. Peter, S. (1984) 'Patterns of object relations in neurotic, borderline and schizophrenic patients', *Psychiatry* 47: 77–92.

Levy, K. N. (2000) 'Attachment style, representations of self and others, and affect regulation: implications for the experience of depression', *Dissertation Abstracts International* 60(9-B): 4895.

—— Blatt, S. J. and Shaver, P. R. (1998) 'Attachment styles and parental representations', *Journal of Personality and Social Psychology* 74: 407–19.

Mahler, M. S. (1968) *On Human Symbiosis and the Vicissitudes of Individuation*, New York: International Universities Press.

—— Pine, F. and Bergman, A. (1975) *The Psychological Birth of the Human Infant: symbiosis and individuation*, New York: Basic Books.

Marziali, E. and Oleniuk, J. (1990) 'Object representations in descriptions of significant others: a methodological study', *Journal of Personality Assessment* 54: 105–15.

Morgan, C. D. and Murray, H. A. (1935) 'A method of investigating fantasies: the Thematic Apperception Test', *Archives of Neurology and Psychiatry* 34: 289–306.

Murray, H. A. (1943) *Thematic Apperception Test*, Cambridge, MA: Harvard University Press.

Osgood, C. E., Suci, G. J. and Tannenbaum, P. H. (1957) *The Measurement of Meaning*, Urbana, IL: University of Illinois.

Piaget, J. (1937) *The Construction of Reality in the Child*, trans. M. Cook, New York: Basic Books, 1954.

Porcerelli, J. H. and Dietrich, D. R. (1994) 'Dietrich Object Relations and Object Representations Scale: convergent and discriminant validity', *Psychoanalytic Psychology* 11: 101–13.

Posner, D. L. (2000) 'Relationship among attachment style, empathy, object representations, and alexithymia', *Dissertation Abstracts International* 60(10-B): 5231.

Quinlan, D. M., Blatt, S. J., Chevron, E. S. and Wein, S. (1992) 'The analysis of descriptions of parents: identification of a more differentiated factor structure', *Journal of Personality Assessment* 59: 340–51.

Rapaport, D. (1950) 'On the psychoanalytic theory of thinking', *International Journal of Psycho-Analysis* 31: 161–70.

Ritzler, B., Zambianco, D., Harder, D. and Kaskey, M. (1980) 'Psychotic patterns of the concept of the object on the Rorschach test', *Journal of Abnormal Psychology* 89: 46–55.

Rosenbaum, S. C. (1998) 'Gender differences in fear of power: the relationship between internal representations of mothers and attitudes toward authority', *Dissertation Abstracts International* 59(5-B): 2431.

Rosenberg, S. D., Blatt, S. J., Oxman, T. E. and McHugo, G. J. (1994) 'Assessment of object relatedness through a lexical content analysis of the TAT', *Journal of Personality Assessment* 63: 345–62.

Rothstein, D. N. (1997) 'Object relations and attachment: a comparison of Rorschach responses and adult attachment classifications', *Dissertation Abstracts International* 58(5-B): 2698.

Schafer, R. (1968) *Aspects of Internalization*, New York: International Universities Press.

Searles, H. (1965) *Collected Papers on Schizophrenia and Related Subjects*, New York: International Universities Press.

Spear, W. E. and Lapidus, L. B. (1981) 'Qualitative differences in manifest object representations: implications for a multidimensional model of psychological functioning', *Journal of Abnormal Psychology* 90: 157–67.

Werner, H. (1948) *Comparative Psychology of Mental Development*, rev. edn, G. Murphy (ed.) and E. B. Garside (trans.), New York: International Universities Press.

—— and Kaplan, B. (1963) *Symbol Formation: an organismic-developmental approach to language and the expression of thought*, New York: Wiley.

Westen, D. (1991) 'Clinical assessment of object relations using the TAT', *Journal of Personality Assessment* 56: 56–74.

White, M. D. (2001) 'Differences in object representations among adult attachment styles', *Dissertation Abstracts International* 61(8-B): 4436.

Winnicott, D. W. (1965) *The Maturational Processes and the Facilitating Environment*, London: Hogarth Press.

Chapter 10

Object relations and the Rorschach

Howard D. Lerner

The past several decades have seen enormous changes in the psychoanalytic understanding of the individual, and central to this development have been equally important changes in the use of projective techniques. From a relatively narrow but solid base established initially by Rapaport, Gill and Schafer (1968) and subsequently advanced by Schafer, Holt, and Mayman, recent advances in both psychoanalytic theory and the psychoanalytic understanding of psychopathology and of treatment have provided new formulations for significant and exciting theoretical, clinical and research efforts. Examples include the investigation and systematic assessment of core psychoanalytic concepts (e.g., object representation, defense, thought process and boundary representation) with the Rorschach and Thematic Apperception Test (TAT) as well as the development of new and creative assessment procedures like early memories, open-ended descriptions of self and significant others, and semi-structured object relations profiles. Collectively these endeavors have operationalized newer, more phenomenological concepts in psychoanalytic theory and provide methodologies and instruments for systematically assessing and evaluating the validity and clinical utility of constructs generated by this expanded body of knowledge.

The purpose of the present chapter is to review the contributions of Sidney Blatt to the study of object relations through the use of the Rorschach. Psychological tests in general and the Rorschach in particular have played a central role in Blatt's wide-ranging research on psychoanalytic concepts. In fact, Blatt has consistently been concerned about the frequent failures of many research studies to use projective techniques in ways that can meaningfully test clinical hypotheses. His work debunks the myth that projective tests provide unreliable and invalid data that have little to contribute to research. In recent years, two somewhat divergent approaches to the use of the Rorschach in both clinical practice and research may be discerned. On the one hand, an atheoretical and highly empirical *sign* approach focuses on a myriad of traditional Rorschach scores and ratios. This approach approximates an application of psychometric principles and values to projective data. On the other hand, Blatt and Lerner (1983a, 1983b), Blatt and Berman (1984), and P. Lerner (1998) have advocated a *conceptual* approach geared toward integrating the plethora of isolated Rorschach scores into a small number of discreet and theoretically relevant variables.

Throughout the course of his work on the Rorschach and object relations, Blatt's research demonstrates how Rorschach scales representing composite variables can offer a superordinate organization of projective test data that is rooted in a conceptual model. This higher-order organization provides a framework for integrating multiple dimensions of Rorschach responses in ways that are clinically relevant, reliable and the focus of extensive validation and research. In what follows, I will review Sidney Blatt's contributions to object relations, with an emphasis on *object representation* as a central concept. Second, I will illustrate how this concept was formulated and operationalized. Next, the wide range of Blatt's research, along with the research he inspired will be reviewed, with the purpose of illustrating his creative use of the Rorschach. Fourth, his view of Rorschach research and the test itself as a measure of representation will be outlined. Finally, I will offer a personal view of Sidney Blatt as a teacher, mentor, and colleague.

The concept of object representation

Freud (1923, 1940) in his formulations about the development of the superego discussed the process of internalization. He stated, ". . . a portion of the external world, has, at least partially, been abandoned as an object and has instead, by identification, been taken into the ego and thus become an integral part of the internal world. This new psychical agency continues to carry on the functions which have hitherto been performed by the people (the abandoned objects) and the external world . . . ." (Freud 1940: 205) This view of internalization was subsequently extended beyond superego formation to include all processes in which interactions with the environment are transformed into internal regulators and are assimilated as characteristics of the self. Many theorists and researchers have studied how the internalization of object relations provides a primary basis for the development of intrapsychic structure (e.g., Blatt 1974; Blatt, Wild and Ritzler 1975; A. Freud 1952; Glover 1950; Hartmann 1950; Kernberg 1975; Mahler 1968). Object relations result in the formation of internal structures (ego functions and cognitive structures such as object and self representations) that regulate and direct behavior. As Blatt and Lerner (1983a) note, psychoanalytic theory and research progressively focused upon the complex interactions among early formative interpersonal relationships and their consequences for the formation of intrapsychic structures that constitute the representational world.

One of Blatt's major contributions has been to show how an understanding of the development of the concept of the object (of the self and others) could be greatly facilitated by an integration of psychoanalytic theory with the formulations of cognitive developmental psychologists, particularly Piaget (1954) and Werner (1948). Blatt has demonstrated how according to developmental psychological theory, all thinking involves a series of mental operations that are the result of the internalization of action sequences. The development of mental representation begins early in childhood and proceeds through four basic stages to intellectual maturity in adulthood: sensorimotor, preoperational, concrete operational, and formal operational. Development, for Piaget and Werner, consists of a progressive unfolding of cognitive structures according to innate principles of functioning in which new cognitive schemas evolve out of earlier cognitive structures.

Blatt criticized the formulations of cognitive developmental psychologists because they were based primarily on the study of children in states of relative quiescence and as the child responded primarily to inert objects. In contrast, according to Blatt, psychoanalytic theorists offered formulations of the child's development of cognitive structures on the basis of the study of children in states of relative arousal within an interpersonal relationship. According to Blatt (1978), it is the internalization of the mother's organized and predictable responses to the individual that provides the basis for the establishment of cognitive structures.

Blatt has consistently defined object representation as referring to the conscious and unconscious mental schemas – including cognitive, affective, and experiential components – of objects encountered in reality. Beginning as vague, diffuse, variable, sensorimotor experiences of pleasure and unpleasure, these schemas gradually expand and develop into differentiated, consistent, relatively realistic representations of the self and the object world. Earlier forms of representations are thought to be based more on action sequences associated with need gratification, intermediate forms are based on specific perceptual and functional features, and higher forms are more symbolic and conceptual (Blatt 1974). There is a constant and reciprocal interaction between past and present interpersonal relationships and the development of representations. These schemas evolve from and are intertwined with the internalization of object relations, and new levels of object and self-representation provide a revised organizational landscape for subsequent interpersonal relationships (Blatt 1974).

Assessment of object representation

On the basis of the principle that the interpretation of an ambiguous stimulus is shaped by the organizing characteristics of the individual's representational world, considerable empirical research has investigated the structure and content of diverse phenomena like early memories, manifest dreams, open-ended descriptions of significant figures, and the human response on the Rorschach. Earlier studies of the human response on the Rorschach suggested that an assessment of object relations – of concepts of self and others – was a core issue in personality development (Ames 1966; Mayman 1977; Rapaport *et al.* 1968) and important in making distinctions among diagnostic groups (Fisher and Cleveland 1968; Landis 1970). As Blatt and Lerner (1983a) noted, these studies remained relatively unintegrated because they were not rooted in a broader more comprehensive conceptual framework of personality development, organization and psychopathology. Psychoanalytic object relations theory offered a general framework for integrating these diverse research findings and for highlighting the developmental significance of interpersonal relationships and the formation of psychological structure. Collectively, these earlier studies, as well as the contributions of research groups at Yale and the University of Michigan (initially reviewed by Blatt and Lerner 1983b), have lent impressive support to the construct validity of object representation as a theoretical dimension that provides important information about the developmental level and quality of interpersonal relationships to which individuals are predisposed. Object representations constitute the structure or template that determine the nature of the experience of the self and the object world.

Research studies

Introduction

Blatt and Lerner (1983a) described two primary research groups that contributed to the widening scope of the theory of object representation and to the development of research procedures for assessing this dimension of personality organization. These two research groups, centered at the University of Michigan and Yale University, represented different but not mutually exclusive approaches to the study of object representation. The late Marty Mayman and his colleagues at the University of Michigan focused on the thematic element of object representations and used a variety of projective test procedures to assess these elements, including early memories, manifest dreams, written autobiographies and Rorschach percepts. The evaluation of object representations from these sources has been studied systematically in relation to levels of psychopathology, types of character structure, independent ratings of object relations, and the capacity to profit from psychotherapy. The research group at Michigan has its theoretical roots in the ego psychological theory and test methods of David Rapaport, integrated with theoretical contributions of Mahler and Kernberg.

For over 30 years, Sidney Blatt and his colleagues at Yale University focused primarily on the structural dimensions of object representation.

Their work, also derived from Rapaport, is based on an integration of object relations theory, ego psychology, and developmental cognitive theories. Drawing on projective test data, particularly the Rorschach, but also the TAT, the manifest content of dreams and open-ended descriptions of significant figures, Blatt and his colleagues developed innovative procedures for the assessment of object representations and have studied the relationships of object representation to normal development, as well as to levels and types of psychopathology, especially in schizophrenia, depression, and borderline personality disorder. More recent studies have used the assessment of object representation to measure change during intensive psychotherapy. Their findings also demonstrate that the structure of object representations continues to develop throughout the life cycle into early adolescence and adulthood and that the quality of object representations provides insight into psychotic and depressive experiences that have profound implications for the therapeutic process.

The study of object representations at the University of Michigan

Mayman (1967) conceptualized object representations as templates or enduring internalized images of the self and of others around which the phenomenological world is structured and into which ongoing experiences of others are assimilated. Mayman asserted that Rorschach content, like the manifest content of dreams and early memories, was more than simply an embellished screen that concealed and hinted at deeper and more profound levels of unconscious meaning. He argued that manifest content in its own right could reflect levels of ego functioning, relative capacity for object relations, and the nature of interpersonal strivings.

Mayman (1967) identified several dimensions by which to assess the content of Rorschach responses. His seminal approach to Rorschach research spawned several scales and construct validity studies that further refined the concept of object representation (Urist 1973) and has extended the thematic analysis of object representations to manifest dreams (Krohn 1974) and autobiographical data (Urist 1973). These methods have been used in studies measuring a person's capacity to enter into and benefit from insight-oriented psychotherapy (Ryan 1973; Hatcher and Krohn 1980). Different scales designed to evaluate object representational levels on a developmental continuum have been correlated with each other (Urist 1973) and have been applied and correlated across various databases, including manifest dreams, the Rorschach, early memories, and health–sickness ratings (Krohn and Mayman 1974). Best known among these methods is Urist's (1977) Mutuality of Autonomy (MOA) Scale, a procedure for systematically evaluating Rorschach responses that express interactions between people, animals, and objects.

The hallmark, then, of the Michigan approach to the study of object representation has been an attempt to add a more experiential, phenomeno- logical, and object relational dimension to theory, assessment, and research.

Research studies at Yale University

The contributions of Blatt and his colleagues to the Rorschach literature have revolved around the study of the development of the concept of the object, both in normal and in various clinical populations. Building on their initial investigation of boundary disturbances, Blatt *et al.* (1976) developed the Concept of the Object Scale (COS), a comprehensive and sophisticated method for assessing object representations in Rorschach records. This object relations scale has been used in more Rorschach studies than any other to date. Based on a creative integration of the developmental theory of Werner (1948) and psychoanalytic ego psychology, the system calls for the scoring of human responses along three developmental dimensions: differentiation, articulation, and integration. Within each of these sub- scales, categories were established along a continuum based on develop- mental levels. Differentiation refers to the type of figure perceived and to whether the figure is a quasi-human detail, a human detail, a quasi-human, or a full human figure. For the dimension of articulation, responses are scored on the basis of the number and types of attributes ascribed to the figure. The integration dimension of response is scored in three ways: the internality of the action, the integration of the object and its action, and the nature of the interaction with another object. Responses are also scored along a content dimension of benevolence–malevolence. In an early study (Blatt *et al.* 1976), the scoring system was applied to the Rorschach protocols of 37 normal subjects on four separate occasions over a 20–year period. Results from this longitudinal study revealed that the human responses on the Rorschach consistently change with development, with a marked and progressive increase in the number of well differentiated, highly articulated, and integrated human responses, a significant increase in the attribution of activity that was congruent with important characteristics of the figure, and an increase in the degree to which human objects were seen in constructive and positive interaction.

Blatt *et al.* (1976) then studied the human responses of a sample of 48 seriously disturbed borderline and psychotic adolescents and young adults and compared their responses to the human responses of the normal sample. They found first, that the seriously disturbed inpatients had a significantly greater number of human responses at lower developmental levels (i.e., responses that were more often quasi-human, distorted, unmoti- vated, incongruent, passive, and malevolent). These responses at lower developmental levels, however, occurred primarily on accurately perceived responses. Second, and quite unexpectedly, patients had a significantly greater number of more developmentally advanced responses than did normal participants on inaccurately perceived responses. These findings were replicated by Ritzler *et al.* (1980). According to Blatt, these results, termed *paradoxical representation*, indicate that patients, as compared to normal participants, function at lower developmental levels when in contact with conventional reality, but at higher developmental levels when they give idiosyncratic interpretations of reality. As such, the data indicate that the tendency to perceive reality adequately does not assist psychotic patients to organize their experience more effectively or adaptively. The findings suggest that there are at least two aspects to the psychotic experience. First, a psychotic patient perceives the world as distorted, undifferentiated, fragmented and destructive. The second aspect involves the psychotic patient's capacity to experience the world unrealistically, but within the unrealistic experience, to function more effectively and to perceive the world less malevolently. Blatt, Schimek and Brenneis (1980) outlined the implication of these Rorschach findings for the treatment of severely disturbed patients. Specifically, for psychotic patients, introducing and interpreting reality is experienced as painful and disruptive and will engender retreat and withdrawal. Thus, although it is incumbent upon the therapist to maintain a reality orientation, it is equally important that he or she recognize and empathize with the pain that accompanies this stance. These clinical findings have been substantiated in research studies involving clinical conditions like borderline personality disorders (Spear 1980; H. Lerner and St. Peter 1984), schizophrenia (Johnson 1980; Spear and Schwager, 1980), depression (Fibel 1979), opiate dependence (Blatt *et al.* 1984), and anorexia (Sugarman, Quinlan and Devenis 1982).

H. Lerner and St. Peter (1984) applied the COS to samples of patients from different clinical groups: outpatient neurosis, outpatient borderline personality disorders, hospitalized borderline personality disorders, and hospitalized schizophrenia. Overall, strong support was found for the general proposition that impairments in level of object representation, as indicated by the assessment of the developmental-structural properties of human responses given to the Rorschach, showed distinct patterns in groups differing in type and severity of psychopathology. Several other informative and unexpected findings were obtained. Subdividing the responses into those accurately perceived and those inaccurately perceived, the investigators found an inverse relationship between developmental level of the concept of the object and degree of psychopathology. That is, the less severe the psychopathology, the higher the developmental level of the patient's concept of the object. This inverse relationship, however, did not hold for the inaccurately perceived response. Here, quite surprisingly, the hospitalized borderline group achieved the highest levels of human differentiation, articulation, and integration. Because response accuracy is taken as an indicator of quality of reality testing, this finding prompted the authors to question the relationship between reality testing and object relations and led them to compare the protocols of the two borderline groups.

It was found that, although the outpatient borderline group produced more accurate and less inaccurate human responses than did their hospitalized counterparts, their responses tended to involve quasi-human rather than whole human figures (H. Lerner and St. Peter 1984). In other words, although outpatient borderline patients were able to perceive objects accurately, the perception was accompanied by a distancing and dehumanizing of the object. The hospitalized borderline patients, by contrast, were unable to distance their objects, and as a consequence, their reality testing suffered. In reviewing the thematic content of the human responses, the investigators found that the hospitalized borderline patients, in comparison with the three other groups, offered the most malevolent content and were the only group to produce inaccurately perceived malevolent responses. Conceptually, these patients may be understood in terms of their inability to defend against or escape from internal malevolent objects. Other investigators have applied modified versions of the concept of the object scale and specific subscales (e.g., Fritsch and Holmstrom 1990; Greco and Cornell 1992).

Throughout his research in psychopathology, Blatt has steadfastly argued for the significance of assessing impairments in object representations and the role they play in predisposing an individual to particular forms of psychopathology. Considerable clinical and research evidence suggests not only that the content and structure of object representations are essential dimensions in specific forms of psychopathology but that, in addition, the changes in structure of object representations parallel changes observed in treatment (H. Lerner 1983; P. Lerner 1986). With the use of the COS in a wide range of studies, the concept of object representation may be regarded as a core structure for investigating the multitude of factors that influence normal psychological growth, the development of psychopathology, and the changes that take place in the psychotherapeutic process.

Boundary representation

Blatt was one of the first theorists to broaden the conceptual basis of several of Rapaport's deviant verbalization scores (Blatt and Ritzler 1974; Blatt et al. 1975; Blatt and Lerner 1983a). In a creative attempt to bridge the notion of thought organization with object relations, Blatt evoked the superordinate concept of *boundary disturbance* and then applied it to several of Rapaport's categories. Boundaries are thought of as early cognitive structures that are fundamental to both cognitive development and, as part of the internalization process, to the formation of the representational world.

Blatt theorized that, in development, representations of independent objects (including self and non-self) are initially merged and fused. The earliest boundary differentiation is that between independent objects. Once the distinction between independent objects has been established, the developing child then differentiates the actual object from his or her internal representations of the object. A third boundary to be established is the differentiation between the external object and one's own associations and reactions to it – that is, between inside and outside and between fantasy and reality.

Blatt and Ritzler (1974) operationally defined the concept of boundary disturbance in terms of three of Rapaport's deviant verbalization scores – contamination, confabulation, and fabulized combination. Accordingly, disturbances in maintaining the boundary between independent objects are reflected in the Rorschach contamination score, a response in which there is a fusing of separate percepts and concepts. Disturbances in maintaining the boundary between inside and outside are reflected in the confabulation response. Here, there is a loss of the distinction between an external percept and personal associations and reactions to the perception. What initially may have been an accurate perception becomes compromised by excessive personal elaborations and associations. A third and less severe type of boundary disturbance is found in the fabulized combination response. In these responses, independent percepts maintain their separateness but are illogically and unrealistically combined, usually on the basis of their spatial contiguity. Although each image maintains its individuality and integrity, the boundary disturbance is reflected in the drawing of the inappropriate relationship.

Blatt and Ritzler (1974) initially found boundary disturbance indices to be related to disturbances in a variety of ego functions (reality testing, quality of interpersonal relations, nature of object representations) in a mixed schizophrenic and borderline sample. The authors found that poorly articulated boundaries occurred most frequently in the more disturbed, chronic patients, who had impoverished object relations, impaired ego functions, and a lifelong pattern of isolation and estrangement.

Because different forms of psychopathology can be understood in terms of an impairment of the capacity to sustain specific boundaries, several studies have attempted to identify the particular boundary disturbance in the borderline patient. H. Lerner, Sugarman and Barbour (1985) devised a Boundary Disturbance Scale based on the work of Blatt and Ritzler (1974). The six-point weighted scale consists of three developmentally ordered types of boundary disturbances and six Rorschach indices of assessing the disturbance. The least severe of the boundary disturbances is termed *boundary laxness* and is indicated by the fabulized combination. More severe is the inner–outer boundary disturbance, which is indicated by the confabulation-tendency and the confabulation response. The third and most severe of the boundary disturbances is disruption of the self–other boundary. Rorschach indices of this disturbance include the contamination-tendency, the incongruous combination and the contamination response. H. Lerner *et al.* (1985) found that independently diagnosed borderline patients could be distinguished from both schizophrenic and neurotic patients on the basis of level of boundary disturbance. Borderline patients were found to experience difficulty maintaining the inner–outer boundary as assessed through the confabulation response of the Rorschach; that is, these patients had difficulty distinguishing between an external object and their own affective reactions to that object. By contrast, the schizo-phrenic patients experienced difficulty in maintaining the developmentally earlier boundary between self and other, as reflected in the contamination response.

In a study involving boundary disturbances in depressive, borderline, and schizophrenic inpatients, Wilson (1985) obtained findings strikingly similar to those of H. Lerner and associates (1985). He too found that the borderline patients scored significantly higher on the Rorschach indices of laxness and (moderately severe) inner–outer boundary disturbance. The schizophrenic patients, in comparison, scored significantly higher on meas-ures of self–other boundary disturbance. Overall, these studies demonstrate the following: (a) there is a direct relationship between severity of psy-chopathology and severity of boundary disturbance; (b) specific types of psychopathology are characterized by specific types of boundary disturbance; and (c) the confabulation response and the contamination response are reliable and useful indicators of specific types of boundary disturbances.

Object representation and the therapeutic process

Blatt and Lerner (1983a, 1983b) and H. Lerner (1983) observed that object relations theory and Rorschach methods for the assessment of object relations have important implications for the understanding and study of the therapeutic process. An accumulation of data suggests convincingly that a comprehensive assessment of the concept of the object and boundary representation on the Rorschach deepens our understanding of psycho-pathology as modes of interpersonal relationships that are based on parti-cular distortions of the concept of the self and the object world, rather than as an array of overt symptoms. According to Blatt and Lerner (1983a: 240),

> If the representational world and the sense of reality are established through the internalization of significant interpersonal interactions, then these concepts should have relevance for understanding, and possibly assessing, significant dimensions of the therapeutic process.

Formulations about therapeutic actions in psychoanalysis and psychoanalytic psychotherapy increasingly emphasize the therapeutic matrix as a significant interpersonal relationship in which the therapist is the mediator in the patient's development of increasing levels of organization.

The most extensive and comprehensive study using the Rorschach as a measure of patient change during long-term intensive inpatient treatment is found in the work of Blatt *et al.* (1988). The sample comprised 90 seriously disturbed adolescents and young adults, aged 18–29 years, hospitalized in the Austen Riggs Center, an inpatient facility with a therapeutic community, in which the patients were seen in intensive, psychoanalytically oriented psychotherapy at least four times per week. On the basis of ratings of initial case records, the patients were subdivided into two groups defined by the nature of their psychopathology. In accordance with Blatt's (1974) distinction between anaclitic and introjective depression, one group included patients whose psychopathology was primarily anaclitic; that is, their major issues centered around themes of affection, intimacy, and attempts to establish need-satisfying interpersonal relationships. The second group comprised patients with introjective psychopathology. These individuals were thought of as overideational and preoccupied with concerns like anger, aggression, and self-definition.

The data involved two independent sets of observations, case records, and psychological tests, including the Rorschach. The data were obtained initially after the first six weeks of hospitalization and again one year later. Rorschachs were scored along several dimensions, including thought disorder, the COS, and the MOA Scale. Several significant and important findings were obtained. Collectively, the entire sample demonstrated significant improvement in social behavior and a reduction in clinical symptoms, as judged by both ratings from the case records and a significant decline in thought disorder on the Rorschach. Both groups exhibited a significant increase in the amount of adaptive fantasy and a significant decrease in the level of malevolence attributed to interactions, as reflected on the MOA Scale. In general, the Rorschach variable of object representation was found to be a more sensitive indicator of change in anaclitic patients than in introjective patients. Strong evidence was found that the therapeutic changes in patients are mainly congruent with features most salient in their personality organization. For example, in the more ideational introjective patients, changes were noted primarily in clinical symptoms and in cognitive functioning as assessed by the Rorschach thought disorder indices. By contrast, in the more interpersonally oriented anaclitic patients, changes were found primarily in case record ratings of interpersonal relationships and in a decrease in inaccurately perceived human forms on the Rorschach.

The Rorschach, when used by itself or as part of a battery, is sensitive to therapeutic changes. In using the Rorschach, investigators have employed both conventional scores and ratios (Weiner and Exner 1991; Exner and Andronikof-Sanglade 1992) and innovative scales (Diamond *et al.* 1990; Blatt *et al.* 1988). In these studies, the Rorschach has been used to assess treatment outcome; however, in turn, implicit in the Rorschach findings are important implications for psychotherapy research. For example, in the studies of Diamond *et al.* (1990) and Blatt *et al.* (1988), it was found that patients differ with respect to rate and configuration of change. Both the extent and nature of change are influenced by types of psychopathology and salient features of the patient's personality organization. Unfortunately, much of the research in psychotherapy outcome has assumed that all patients are the same and that they all change along the same dimensions (Blatt *et al.* 1988). Findings from these studies clearly indicate that future research in psychotherapy, both in design and methodology, must take into account differences among patients.

The Rorschach as a representational test

The need to move beyond the Rorschach's application to understand the nature of the task itself has been addressed by virtually all the prominent Rorschach theorists, past and present. As P. Lerner (1998) observes, the controversies stirred all go back to Herman Rorschach himself, who never completed the theoretical foundations of his experiment (Rorschach 1921). Early theorists, including Rorschach, emphasized perceptual processes, with varying importance given to associative processes in the task of taking the Rorschach. Rorschach viewed perception as an interpretive process that included sensation, memory, and association. Thus, when shown an inkblot, the participant registers sensations, organizes them into images on the basis of past experiences, and then ascribes meaning to the images by associating them with analogous memory engrams. Rapaport, Gill and Schafer (1945–6) attributed a key role to perception, although he assigned much significance to the associative process. Exner (1991) is perhaps the most prominent contemporary Rorschach theorist who conceives of the task as fundamentally perceptual. Using several studies pertaining to patterns of visual scanning of the blots, stimulus characteristics of the blots, response frequencies, set influences, and the impact of personality and cognitive style on differences on responses, he subdivided the response process into three phases: encoding and classification, rank ordering and discarding, and final selection and articulation.

Blatt (1990) was the first contemporary theorist to draw attention to the importance of representational processes as central to the Rorschach. He argues, that because Rorschach himself developed the method at a time when the scientific zeitgeist emphasized perceptual processes and behavioral responses, it was inevitable he would consider his technique as "a test of perception." In contrast to this view, Blatt notes that perception and representation are interrelated. Regarding the Rorschach, he (Blatt 1990: 402) argues:

> Interpretations of a Rorschach protocol as a perceptual test are still valid, but they are insufficient. The use of the Rorschach as a method of personality assessment can be greatly enhanced if we also consider responses not just as a perceptual experience but rather as [also] indicating cognitive-representational processes.

Blatt suggests that aspects of Rorschach responses be viewed along a continuum from perception to representation. At the perceptual end of the continuum are responses to form, color, and shading. Form level, the accuracy of fit of percept to stimulus, occupies a midpoint, reflecting a blend of perceptual and representational processes. At the representational pole are movement responses and content, Rorschach variables reflective of an individual's cognitive constructions and meaning systems. Both Blatt (1990) and Leichtman (1996) suggest that a representational conception of the Rorschach provides a stronger rationale for certain scoring categories, such as form level ratings. A representational perspective broadens the view of the nature of the Rorschach stimuli. As P. Lerner (1998) suggests, a perceptual conception highlights the ambiguity of the stimuli; a representational conception emphasizes the plasticity of the stimuli. Representational theory introduces a change in the logic of the Rorschach inference process. Whereas the earlier assumption that Rorschach percepts reflect a characteristic way of perceiving, a newer representational conceptualization holds that inferences from test responses "are based on the premises that there are consistencies in how individuals represent their experience across different symbolic modalities and different situations" (Leichtman 1996: 180). Here, emphasis is placed on the ways in which an individual experiences and represents his or her world.

Sidney Blatt: an appreciation

The concept of internalization has occupied a preeminent position in the psychoanalytic literature since Freud's initial formulation of this idea. This concept has been discussed from such perspectives as the importance of inadequate or distorted internalizations in psychopathology, the place of internalization in the treatment process, the function of internalizing mechanisms like defenses, and the role of internalization in growth and development. It is within this latter perspective, internalization as a vehicle for growth and development, that I would like to share some thoughts about Sidney Blatt. I have been blessed with wonderful training. My post-doctoral training at Yale was by far the most meaningful growth experience of my career. Being immersed in clinical and diagnostic work with hospitalized patients provided the opportunity to conduct research, to attend stimulating seminars, and to receive superb supervision. This training experience was provided by Sid Blatt. What was most significant was the opportunity to conduct research and to integrate clinical work with the rigors of quantitative methods, statistics, and, in terms of the Rorschach, the opportunity to analyze a large number of protocols. It is one thing to be exposed to norms based on large samples and something quite different to immerse oneself in reading hundreds of protocols generated by patients exhibiting a wide range of psychopathology. Sidney Blatt is at once a brilliant scholar, a prolific researcher, and a respected colleague. We engaged in collaborative efforts that led to several publications. He was a wonderful mentor and role model. Sid never made me feel stupid, and he could move with ideas in enormously fascinating and creative ways. He was immensely generative, facilitative, and supportive. I have identified deeply with his exuberance and enthusiasm for ideas. Through the course of my training, the accumulated history, continuity, and body of knowledge that have been transmitted to me has been in the context of a psychological ambience, a relationship that conveyed to me the ideals, attitudes, and personal qualities of my mentor, and such relationships happen to be essential for our profession. These goals and ideals cannot be achieved by cognitive teaching and learning alone. I identified with far more than Sid's knowledge and skills. I internalized his entire being, his values, ideals, passions, and attitudes, including his attitude toward me.

Internalization, intense learning, presupposes a clear distinction between self and other concerning personhood and clarity concerning respective roles, functions, responsibilities and goals. A mutually shared goal of training also involves the student's eventual sense of greater autonomy. Knowledge and skills originating in the mentor become progressively a part of and accessible to the student. Eventually, students are increasingly able to do for themselves those functions they originally looked to their mentors to perform. Therefore, my experience with Sidney Blatt can be judged not simply in terms of external criteria, such as amassing funds of information or functioning more competently, but also in terms of internal criteria like important shifts in my sense of self, progression toward a professional identity, and greater awareness and sensitivity in experiencing and relating to others. Through the internalization process, I have learned that teachers, supervisors, and mentors need never die; rather they can live on in our memories forever. There are several we believe in; however, if we are lucky, there are a few who also believe in us. Those individuals, such as Sid Blatt, are not only remembered, but cherished.

References

Ames, L. (1966) 'Longitudinal survey of child Rorschach responses: older subjects aged 10 to 16 years', *Genetic Psychology Monograph* 62: 185–229.

Blatt, S. J. (1974) 'Levels of object representation in anaclitic and introjective depression', *Psychoanalytic Study of the Child* 29: 107–57.

—— (1978) 'Paradoxical representations and their implications for the treatment of psychosis and borderline states', paper presented to the Institute for Psychoanalytic Research and Training, New York City, NY, May 18, 1978.

—— (1990) 'The Rorschach: a test of perception or an evaluation of representation', *Journal of Personality Assessment* 55: 394–416.

—— and Berman, W. (1984) 'A methodology for the use of the Rorschach in clinical research', *Journal of Personality Assessment* 48: 226–39.

—— —— Bloom-Feshbach, S., Sugarman, A., Wilber, C. and Kleber, H. (1984) 'Psychological assessment in opiate addicts', *Journal of Nervous and Mental Disease* 172: 156–65.

—— Brenneis, C., Schimek, J. and Glick, M. (1976) 'A developmental analysis of the concept of the object on the Rorschach', unpublished manuscript, Yale University, New Haven, CT.

—— Ford, R., Berman, W., Cook, B. and Meyer, R. (1988) 'The assessment of change during the intensive treatment of borderline and schizophrenic young adults', *Psychoanalytic Psychology* 5: 127–58.

—— and Lerner, H. (1983a) 'Investigations in the psychoanalytic theory of object relations and object representations', in J. Masling (ed.) *Empirical Studies of Psychoanalytic Theory*, vol. 1, Hillsdale, NJ: Analytic Press, pp. 189–249.

—— and —— (1983b) 'The psychological assessment of object representations', *Journal of Personality Assessment* 47: 7–28.

—— and Ritzler, B. (1974) 'Thought disorder and boundary disturbances in psychosis', *Journal of Consulting and Clinical Psychology* 42: 370–81.

—— Schimek, J. and Brenneis, C. B. (1980) 'The nature of the psychotic experience and its implications for the therapeutic process', in J. Strauss, M. Bowers, T. W. Downey, S. Fleck, S. Jackson and I. Levine (eds) *The Psychotherapy of Schizophrenia*, New York: Plenum, pp. 101–14.

—— Wild, C. and Ritzler, B. (1975) 'Disturbances of object representations in schizophrenia', *Psychoanalysis and Contemporary Thought* 4: 235–88.

Coates, S. and Tuber, S. (1988) 'The representation of object relations in the Rorschach of extremely feminine boys', in H. Lerner and P. Lerner (eds) *Primitive Mental States and the Rorschach*, Madison, CT: International Universities Press, pp. 647–64.

Diamond, D., Kaslow, N., Coonerty, S. and Blatt, S. (1990) 'Changes in separation-individuation and intersubjectivity in long-term treatment', *Psychoanalytic Psychology* 7: 363–98.

Exner, J. (1991) *The Rorschach: A Comprehensive System* vol. 2, 2nd edn, New York: Wiley.

—— and Andronikof-Sanglade, A. (1992) 'Rorschach changes following brief and short-term therapy', *Journal of Personality Assessment* 59: 59–71.

Fibel, B. (1979) 'Toward a developmental model of depression: object representation and object loss in adolescent and adult psychiatric patients', unpublished doctoral dissertation, University of Massachusetts, Amherst, MA.

Fisher, S. and Cleveland, S. (1968) *Body Image and Personality* 2nd rev. edn, New York: Dover Publications.

Freud, A. (1952) 'The mutual influences in the development of ego and id', *Psychoanalytic Study of the Child* 7: 42–50.

Freud, S. (1923) 'The ego and the id', in J. Strachey (ed. and trans.), *The Standard Edition of the Complete Psychological Works of Sigmund Freud*, vol. 19, London: Hogarth Press, 1961, pp. 12–50.

—— (1940) 'An outline of psychoanalysis', in J. Strachey (ed. and trans.), *The Standard Edition of the Complete Psychological Works of Sigmund Freud*, vol. 23, London: Hogarth Press, 1961, pp. 215–93.

Fritsch, R. and Holmstrom, R. (1990) 'Assessing object representations as a continuous variable: modification of the concept of the object on the Rorschach scale', *Journal of Personality Assessment* 55: 319–34.

Glover, E. (1950) 'Functional aspects of the mental apparatus', *International Journal of Psycho-Analysis* 31: 125–31.

Greco, C. and Cornell, D. (1992) 'Rorschach object relations of adolescents who committed homicide', *Journal of Personality Assessment* 59: 574–83.

Hartmann, H. (1950) 'Comments on the psychoanalytic theory of the ego', in *Essays in Ego Psychology: selected problems in psychoanalytic theory*, New York: International Universities Press, 1964, pp. 115–41.

Hatcher, R. and Krohn, A. (1980) 'Level of object representation and capacity for intensive psychotherapy in neurotics and borderlines', in J. Kwawer, H. Lerner, P. Lerner and A. Sugarman (eds) *Borderline Phenomena and the Rorschach Test*, New York: International Universities Press, pp. 299–320.

Johnson, D. (1980) 'Cognitive organization in paranoid and non-paranoid schizophrenia', unpublished doctoral dissertation, Yale University, New Haven, CT.

Kernberg, O. (1975) *Borderline Conditions and Pathological Narcissism*, New York: Aronson.

Krohn, A. (1974) 'Borderline empathy and differentiation of object representations: a contribution to the psychology of object relations', *International Journal of Psychoanalytic Psychotherapy* 3: 142–65.

—— and Mayman, M. (1974) 'Object representations in dreams and projective tests', *Bulletin of the Menninger Clinic* 38: 445–66.

Landis, B. (1970) 'Ego boundaries', *Psychological Issues* 6 (4), Monograph No. 24, New York: International Universities Press.

Leichtman, M. (1996) *The Rorschach: a developmental perspective*, Hillsdale, NJ: Analytic Press.

Lerner, H. (1983) 'An object representation approach to psychostructural change: A clinical illustration', *Journal of Personality Assessment* 47: 314–23.

—— and St. Peter, S. (1984) 'Patterns of object relations in neurotic, borderline and schizophrenic patients', *Psychiatry* 47: 77–92.

—— Sugarman, A. and Barbour, C. (1985) 'Patterns of ego boundary disturbances in neurotic, borderline and schizophrenic patients', *Psychoanalytic Psychology* 2: 47–66.

Lerner, P. (1986) 'Experiential and structural aspects of the (c) Rorschach response in patients with narcissistic personality disorders', in M. Kissen (ed.) *Assessing*

Object Relations Phenomena, New York: International Universities Press, pp. 333–48.

Lerner, P. (1998) *Psychoanalytic Perspectives in the Rorschach,* Hillsdale, NJ: Analytic Press.

Mahler, M. (1968) *On Human Symbiosis and Vicissitudes of Individuation,* vol. 1, New York: International Universities Press.

Mayman, M. (1967) 'Object representations and object relationships in Rorschach responses', *Journal of Projective Techniques and Personality Assessment* 31: 17–24.

—— (1977) 'A multidimensional view of the Rorschach movement response', in M. Rickers-Ovsiankina (ed.) *Rorschach Psychology,* 2nd edn, Huntington, NY: Krieger, pp. 229–50.

Piaget, J. (1954) *The Construction of Reality in the Child,* trans. M. Cook, New York: Basic Books.

Rapaport, D. (1950) 'The theoretical implications of diagnostic testing procedures', *Congres International de Psychiatric* 2: 241–71.

—— Gill, M. and Schafer, R. (1945–6) *Diagnostic Psychological Testing,* Chicago, IL: Yearbook Publishers.

—— —— and —— (1968) *Diagnostic Psychological Testing,* rev. edn, R. R. Holt (ed.), New York: International Universities Press.

Ritzler, B., Zambianco, D., Harder, D. and Kaskey, M. (1980) 'Psychotic patterns of the concept of the object on the Rorschach', *Journal of Abnormal Psychology* 89: 46–55.

Rorschach, H. (1921) *Psychodiagnostik*; trans. P. Lemkau and B. Kronenberg, *Psychodiagnostics,* 6th edn, New York: Grune and Stratton, 1964.

Ryan, E. (1973) 'The capacity of the patient to enter an elementary therapeutic relationship in the initial psychotherapy interview', unpublished doctoral dissertation, University of Michigan, Ann Arbor, Michigan.

Ryan, R., Avery, R. and Grolnick, W. (1985) 'A Rorschach assessment of children's mutuality of autonomy', *Journal of Personality Assessment* 49: 6–12.

Spear, W. (1980) 'The psychological assessment of structural and thematic object representations in borderline and schizophrenic patients', in J. Kwawer, H. Lerner, P. Lerner and A. Sugarman (eds) *Borderline Phenomena and the Rorschach Test,* New York: International Universities Press, pp. 321–42.

—— and Schwager, E. (1980) 'New perspectives on the use of psychological tests as a measure of change over the course of intensive inpatient psychotherapy', paper presented at the Society for Personality Assessment, Tampa, Florida.

—— and Sugarman, A. (1984) 'Dimensions of internalized object relations in borderline and schizophrenic patients', *Psychoanalytic Psychology* 1: 113–30.

Sugarman, A., Quinlan, D. and Devenis, L. (1982) 'Ego boundary disturbance in juvenile anorexia nervosa', *Journal of Personality Assessment* 46: 455–61.

Tuber, S. (1983) 'Children's Rorschach scores as predictors of later adjustment', *Journal of Consulting and Clinical Psychology* 51: 379–85.

Urist, J. (1973) 'The Rorschach test as a multidimensional measure of object relations', unpublished doctoral dissertation, University of Michigan, Ann Arbor, Michigan.

—— (1977) 'The Rorschach test and the assessment of object relations', *Journal of Personality Assessment* 41: 3–9.

Weiner, I. and Exner, J. (1991) 'Rorschach changes in long-term and short-term psychotherapy', *Journal of Personality Assessment* 56: 453–65.

Werner, H. (1948) *Comparative Psychology of Mental Development*, rev. edn, G. Murphy (ed.) and E. B. Garside (trans.), New York: International Universities Press.

Wilson, A. (1985) 'Boundary disturbance in borderline and psychotic states', *Journal of Personality Assessment* 49: 346–55.

Chapter 11

The Rorschach method

A starting point for investigating formal thought disorder

Philip S. Holzman

Although the disturbances of thinking that accompany schizophrenia are arguably the most dramatic identifiers of this illness, they stubbornly resist the efforts of contemporary neuroscience to uncloak their mysterious origins and their basic nature. The two pioneering systematizers of schizophrenic disorders, Kraepelin and Bleuler, assigned to the thought disturbances of schizophrenia the role of a telltale indicator that identifies this syndrome. About a century later, we find ourselves only marginally further towards understanding their mechanisms. With the help of the newly invented and sharpened measuring tools of cognitive neuroscience, however, moving beyond the old established frontier is now closer to realization.

Three aspects of formal thought disorder

A few facts about formal thought disorder are clear. First, the disruption in thinking occurs principally in the *forms* of thought rather than in the *content* of thoughts. That is, strained logic, word misusages as well as new word coinages or invented words, and fused, composite, and incoherent ideas are among the many aspects of schizophrenic thinking. The content of thoughts, however, no matter how delusional they may eventually be shown to be, may still be realistic, whether they are counterfactual proposals, creative or imaginative new ideas, a passage from postmodern literary criticism, or a philosophical treatise. For example, in these days of electronic miniaturization, the idea of the bugged Martini olive is no longer a crazy one. Nor, after 11 September 2001, is a portent of the destruction of another World Trade Center necessarily the product of a paranoid apocalyptic imagination. David Rapaport, one of my most influential teachers, was fond of the aphoristic version of this point. About the difficulty in distinguishing a delusion from a thought based solidly in reality, he often quipped, "Just because you call me a son of a bitch, it doesn't mean I'm not a son of a bitch."

Second, formal thought disorder is not specific to schizophrenic conditions. Other psychiatric disorders, such as mania, obsessional thinking, and paranoia, betray their presence in the formal qualities of their thought products. A feature of many approaches to the nature of formal thought disorder has been a quest to discover its single essence. Chapman and Chapman (1973) identified several qualities of schizophrenic thinking, such as a tendency to yield to the strongest, most recent, or most familiar meaning of words, a loss of the ability to reason in abstract terms, over-inclusive thinking, and attentional impairment. Johnston and I examined these and other qualities of schizophrenic thinking and concluded that none of them is specific to schizophrenia (Johnston and Holzman 1979), although all of them do occur in schizophrenia. Other conditions, such as major affective disorders (particularly mania), conditions that result from brain lesions in various brain loci, and acute psychological trauma, also show characteristic thought disruptions. All of these disruptions can occur with different degrees of severity, and their prevalence can vary with the acuteness and chronicity of the disorder. Their one single essence will continue to elude us because there is no single form of psychotic thought disorder.

Another insistent feature of thought disorder is its variability from moment to moment. That is, thought disruptions are intermittent. They do not occur regularly and continuously. Both their intensity and their prevalence fluctuate. They also vary in their form from moment to moment. In these respects, they are like many other dysfunctions in schizophrenic patients. This aspect of schizophrenic response deserves special study because it sets itself apart from brain disorders in which intermittency is not the rule. Hippocampal damage, for example, wreaks its havoc on memory with hardly any intermittency; certain lesions of the primary visual cortex will destroy vision with no remission. The measurement of this insistent variability becomes important for appreciating many aspects of schizophrenic behavior, including that of thought disorder (Matthysse *et al.* 1999).

Familial aspects of formal thought disorder

There is yet another important aspect of schizophrenic thinking. Many of the clinically unaffected biological relatives of schizophrenic patients show mildly peculiar thought processes. Bleuler called such people *latent schizophrenics*, a term that was later expanded into the *schizophrenia spectrum*. Whether the thought slippage alone that is present in these nonpsychotic relatives is associated with a diagnosable condition is doubtful because most of these same biological relatives of schizophrenic patients manifest no schizophrenic symptoms, such as interpersonal aversiveness, blunted affect, or unconventional ideas. In our sample of about 500 relatives, however, almost half tend to show one or several behavioral traits that have no obvious relation to schizophrenic symptoms. For example, a disorder of smooth pursuit eye movements (Holzman *et al.* 1974) and impairments in spatial working memory (Park, Holzman and Goldman-Rakic 1995) occur at higher frequencies in these unaffected biological relatives of schizophrenic patients than does schizophrenia itself. These traits do occur in the general population, but that prevalence is much lower than in the families of schizophrenic patients.

Although the familiality of these traits raises the issue of genetic transmission of schizophrenia, their presence bolsters the view that it is not schizophrenia *qua* psychosis that is inherited but some disposition whose essential character we have not yet discovered. In contrast to the prevailing Zeitgeist prior to the 1970s, which belittled the role of biological factors – especially genetic determinants – in psychiatric disorders, it is no longer heretical today to discuss the genetics of schizophrenia or to regard schizophrenia as a complex disease that, like many diabetic or hypertensive conditions, has significant genetic determinants. This change in how one views the role of biological factors in the etiology and pathogenesis of schizophrenia owes much to the work of Kety and his colleagues in their adoption studies carried out in the 1960s (e.g., Kety, Rosenthal and Wender 1978; Kety *et al.* 1976).[1]

Understanding the nature of thought disorder

Thus far, I have argued that formal thought disorder comprises many kinds of slippages in thinking, and therefore no single indicator of its presence will prove to be pathognomonic. A scoring system that takes account of the multifaceted nature of thought disorders will more likely have the power to detect people whose thinking shows intermittent disruptions; such a system can put us on the path to understanding the nature and etiology of these strange slippages. The realization that a global system offered the most fruitful starting point for the study of this mercurial phenomenon led to the construction of the Thought Disorder Index (TDI; Johnston and Holzman 1979). The Rorschach test, which tends not to rely on practiced and overlearned responses, seemed most likely to yield the wide sample of thought disturbances that we sought.

The TDI, assessed from Rorschach test responses, provides a global measure of formal thought disorder. It presumes that there are different types of disordered thinking, some of which are more serious indicators of pathology than are others. The TDI is a descendant of an earlier study of diagnostic psychological testing by Rapaport, Gill and Schafer (1968). These authors, working at the Menninger Clinic, where they tested patients from different diagnostic groups, collected and categorized numerous verbalizations they considered to be deviant, and they determined the degree to which patients in different psychiatric groups produced each type of verbalization. The authors made no claim for either the completeness or the internal consistency of their list. They admitted that the distinctions they made were not easy for all clinicians to make. They presented their work as only a good starting point for constructing a catalogue of deviant verbalizations as one way to begin to bring conceptual order into the range of pathological verbalizations that emerge during either a psychiatric interview or a psychological testing situation.

Rapaport *et al.* (1945–6) divided the pathological verbalizations into two categories. The first, tied to the nature of responses given during the Rorschach test, was based on how reality-rooted the response was. An example of a response poorly anchored in reality is this description of Card I: "A termite with closed eyes." Here the perceptual justification for this response is weak at best. The second category, how the person verbalized the response, took note of whether the *verbalization* was rooted in reality. Deviant communication of a response reflects the *end product* of pathological thoughts, rather than the thoughts themselves. Verbalizations denoted as *peculiar*, *queer*, or *confused* occur *after* the initial thought has been formed and betray the thought slippage through the vehicle of the odd language. In constructing the TDI, Johnston and I began with the Rapaport *et al.* (1945–6) scheme and its modification by Watkins and Stauffacher (1952). We studied more than thirty kinds of thought slippage. The present TDI comprises 23 categories of thought disorder. Although in principle, one can score thought disorder from any extended verbal sample, we now rely on responses to the Rorschach. These categories are presented with a few examples in Table 11.1. They are also arranged on a four-point scale of severity.

Normal and abnormal thinking

For the most part, when normal people respond to a Rorschach card, they understand that their responses should have sufficient justification in the organization of the blots; that is, the normal person follows an implicit instruction to stay within conventional everyday logic. Rapaport and colleagues stated,

> Just as they should not give responses they cannot confirm by reference to the inkblot, so their responses should not be so dominated by the perceptual configurations of the inkblot that they are no longer subject to critical control, and thus become absurdly combined or absurdly integrated.
>
> (Rapaport *et al.* 1968: 429)

It is the same with the language the subject uses to convey the response to the examiner; the normal subject understands that language must be understandable and not elliptical. Matthysse observed that,

Table 11.1 TDI categories and levels of severity with selected examples

Level	Category number	Category description and examples
0.25		
	1	Inappropriate distance
		A Loss or increase of distance (*I'm afraid of what else it could be . . . It scares me when I think of what else it could be*)
		B Excessive qualifications
		C Concreteness (*some kind of fancy military jet flying up the card*)
		D Overspecificity (*a four-legged lamb*)
	2	Vagueness (*Nothing but two figures on each side, I don't know what kind of figures. They don't look like people. They just looked like two smears*)
	3	Flippant response
	4	Peculiar verbalizations and responses
		A Peculiar expressions (*the posterior pronunciations*)
		B Stilted, inappropriate language (*It's a piece of animation*)
		C Idiosyncratic word usage (*There's a segregation between mouth and nose*)
	5	Word-finding difficulty
	6	Clangs
	7	Perseverations
	8	Incongruous combinations
		A Composite response (*a bear with a duck's face*)
		B Arbitrary form-color responses (*an orange pelvic bone*)
		C Inappropriate activity response (*a beetle crying*)
0.50		
	9	Relationship verbalization (i.e., an allusion to an earlier card) (*that being the mandibles in the very first picture*)
	10	Idiosyncratic symbolism (*the red is trouble*)
	11	Queer responses
		A Queer expressions (*inward type of photograph of a flower's reproductive cells*)
		B Queer imagery (*idealized fire*)
		C Queer word usage (*pestals on a flower*)
	12	Confusion (*some people smoking matches and burning cigarettes*)
	13	Looseness (*because it's black, dark, darkness, lovemaking*)
	14	Fabulized combinations, impossible or bizarre (*Two crows with afros and they're pushing two hearts together. Two fetal bears on a coral reef*)
0.75		
	15	Fluidity (*The head of a rocket or the head of a bear or the head of a bird . . . looked like something was becoming something else*)
	16	Absurd responses (*This is sticking out here. Remember that's the-uh-cure there. It's our cure, it's called. All together we can fly and understand God. Altogether we are the butterfly*)

Table 11.1   (Continued)

Level	Category number	Category description and examples
	17	Confabulations A Details in one area generalized to a larger area B Extreme elaboration (*The light bulb is – I think it's man-made. And the pink is down here and it gives energy for the light bulb . . . and the vapors from the pink . . . cause the green and the orange to . . . be there . . .*)
	18	Playful confabulation (*An evil witch doing a square dance . . . She had her dress like this and she was doe-see-doeing*)
	19	Autistic logic (*I see something rather like an appendix. Looked to me totally useless, so I thought of the appendix*)
	20	Fragmentation (*a leg, and arm, a face, hot cha cha*)
1.0		
	21	Contamination (*This is definitely a man . . . a man butterfly, a butterfly with a man's face – could be a dark cloud that's dark because it swallows up all . . . ah . . . the dark particles – man butterfly . . . it could be a cloud-like man-butterfly*)
	22	Incoherence (*A duck . . . their disarrangements. They follow out together, they follow one another. The two toes together, meeting one another. They jacked up in back, like spinal cord being broken*)
	23	Neologisms (*That's tevro or neoglyphics*)

Thinking is so easy for normal people. Our thoughts effortlessly conform to an extraordinarily complicated set of syntactic, semantic, and logical constraints, as well as to whatever additional requirements must be satisfied so that they are judged 'sane.' There is no struggle to make them conform. We do not seem to calculate before we think, nor do we filter out ill-formed thoughts just before speaking. . . . Normal thinking demands no special concentration and takes hardly any time.

(Matthysse 1987: 173)

But for schizophrenic patients, these constraints seem not to be effective in steering thoughts. The tasks for a science of psychopathology require, first of all, that judgments of whether thoughts are disordered must be reliably made. Second, after identifying what are disordered thoughts, one must then try to discover their causes.

The first of these tasks, that of reliably identifying the range of thought disorders, is the easier one. Recognizing what is an occurrence of thought disorder is a less subjective judgment than it may first appear to be. Both the TDI scorer's judgment of the actual possibilities of the spatial arrangement of the Rorschach inkblots and the peculiarity of the words used by a patient to convey that responses are based upon knowledge of the prototypicality of these products. Assessment of prototypicality is an area of social psychology explored by Rosch (1973), who noted that, as with any set of objects that represents a category, experience with seeing a range of objects subsumed under that category trains the observer to distinguish the modal response from the deviant one. For most of us, German Shepherds are better prototypical dogs than Chihuahuas. We can and we constantly do make judgments about the adequacy and typicality of many things, and so it is with words and their meanings.

Establishing reliability of judging whether a percept or a verbalization is or is not an example of disordered thinking requires training and exposure to many examples of Rorschach responses. As with most qualitative judgments, consensus scoring in groups of well-trained scorers can improve reliability, and periodic review and recalibration have become part of a standard TDI scoring procedure in our laboratory. Coleman *et al.* (1993) demonstrated that, among four teams of trained raters, the intraclass correlation was 0.74, and the Spearman rank correlations among the six possible pairs of rating teams ranged from 0.80 to 0.90.

The TDI as a clinical tool

As a clinical tool, the TDI has been used within psychiatric hospitals and clinics to detect the presence of thought disorder and thus help in the differential diagnostic work that must precede the prescription of proper treatment. Prior to the mid-1950s, it hardly mattered what diagnosis was assigned to a patient because there were no truly rational treatments. Today, however, it does matter whether a patient is assigned the diagnosis of bipolar disorder or schizophrenia because of pharmacological choices available now. In its clinical application, the TDI has shown itself capable of making valid distinctions between bipolar disorders (manic psychosis, for example) and schizophrenia in adult and in adolescent patients (Makowski *et al.* 1997; Solovay, Shenton and Holzman 1987), and thus has become an important adjuvant to a treatment decision. Furthermore, the TDI has been successfully used to distinguish variant forms of schizoaffective disorder (see, e.g., Shenton, Solovay and Holzman 1987). Moreover, it is able to track clinical changes, such as improvement following administration of specific treatments, even before clinicians are able to notice changes (Hurt, Holzman and Davis 1983). Because the TDI requires verbatim transcripts and can be reviewed for instances of thought slippage, it is able to provide subtle instances of thought disorder that have eluded detection even by experienced clinicians. The TDI can thus assume a rightful place as a valid measure of clinical state.

The TDI as a research tool

My colleagues and I believe that to identify the fundamental constituents of schizophrenia, one must first parse that complex set of behaviors into simpler components that in turn can more easily be traced to known biological processes in the central nervous system. This admittedly reductionistic approach promises to lead to underlying cellular and genetic processes that contain the relevant conditions for developing clinical schizophrenia. The steps must be short, but they offer the scientist a path from the broad and bewildering symptoms of this psychotic disorder to more empirically based neuroscience.

First, one must be clear about whether we are investigating a thought disorder or whether the phenomenon in question is a language or a speech disorder. The three possibilities point to different paths for studying brain abnormalities: of language, of speech, or of thought. That is, different brain networks are implicated in these three different processes. The scale's name, the Thought Disorder Index, establishes our position on this issue: the abnormalities the scale identifies are those of *thought*, and not of *language* or of *speech*.

Although the language of schizophrenic patients often appears to be abnormal, language is usually the medium through which thoughts are conveyed. It is therefore usually transparent, and we tend to look through the language to the thought, although language itself can become the object of an examination, as for example, when a literary critic examines the style of a writer or when we try to learn another language (see Heider, 1959).

Additionally, schizophrenic patients do not speak a shared language. There is no such thing as a schizophrenic language. Schizophrenic patients have the same difficulties anyone has in understanding what another schizophrenic patient is trying to say (Hunt and Walker 1966). Furthermore, language and thought are also conceptually separable as domains of disorder; language disorders can exist without thought disorders, and vice versa. For example, the congenitally deaf are generally able to read a written language at no better than a fifth-grade level, and their language is laden with syntactic and grammatical errors. However, when they communicate in sign language, their formal thinking shows no impairment in organization. And there are cases of thought disorder with no language disorder, as in pure paranoia; there flagrant thought disorder, in the form of systematized delusions, occurs with no trace either of a language disorder or of peculiar word misusages.

One can demonstrate that the basic properties of speaking a language – morphology, phonotactics, and syntactics – are preserved in schizophrenic patients. Schizophrenic patients do not violate the rules of linguistic inflection – the tolerable linguistic sound clusters – or the word order rules of their language. Even when they invent words, as in neologisms, they do not violate the phonotactic rules of the language they are speaking. Language use, moreover, is a manifestation of human thinking processes. The oddness of schizophrenic communication comes not from grammatical or syntactical errors. The schizophrenic patient's communications are odd because their meaning appears strange to us. An example will make this point clear. Consider the sentence, "Him goed to Donny's house." Compare it with, "She took the loaded hair under the sense." The first sentence, although grammatically and morphologically poor, is understandable. The second, although grammatically, syntactically, and morphologically correct, is not understandable; it strikes the reader as strange. Cruse (1986) noted that we do not communicate with isolated words; that is, words are not, in and of themselves, the bearer of messages. One must have a string of words that is at least a phrase or a simple sentence for one to judge whether the utterance is semantically odd. In Cruse's view, with which I agree, the meaning of a word is reflected in the context in which it is used.

Having taken the position that both thought organization and functioning are impaired in schizophrenia, I can begin a causal investigation with the impairments denoted by the TDI. Previous studies using the TDI established that schizophrenic patients produce thinking disturbances on only some of the 23 categories of thought disorder (Kestnbaum Daniels *et al.* 1988; Shenton *et al.* 1987; Solovay *et al.* 1987). The initial step after having taken this position is to quantify the degree of oddness. With respect to the total TDI score, both manic and schizophrenic patients produce considerably more thought-disordered responses than do normal people, but those two patient groups do not differ from each other. Thus, psychotic patients, regardless of the type of psychosis, tend to produce essentially equal quantities of thought-disordered utterances.

The two major groups of psychotic patients, however, arrive at their high TDI levels differently. In a set of studies that applied factor analytic and discriminant function statistical techniques to the utterances of 97 psychotic patients, my colleagues and I determined that the groups of manic and schizophrenic patients produced different profiles of thought disorder. Those whose psychosis was independently determined to be a manic disorder showed weighting on a factor called Expansive Thinking, which included the TDI categories of *playful confabulation, incongruous combinations, flippant responses,* and *fabulized combinations.* Clear combinatory thinking and jocularity are the hallmarks of the manic thought disorder. Combinatory thinking reflects a tendency to group percepts, ideas, or images in an incongruous, unrealistic, or inappropriate manner that at times can be imaginative and creative but that may be extravagant and take on extreme counterfactual qualities, as occurs in many manic episodes.

The schizophrenic patients showed high loadings on factors labeled Unconventional Verbalizations, which included the categories of *peculiar and queer verbalizations, absurd responses,* and *neologisms,* and Disorganization, which comprises *word-finding difficulty, confusion,* and *incoherence.* Disorganized thinking reflects confusion in thinking that extends to disorganization. Unconventional verbalizations reflect the use of odd words and phrases that, unlike that of poets and other creative writers, is not under voluntary control.

The two major psychotic groups, however, did not differ with respect to the number of responses produced in the Associative Looseness factor, which comprised the following categories from the TDI: *inappropriate distance, clangs, perseveration, relationship verbalizations, looseness,* and *fluidity.* The group of responses subsumed under the rubric of associative looseness reflects a tendency for utterances to be guided more by internal sets and shifts of set than by the social constraints of the task, in this case the completion of the demands of the Rorschach test. The massing of these responses suggests poor control over inhibitory efforts, which is characteristic of both manic and schizophrenic patients.

To clinicians, it comes as no surprise that the TDI reveals what they have known all along: manic thought disorder manifests itself as loosely tied together ideas that are too easily and excessively combined and elaborated. Schizophrenic thought disorder shows very little of the playful, showy, elaborately ideationally loose productions of the manic type. Rather, fluid thinking, interpenetrations of one idea by another, unstable referents of words, and fragmented and elliptical communications give the impression of inner confusion that is often not explicitly verbalized. In many instances, listeners are also confused by what they hear. And there is a set of thinking disorders that is common to both psychoses. What the TDI has done, however, is to establish a schema and initial sorting of the form varieties of thought disruption in psychosis. This schema serves as a launching point for systematic research into the brain functions that underlie these anomalies.

Thus, the catalog of thought disturbances yielded by the TDI encourages one to distinguish between manic and schizophrenic psychoses. Specific studies support the Kraepelinian position that schizophrenia and manic-depressive conditions are two different conditions (e.g., Shenton *et al.* 1987; Solovay *et al.* 1987). Efforts to elide the distinctions between these conditions seem to us to have been based too rigidly on symptom assessments that both Kraepelin and Bleuler warned might mislead the investigator. The position I take here does not suggest that mania and schizophrenia are homogeneous conditions. Indeed there are many indications that these conditions are heterogeneous in terms of their pathogenesis, pathophysiology, and even their genetic etiology.

Examples of research on formal thought disorder

The TDI has been useful as a tool for launching new research probes into the nature of thought disorders. Earlier I argued that language and speech are not impaired in the functional psychoses, where the capacity to vocalize human sounds and to use and understand language is normal. The impairments lie in instances of impaired language *performance*, rather than in language *competence*, to borrow Chomsky's (1969) useful distinction. The impairments in performance reveal the cogwheeling, blending, and integrating of thought with language. This view suggests that a productive research approach is to scrutinize how concepts, ideas, and images are organized, accessed, and placed at the disposal of language for communication. Some examples of research on formal thought disorder using the TDI follow.

Psycholinguistic approaches to thought disorder

When a phrase strikes the listener as odd or peculiar, there is a clash between the word and the meaning that is implied in the usage. When a patient remarks that an area of a Rorschach card looks like "potential ears" or "two pointed obtrusions," the listener is surrounded by an aura of ambiguity about the intended meaning. The patient has used real, recognizable English words, but the semantic accuracy of the phrases in which those words appear is sufficiently off the mark that one is not quite sure what the speaker intends to say. One can, of course, make an effort to understand the speaker's intention by looking through the phrases to the presumed meaning and thereby ignore most of the peculiarities. My colleagues and I directed our research efforts towards reducing these linguistic anomalies to simpler processes that can be parsed into components that yield to research dissection. As a start, Debra Titone of our laboratory entertained the hypothesis that, in light of the prevalence of these peculiar and queer word usages, schizophrenic patients would be comparatively insensitive to contextual constraints. The resulting study was an examination of lexical ambiguity in schizophrenia.

Many aspects of language convey ambiguity and uncertainty about meaning. In English, for example, the words "sun" and "son" are homonyms, and only when they are used in a sentence is one able to decide whether the speaker is referring to one's male offspring or to the solar disk. There are many examples of such ambiguities in English, and Chapman, Chapman and Daut (1976) reported that schizophrenic patients showed a significant tendency to attend to the more frequent or the more usual meaning of a word than normal subjects did. That is, although the word "pen" can be used to denote a writing implement (the stronger or more usual meaning), it can also be used to denote an enclosure for animals (the weaker or less frequent meaning). Titone and colleagues used a semantic priming task that allowed them to assess how schizophrenic patients process the relevant and irrelevant meanings of words (Titone, Levy and Holzman 2000). Schizophrenic patients and controls listened to 64 noun-noun homonyms that were placed within phrase contexts that were biased toward the less frequent meaning of the words. Immediately after the presentation of the spoken prime, the subjects viewed targets that were related to either the dominant or the subordinate meaning of the word. The task was to decide whether the targets are a word or a nonword, and to press a button upon making a decision. The context settings were constructed so that homonyms were set within sentences that were either moderately biased or strongly biased toward the subordinate meaning. The result of this biasing procedure made the subordinate meaning always contextually relevant and the dominant meaning always contextually irrelevant. Thus, subjects responding to the subordinate meanings of targets were detecting the relevant information in the sentence.

The results showed that when the context was strongly biased toward the subordinate meaning of the homonym, both schizophrenic patients and controls showed priming of the subordinate meaning. When, however, the context was only moderately biased toward the subordinate meaning, the schizophrenic patients showed priming of the dominant target, thereby indicating a failure to inhibit the inappropriate meaning. Here, then, is evidence that although schizophrenic patients are able to use context for controlling behavior, the clues to context must be stronger in the patients than in normal participants in order to inhibit inappropriate responses. The involvement of impaired inhibitory processes in linguistic usage now directs a search for the source of one aspect of the formal thought disorder of schizophrenia not only to brain areas that control language use but also to inhibitory processes that implicate prefrontal areas.

Thought disorder and brain morphology

Shenton and colleagues (1992), using structural magnetic resonance imaging scans, found that three regions in the temporal lobes of chronically ill schizophrenic patients showed reduced tissue, although there were no global differences in absolute brain volume. The tissue reduction was particularly striking in the left superior temporal area, located in the auditory association cortex, and was highly negatively correlated with the amount of thought disorder as measured by the TDI: the greater the thought disorder, the smaller the superior temporal gyrus volume. An earlier, independent study had shown that the severity of auditory hallucinations was related to a tissue reduction in that same area (Barta et al. 1990). These studies strongly suggest that the superior temporal gyrus, the cingulate, and the hippocampus are implicated in disturbances of effective thinking, in addition to the frontal areas that control inhibitory processes. Now that the technology is available for observing brain activation while mental processes are actually occurring, with the use not only of functional magnetic resonance scanning but also of magnetoencephalography, we can look forward to more data about the functioning network of brain areas when thinking is normal and when it is disturbed.

Thought disorder in psychometrically selected schizotypes

A study undertaken at Cornell University examined the presence of thought disorder, as measured by the TDI, in normal college students who were selected for having experiences of perceptual aberrations (Holzman, *et al.* 1996). The participants were identified on the basis of their scores on the Perceptual Aberration Scale (PAS) constructed by Chapman, Chapman and Raulin (1978). Poor motivation, inattention, medication effects, generalized performance deficits, and social withdrawal, all of which influence to some extent studies of schizophrenic patients, will less influence a study of people with these very mild schizophrenic-like symptoms. Thus, my colleagues and I assumed that potentially *psychosis-prone* individuals within the general population, like the relatives of schizophrenic patients, might bear schizophrenic traits even though none were currently ill and most will never become psychotic.

The participants were first year undergraduates at Cornell University who completed the PAS. None of the students had a diagnosis of any psychotic disorder at the time of testing, as determined by individual screening, and all were in good academic standing. However, those with high PAS scores had mean total TDI scores at the upper limit of normal subjects (8.83), and those with low PAS scores had mean TDI scores of 3.65. The high PAS students also showed a significantly greater number of responses that were scored as peculiar and queer verbalizations, autistic logic, and ideational looseness, all categories that are associated with schizophrenia. The presence of similar qualities of thought disorder in schizophrenic patients, psychometrically selected schizotypes, and unaffected first-degree relatives of schizophrenic patients suggests that this quality of thought disorder is common to several groups with an increased liability for schizophrenia.

Use of the TDI in linkage studies

The increased amount of thought disorders that appear in the relatives of schizophrenic patients suggest that this aspect of cognitive dysfunction can be effectively used to identify gene carriers to help in linkage studies. Vuchetich and colleagues (2001) conducted a segregation analysis of the inheritance of thought disorder in five large Danish families selected for the presence of schizophrenia. They found strong evidence of a major gene effect on the expression of thought disorder (as measured by the TDI), particularly the categories of peculiar and queer verbalizations. The presence of formal thought disorder can now be useful as an endophenotypic indicator that can increase the power of linkage analyses in a search for genes implicated in the transmission of schizophrenia. Many studies have shown that the recurrence risk[2] for clinical schizophrenia is rather low, probably not more than about 6 per cent (Tsuang, Winokur and Crowe 1980). When compared with morbidity risks for diseases that show a dominant or recessive pattern of transmission, such as Huntington's disease and cystic fibrosis, where linkage strategies have been spectacularly successful, the rates for schizophrenia itself are far too low to afford the needed power to conduct similar traditional linkage studies. The strategy in the case of diseases with a low recurrence risk rate like schizophrenia is to try to broaden the phenotype to include traits that have a higher recurrence risk. This is the rationale for our use of eye tracking dysfunctions as a pleiotropic expression of schizophrenia (Matthysse, Holzman and Lange 1986; Matthysse and Parnas 1992).

Conclusions

The most striking symptoms of schizophrenia are among those that have eluded our research grasp for so long. Here I have argued that first steps in the effort to probe the essence of the thought disorder must begin by describing it in a heuristic manner and then subject the processes we have identified to simpler processes that themselves can be referred to central nervous system processes that will yield information about how tangled thoughts come about. In this effort, I have argued that the basic phenomenon is a thought disorder and not a language or a speech disorder. With the use of the TDI, my colleagues and I identified different kinds of thought disorder, some of which characterize schizophrenic thinking and some manic thinking. I have presented several examples of research stemming from inquiries into thought disorder. These research examples, in turn, require systematic reduction to their simpler components, which then can be related to the ways in which the brain processes information, thus making the subject of formal thought disorder available to the powerful, new tools of contemporary cognitive neuroscience and of genetics.

Notes

1 This biological view of schizophrenia and its associated disorder of thinking should not be construed as antithetical to a more conflict-based theory of these same phenomena, such as that offered by Professor Sidney Blatt. Discussion of the congruencies and differences between these points of view requires and deserves more than the space allotted to this contribution. It is noteworthy that Freud reserved a biological basis for the dynamic psychological processes included within psychoanalytic theory (see, e.g., Freud 1914, p. 78, as only one instance of his view that "all of our provisional ideas in psychology will presumably some day be based on an organic substructure.").
2 "Recurrence risk" denotes the percentage of biological relatives (here the reference is to first-degree relatives) of a person with schizophrenia who, themselves, are clinically schizophrenic.

References

Barta, P. E., Pearlson, G. D., Powers, R. E., Richards, S. S., and Tune, L. E. (1990) 'Auditory hallucinations and smaller superior temporal gyral volume in schizophrenia', *American Journal of Psychiatry* 147: 1457–62.

Chapman, L. J. and Chapman, J. P. (1973) *Disordered Thought in Schizophrenia*, New York: Appleton Century Crofts.

—— —— and Daut, R. L. (1976) 'Schizophrenic inability to disattend from strong aspects of meaning', *Journal of Abnormal Psychology* 85: 35–40.

—— —— and Raulin, M. L. (1978) 'Body-image aberration in schizophrenia', *Journal of Abnormal Psychology* 87: 399–407.

Chomsky, N. (1969) *The Acquisition of Syntax in Children from 5 to 10*, Cambridge, MA: MIT Press.

Coleman, M. J., Carpenter, J. T., Waternaux, C., Levy, D. L., Shenton, M. E., Perry, J., Medoff, D. and Holzman, P. S. (1993) 'The Thought Disorder Index: a reliability study', *Psychological Assessment* 3: 336–42.

Cruse, D. A. (1986) *Lexical Semantics*, Cambridge, England: Cambridge University Press.

Freud, S. (1914) 'On narcissism: An introduction', in J. Strachey (ed. and trans.) *The Standard Edition of the Complete Psychological Works of Sigmund Freud* vol. 14, London: Hogarth Press, pp. 69–102.

Heider, F. (1959) 'On perception, event structure, and the psychological environment', *Psychological Issues*, 1 (Whole No. 3).

Holzman, P. S., Coleman, M. J., Levy, D. L. and Lenzenweger, M. F. (1996) 'Thought disorder, perceptual aberrations, and schizotypy', *Journal of Abnormal Psychology* 105: 469–73.

—— Proctor, L. R., Levy, D. L., Yasillo, N. J., Meltzer, H. Y. and Hurt, S. W. (1974) 'Eye tracking dysfunctions in schizophrenic patients and their relatives', *Archives of General Psychiatry* 31: 143–51.

Hunt, W. A. and Walker, R. E. (1966) 'Schizophrenics' judgments of schizophrenic test responses', *Journal of Clinical Psychology* 22: 118–20.

Hurt, S. S., Holzman, P. S. and Davis, J. M. (1983) 'Thought disorder: the measurement of its changes', *Archives of General Psychiatry* 40: 1281–5.

Johnston, M. H. and Holzman, P. S. (1979) *Assessing Schizophrenic Thinking*, San Francisco: Jossey-Bass.

Kestnbaum Daniels, E., Shenton, M. E., Holzman, P. S., Benowitz, L. I., Coleman, M. J., Levin, S. and Levine, D. (1988) 'Patterns of thought disorder associated with right cortical damage, schizophrenia, and mania', *American Journal of Psychiatry* 145: 944–9.

Kety, S. S., Rosenthal, D. and Wender, P. H. (1978) 'Genetic relationships within the schizophrenia spectrum: evidence from adoption studies', in R. L. Spitzer and D. F. Klein (eds) *Critical Issues in Psychiatric Diagnosis*, New York: Raven Press, pp. 213–23.

—— —— —— and Schulsinger, F. (1976) 'Studies based on a total sample of adopted individuals and their relatives: why they were necessary, what they demonstrated and failed to demonstrate', *Schizophrenia Bulletin* 2: 413–28.

Makowski, D. G., Waternaux, C., Lajonchere, C., Dicker, R., Smoke, N.,

Koplewicz, H., Min, D., Mendell, N. R. and Levy, D. L. (1997) 'Thought disorder in adolescent onset schizophrenia', *Schizophrenia Research* 23: 147–65.

Matthysse, S. (1987) 'Schizophrenic thought disorder: a model-theoretic perspective', *Schizophrenia Bulletin* 13: 173–84.

—— Holzman, P. S. and Lange, K. (1986) 'The genetic transmission of schizophrenia: application of Mendelian latent structure analysis to eye tracking dysfunctions in schizophrenia and affective disorder', *Journal of Psychiatric Research* 20: 57–65.

—— Levy, D. L., Wu, Y., Rubin, D. B. and Holzman, P. S. (1999) 'Modeling intermittent degradation in schizophrenic performance', *Schizophrenia Research* 40: 131–46.

—— and Parnas, J. (1992) 'Extending the phenotype of schizophrenia: implications for linkage analysis', *Journal of Psychiatric Research* 26: 329–44.

Park, S., Holzman, P. S. and Goldman-Rakic, P. S. (1995) 'Spatial working memory deficits in the relatives of schizophrenic patients', *Archives of General Psychiatry* 52: 821–8.

Rapaport, D., Gill, M. M. and Schafer, R. (1945–6) *Diagnostic Psychological Testing*, Chicago, IL: Yearbook Publishers.

—— —— —— (1968) *Diagnostic Psychological Testing*, (rev. edn, ed. R. R. Holt), New York: International Universities Press.

Rosch, E. (1973) 'On the internal structure of internal and semantic categories', in T. E. Moore (ed.) *Cognitive Development and the Acquisition of Language*, New York: Academic Press, pp. 111–44.

Shenton, M. E., Kikinis, R., Jolesz, F. A., Pollak, S., LeMay, M., Wible, C. G., Hokama, H., Martin, J., Metcalf, D., Coleman, M. and McCarley, R. W. (1992) 'Abnormalities of the left temporal lobe and thought disorder in schizophrenia', *New England Journal of Medicine* 327: 604–12.

—— Solovay, M. R. and Holzman, P. S. (1987) 'Comparative studies of thought disorder: 2. schizoaffective disorder', *Archives of General Psychiatry* 44: 21–30.

Solovay, M. R., Shenton, M. E. and Holzman, P. S. (1987) 'Comparative studies of thought disorder: 1. mania and schizophrenia', *Archives of General Psychiatry* 44: 13–20.

Titone, D., Levy, D. L. and Holzman, P. S. (2000) 'Contextual insensitivity in schizophrenic language processing: evidence from lexical ambiguity', *Journal of Abnormal Psychology* 109: 761–7.

Tsuang, M. T., Winokur, G. and Crowe, R. R. (1980) 'Morbidity risks of schizophrenia and affective disorders among first degree relatives of patients with schizophrenia, mania, depression and surgical conditions', *British Journal of Psychiatry* 137: 497–504.

Vuchetich, J. P., Levy, D. L., Holzman, P. S., Perlt, D., Parnas, J. and Matthysse, S. (2001) 'Evidence for a major gene effect on thought disorder in schizophrenia pedigrees', *Schizophrenia Research* 49: 79.

Watkins, J. G. and Stauffacher, J. C. (1952) 'An index of pathological thinking in the Rorschach', *Journal of Projective Techniques* 16: 276–86.

Part IV

Psychotherapy and the treatment process

Some reflections on the therapeutic action of psychoanalytic therapy[1]

Peter Fonagy and Mary Target

Sidney Blatt deserves several Festschrifts. His stature in the field is almost unique. His capacity to bridge the world of Yale psychology (one of the most highly cited departments of psychology in the world) and the world of psychoanalysis leaves all of us with a brilliantly lighted path to follow. In this tribute to his work, we will look at some of our ideas on the nature of therapeutic change, a topic to which Sid devoted considerable attention throughout his career. His pivotal paper with Behrends (Blatt and Behrends 1987) has been a guiding inspiration in our pursuit of a developmental model of psychic change. His most recent writings with Ken Levy (Levy and Blatt 1999; Levy, Blatt, and Shaver 1998) on attachment and with John Auerbach on self-reflexivity (Auerbach and Blatt 1996, 2001) have brought us particularly close. His paper with Blass on attachment and separateness (Blatt and Blass 1990) has helped many in the field to organize their ideas about developmental psychoanalytic approaches and was one of the core influences on our recent monograph (Fonagy and Target 2003). We have had the opportunity to work with Sid as a teacher, and his work in that context, as we suspect in the clinical, is a masterly bridging of the dialectic interaction between the two developmental lines, attachment and separateness, to which he has drawn attention. He is able at once to provide impetus for independence while offering himself as generously as any teacher ever has, as a resource, as an example, and as an ideal. We have learned an enormous amount from Sid Blatt, from his writings, but even more from his approach to his subject matter, characterized by commitment, dignity, enthusiasm, open-mindedness and generosity. He has given all of us so much and deserves so much more than we are able to give him in return.

It would be a brave or foolhardy person who would announce a definitive model of therapeutic action. In this chapter, we shall present a personal heuristic that helps *us* understand how patients progress through psychoanalytic treatment. Obviously, it is our hope that the distinctions identified may be useful beyond providing signposts to everyday clinical work, but the basic objective is not one of adding a new theory to an already overburdened literature. Rather, it is to link characteristic aspects of change to phases of an analytic process and to distinguish some putative psychological components of the process of change in psychoanalysis that might be helpful in our attempts at defining with greater rigor what a psychoanalytic process is.

We shall distinguish three types of psychic change linked to each other loosely across the course of treatment, each working through a focus on the relationship with the therapist. They are: (a) intersubjective shifts, (b) changes of mental processes, and (c) changes in mental representations. To illustrate these three types of change, we would like to introduce a patient whom one of us[2] saw in analysis some years ago: Mr. A.

Introducing Mr. A

Mr. A started his analysis in a rage of which Kohut (1972) himself would have been proud. The couch was invented to humiliate and belittle people who needed help. The analyst's silence was a deliberate mockery. My talking about "working together" on his problems was a calculated insult. I wanted to work "on him" or more likely "in him." Working with him suggested a partnership that was clearly a million miles from his perception of my intention in recommending the couch. His assessment with Professor X had been civilized and urbane, whilst he could tell that I was a second-rater who lived in the shadows of great men. The paper tissue on the pillow provided a magnet around which the iron filings of his shame and sense of being ridiculed were all aligned. Did I think that he would infect my other patients? Did I think he had head lice? Or, even worse, did I delude myself into some pathetic medical identity by the pretense of sterile conditions?

I knew nothing about Mr. A at this stage, except that he was 32 and well to do. The referral was from a very senior colleague who had seen and liked him and who had pressured me to take him, sight unseen. He came late for his initial interview and said very little about his background, except that his childhood had led to his suffering from anxiety and depression and that he frequently felt an overwhelming sense of inadequacy in competitive relationships with other men.

I was relatively inexperienced; who was I to say that Professor X was wrong in suggesting that Mr. A would be a good case for me to learn to work independently as an analyst. In fact, I recall feeling extremely grateful to my senior colleague after the referral. By the end of Mr. A's first session, however, I was extremely angry with both Mr. A and my senior colleague. In fact I had a formulation. My senior colleague had exactly the same narcissistic problems as Mr. A, so naturally he saw him as a charming man. I would have been happy to leave them both to enjoy the other's company.

For the best part of a whole year of five times weekly analysis, Mr. A kept me in such a furious state. I managed some interpretive work with him, but I found it hard to keep my wish to punish him at bay. One Friday session he was particularly boastful, listing the properties he owned and suggesting that my consulting room could be moved, with advantage, to one of his large houses, which was situated in a neighborhood where many successful psychiatrists practiced. I managed an interpretation about him wanting me close to him over the weekend and also under his control, so he could avoid the humiliation of having to miss me. In response, he assured me that, if that had indeed been his intention, then he would simply have bought the house I was in. But in reality, he was quite fed up with my monotonous whining, was grateful for the respite, and had considered extending it by taking an unscheduled break early the coming week. I persisted in what I realized at the time to be an easily deflected approach. "You are frightened of the helplessness which allowing yourself to become attached to someone faces you with. You don't need to have complete control and buy this house as long as you can arrange to come and go as you please." He responded, hitting hard: "Look, if you could afford to buy this house, then you would not be renting one of its shabbiest rooms. Just because you can't, there is no point in your getting irritated, just because you know I could."

This kind of repartee was typical of my work with him. Working on his experiences in the here and now came naturally to Mr. A, as there appeared to be few people besides himself in whom he was interested. I began to think of him as Teflon man because none of my attempts to reach him appeared to stick. I repeatedly tried to address his sense of shame and vulnerability, which, I believed, partly motivated his defensive behavior. He seemed unable to hear my comments and often, quite rudely, would start talking in the middle of carefully sculptured interventions. He would make me feel alternately enfeebled and angry, and at some level, I was deeply puzzled as to why he was coming.

At this point, I should explain Mr. A's relevance to a discourse on therapeutic action because it is clear little useful analytic work was being done. The challenge that Mr. A set psychoanalytic scholarship, going far beyond my shabby consulting room, was the improvement in his personal happiness and relationships that accompanied our attempt at starting a psychoanalytic process. By the end of treatment, his depression disappeared, his anxieties receded, his collaboration with his male colleagues, including his competitors, improved; he even started what sounded like a reasonable relationship with a woman who was his equal – a radical change from his previous attachments to prostitutes or to the uneducated women he had described as "scrubbers." We would speculate that cases of unaccountable improvement, such as Mr. A, are perhaps more common than psychoanalytic reports of successful treatments might lead us to suspect. But even if there were just one Mr. A, the benefit he gained from his less than adequate treatment might justify scrutiny.

Outcome and process aims

One approach to such a case, perhaps most characteristic of the French school of psychoanalysis, might be that symptomatic improvement is a largely irrelevant aspect of the therapeutic action of psychoanalysis. However, already in 1965, Wallerstein noted that, whilst analysts adopted a therapeutic stance that Bion (1967) later characterized as without memory or desire, behind this lay the dramatic ambition fundamentally to alter the patient's personality organization. A lack of concern with clinical outcome seems curious at a time when evidence-based medicine (Kerridge, Lowe and Henry 1998; Sackett *et al.* 1996) is forcing all mental health practitioners to state their therapeutic goals and the expected outcome of their interventions.

Our position is that it is inappropriate to dismiss symptomatic improvement as irrelevant, particularly because most patients come with precisely this concern. It should also be acknowledged, however, that Mr. A's analysis, despite considerable symptomatic improvement, categorically failed to achieve any of the ambitious goals that psychoanalytic authors have specified. These are normally termed *process aims* and are to be distinguished from *outcome aims* (Kennedy and Moran 1991). What the experience with Mr. A appeared to demonstrate was that process and outcome aims of psychoanalytic therapy were at best loosely coupled and at worst unrelated to one another. Yet if our theory of pathology is to be considered truly comprehensive, improvements that are not specific to the psychoanalytic experience should be accommodated as readily as those changes that we believe ourselves to have instigated. I believe the concept of *intersubjective shifts* accounts for some of these cases of unexplained improvement.

Intersubjective shifts

The lack of a stable sense of self is a central difficulty for narcissistic patients, particularly at the borderline end of this spectrum. By contrast, reflective function is essential to self-organization (Fonagy *et al.* 2002). Reflective function, we believe, is the psychological process that maintains our *intentional stance* – Dennett's (1978) phrase for the interpretation of behavior in terms of underlying mental states (beliefs, desires, wishes, feelings, thoughts, etc.). The symbolic representation of mental states may be seen as a prerequisite for a sense of identity; they form the core of a sense of psychological self (see Figure 12.1a). As Cavell (1993) has thoughtfully demonstrated, self-knowing self-states do not arise intrinsically from within the mind. They are internalized from the other who knows and mirrors the self. At the core of all our selves, then, is an image our object created of us as intentional beings (see Figure 12.1b). For example, Gergely and Watson's (1996) theory of the development of affective understanding posits that infants' understanding of their own emotional experience depends on contingent, marked mirroring by the mother. Infants understand what they are feeling by looking at the mother's face and seeing the emotion there that they feel. They know that they, and not mother, feel it because the mother marks her expression of the affect, clearly designating it as not "real." Recently Auerbach and Blatt (2001) have also advanced the notion that attunement of the caregiver to the infant creates an experience of intersubjectivity that, in normal development, helps in integrating transitional fantasy with realistic cognition.

In Mr. A's case, parental self-absorption probably precluded the development of an authentic, organic self-image built around internalized representations of self-states. His mother was the only parent of any adult patient I have treated who attempted to come to her son's sessions. One day, she simply turned up at the reception desk of my consulting rooms. The receptionist, accustomed to the peculiarities of a psychoanalytic practice, phoned my office in confusion, saying: "Oh, Peter, I don't know what to do! A Mrs. A is here, determined to see you. She says you have her child in treatment. She can't mean Mr. A, can she?" My curiosity drove me downstairs to meet her. When denied access to my consulting room, she insisted on telling me in the hallway about her failed third marriage, which in her view was undoubtedly upsetting her son. I had to draw on all the reserves my analytic training had equipped me with to maintain what passed for neutrality and yet assert the privacy of Mr. A's analytic treatment.

If, as indeed we suspect was the case for Mr. A, the maternal object is unable or unwilling to reflect the child's internal state, or projects her own internal state onto the child, intentional states will not be symbolically bound, and the developmental basis of the self-structure will be absent (see Figure 12.1c). Thus, Koós and Gergely (2001) found that babies whose attachment will be disorganized at 12 months are more likely to look at themselves in the mirror than at their mothers at six months of age, when these two are offered as alternatives. The weakness of a self-image not reinforced by adequate mirroring leaves the child with affect that remains unlabeled and confusing – presumably what Bion (1962) considered unmetabolized or uncontained. The building blocks of reflective function, mentalized self-states, are absent. The turmoil that results will make the child even more desperate to seek closeness, to find some organizing structure for his affect, in whatever form this might be available. The child will be willing to take in reflections from the object that do not map onto anything within his own experience. This will lead to the internalization of representations of the parent's state, rather than of a usable version of the child's own experience. Such internalizations create an *alien experience within the self* that is based on representations of the other within the self. There may be similarities here to the "alien objects" that Britton (1998) has described on the basis of clinical work with patients such as these.

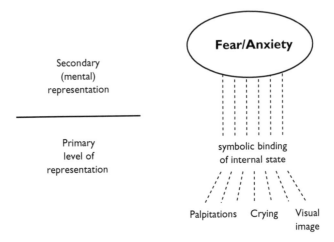

Figure 12.1a   The experience of emotion, such as fear or anxiety, is a second-order representation of the primary representations of constitutional self-states

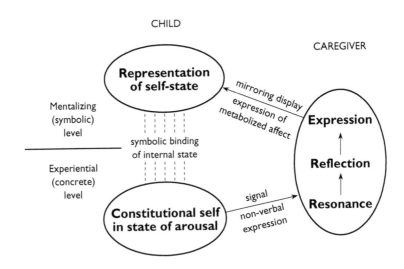

Figure 12.1b   Constitutional self-states are symbolically bound by the internalization of the object's mirroring displays

Self-representation and childhood neglect

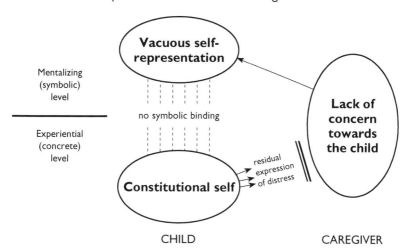

Figure 12.1c   In cases of neglect or abuse, the secondary representation of self-states is not created, and affects are perceived as unmetabolized self states

Figure 12.1   A schematic representation of the development of the experience of affect
Source: Based on Gergely and Watson, 1996

Once internalized, the alien presence interferes with the relationship between thought and identity: Ideas or feelings are experienced as one's own that do not seem to belong to the self. The alien self destroys the coherence of self or identity, a coherence that the intentional stance demands. The experience of consistency can be restored only by constant and intense projection. There is ample evidence for this process in the attachment literature. Children with a history of disorganized attachment to the parent have been shown to develop a pattern of controlling behavior towards their attachment figures. I believe that what we are seeing here is the child's desperately projecting the alien parts of the self back into the parent, forcing the parent to enact the feelings that create incongruence within the child's self-structure. Understanding this process is vital clinically because, in contrast to the neurotic case, the projection is motivated not by superego pressures but by the need to reestablish the continuity of self-experience.

People like Mr. A are reachable, we believe, only at the moment when their externalization of the alien other is felt to be complete. It is this externalization process, and the window of opportunity it offers, that we refer to as an intersubjective shift. The difficulty is that these are not the

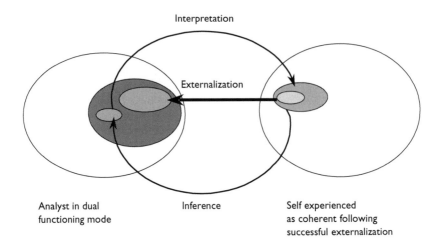

Interpretation

Externalization

Analyst in dual   Inference   Self experienced
functioning mode   as coherent following
                                            successful externalization

Figure 12.2   The process of changing intersubjective representational shifts. The
analyst needs to see and create a coherent representation of the patient's
"true-self" beyond, but concurrently with, countertransference
enactments

moments when one is likely to function effectively as an analyst. Bateman
(1998) described the same phenomenon sensitively in the context of
Rosenfeld's (1964) distinction between thick-skinned and thin-skinned
narcissistic personalities and argued that narcissistic individuals alternate
between thick-skinned (derogatory and grandiose) and thin-skinned
(vulnerable and self-loathing) states. He shows that interpretive work can
be done with such patients only at the dangerous moments when they are
in movement from one state to the other. We think that what Bateman
describes is the successful externalization of the alien self (the derogatory
or self-hating self). The externalization of the persecutory object within the
self leaves the patient able to listen and even experience concern. If we look
at them in the context of an attachment relationship, such patients adopt
the caregiving component of the *controlling-caregiving* pattern referred to
above. Having externalized the alien part of the self, into the parent, they
can then try to look after it, still in a very bossy and controlling way. The
analyst, faced with a more sophisticated version of this process, needs to
be in a dual functioning mode, to infer and create a coherent representation of the patient's true self, separate from but concurrently with any
countertransference enactment (see Figure 12.2). However, this is where
therapy often fails, because as soon as patients hear anything other than
what they projected onto the analytic object, they must once again be
on the alert. They might be risking the return of the laboriously ejected
introject.

Changes in mental processes and the recovery of reflective function

Strangely, whilst psychoanalysts have long recognized that all mind is representation, they have been curiously uninterested in the mechanisms that generate and organize these: mental processes. Mental representations are the products of mental processes; a mental process is the violin from which the melody of mental representation originates.

The notion that mental processes are as vulnerable to the vicissitudes of conflict as mental representation is implicit in many psychoanalytic writings. We believe that patients with severe personality disorder inhibit one particular aspect of the normal development of mental processes – their reflective function (Fonagy and Target 1997). This is the psychological process that maintains our intentional stance. Patients with inhibited reflective function have little reliable access to an accurate picture of their own mental experiences, their representational worlds. In intense relationships that reevoke the attachment context, they inhibit the capacity to recognize thoughts and feelings, instead responding to them within one of two early modes of experience of psychic reality: *psychic equivalence*, in which internal states are mapped onto external reality and assumed to reflect it faithfully, or *pretend*, in which all states of mind are treated as completely separate from everyday reality. They either are gripped by thoughts, as though they were reality, or experience them as utterly inconsequential. Without the capacity to mentalize, they are unable to take a step back and to respond flexibly and adaptively to the symbolic, meaningful qualities of other people's behavior. Instead, they find themselves caught in fixed patterns of attribution, rigid stereotypes of response, nonsymbolic, instrumental use of affect – mental patterns that are not amenable to either reflection or modulation. They inhibit their capacity to think about thoughts and feelings in themselves and in others, prototypically as an adaptation to severe or chronic maltreatment.

Mr. A, as a vulnerable child, confronted with an undoubtedly intrusive and probably extremely self-preoccupied mother, could not bear to develop a coherent image of his own mental state that could have served as the basis for an understanding of others. Although apparently somewhat reflective, his rigidity betrayed his incapacity truly to reason with mental states. The rigidity that imbued his representational world was one of the most striking aspects of Mr. A's treatment. His tendency to hold on to a specific point of view went far beyond that which might be associated with habitual patterns of defense. Like other patients, Mr. A organized the analytic relationship to conform to his unconscious expectations. But, for Mr. A, these expectations were experienced with the full force of reality, and alternative ways of viewing things were either dismissed out of hand or entered into in superficial and meaningless ways. Equally striking was that a lack of consistency between representations apparently caused little distress. The object, cherished as the source of salvation one day, could become the source of damnation the next. And thus his entire representational system seemed both in constant flux and immutable to lasting change.

Britton's (1995) distinction between *knowledge* and *belief* is helpful here. Mr. A did not *believe* in his superiority – he *knew* it. Belief entails uncertainty and the knowledge that a mental state is just a way of constructing experience, not reality itself. Mr. A's knowledge, however, existed only when reinforced by an external reality. He would constantly seek evidence and assurances of his superiority, which having been obtained almost immediately became valueless and effectively nonexistent. More evidence would be demanded. The mere state of knowledge had no permanence; as with infants, his sense of himself was ephemeral. He lived in a world of psychic equivalence (Fonagy 1995; Fonagy and Target 1996; Target and Fonagy 1996), where he believed whatever he thought actually did exist in the physical world. And all that existed in the physical world, Mr. A had certain knowledge of. Although this is perhaps normal for the child of three or four, the persistence of the psychic equivalence mode of relating is a major complication in the establishment of normal object relations. The perception of a reaction in the other is tantamount to its presence, without room for doubt, uncertainty and thus the possibility of alternative understandings.

It is psychic equivalence that reveals the alien self. Normally, mentalized self-narratives obscure the discontinuities of self-organization. Mr. A's intersubjective shifts were triggered by his inability to integrate his alien self-states into a coherent narrative. Forcing the analyst to enact remained the only route to the experience of self-coherence. The psychic equivalence mode of functioning precludes normal interpretative analytic work. Beyond the usual conceptualization of resistance, the requirement of isomorphism between internal and external leaves no room for an alternative analytic perspective. This formulation of course begs the question of how change may be achieved. In our view, change can happen solely through the revival of reflective function.

What brings about change in reflective function?

Mr. A did eventually show change in terms of process aims (his reflective function), as well as outcome aims (feeling better outside analysis). Change was slow and was clearly marked by an initial worsening of his depression as he became increasingly aware of undesirable aspects of his personality. There was no specific point that could be marked with the prefix of "turning." No clever interpretations were made that could be singled out as delivering the change. Yet there was change, perhaps most noticeable in the change of atmosphere of the sessions. After three years of hard work, it became possible to talk with Teflon man.

The ongoing discussions on therapeutic action have generally acknowledged that the psychic change in individuals who manifest developmental deviations, impairments, deficits, or underlying structural deficiencies fits poorly with the neurotic model of therapeutic action. From the late 1970s, many writers have shifted the emphasis from structural change as the focus of therapeutic action to the transaction between patient and analyst as a curative experience and to the early mother–child relationship as the most appropriate analogue for the therapeutic encounter. Developmental processes are invoked by those who link therapeutic action to the holding environment (Modell 1976), separation-individuation (Blatt and Behrends 1987; Stolorow and Lachmann 1978), a sense of union with the primary object (Loewald 1979), social referencing (Viederman 1991), empathy (Emde 1990), or other aspects of developmental processes (Goodman 1977; Schlessinger and Robbins 1983). Recently, Blatt and Auerbach (2000) discussed the complexities of a naïve developmental view in attempting to understand long-term therapeutic change, its quantity, its quality and the patient's resistance.

These developmental models cannot give a satisfactory account of therapeutic action with the difficult patient. Abrams (1990) makes the obvious point that the developmental sequences in psychoanalysis and the biological constraints imposed on normal development make for discrepancies that should invalidate the developmental metaphor. Mayes and Spence (1994) make the important but counterintuitive observation that the developmental metaphor applies more to relatively well-endowed adults who historically probably had the benefit of the kind of caregiving experiences that reemerge in the transference, whilst the group of patients with whom these metaphors are most often used simply do not have the capacities that might make the developmental metaphor applicable.

So what was it that caused a shift in Mr. A's psychic reality? We do not believe there is a single answer to this question. We believe that reflective processes are enhanced by work in the transference, work that highlights differences in perspective between self and other. The transference also focuses the patient on the analyst's mental state as he tries to conceive of the patient's beliefs and desires. The repeated experience of finding himself in the mind of his therapist not only enhances self-representation but also removes the patient's fear of looking. Believing, as opposed to knowing, now allows uncertainty, rather than reliance on rigidity, and ultimately allows vulnerability, from which grandiosity can only afford momentary protection.

In what we believe to be an appropriate use of the developmental metaphor, the analyst performs the function of the object who enters into the child's pretend play, creating a transitional sphere of relatedness. Here hard to bear thoughts and emotions may be played with while also experienced as real; the phobic avoidance of mentalization gradually and tentatively gives way to reflective function. More generally, a degree of flexibility and mutual adaptation is required between patient and analyst. The principal aim of the process must be to make the world of feelings and ideas safe for the patient.

Optimally, the patient's mental work recapitulates that of the analyst. The analyst's thinking, even if initially neither understood nor appreciated by the patient, continually challenges the patient's mind, stimulating a need to conceive of ideas in new ways. What is crucial, then, is the active engagement of one mind with another, inconceivable without empathy, holding, and containment. In our view, attachment to the therapist is the necessary condition that permits the mental proximity that is the essential precondition for this type of change. Yet none of these is directly responsible for the therapeutic action. This leads us on to discussion of our third concept – representational change.

Representational change

It is only when mental processes have been to some measure freed that change in representational structure is possible. Technically, this is a key stumbling block for beginning clinicians who understandably aim to modify specific representations as soon as their insights permit.

Mr. A's analysis illustrates representational change. As the analysis progressed, his picture of himself in dreams gradually shifted from an empty palace of the beginning of the analysis to a frightened mouse in its third year and, two years later, at the end of the analysis, to a man with a physical handicap. Perhaps most striking was the way his images of past figures were revised. He had almost never discussed his parents in his analysis in the first year without denigration but in the second year discovered his father as someone he admired for his tenacity and fair-mindedness. A frequently recalled episode where he had felt humiliated and ridiculed by a grandfather who had played a trick on him gradually took on a far more benign coloring. He now experienced this episode as illustrating the man's wish to surprise and tease him, rather than mock and humiliate.

We could summarize such representational changes under three categories:

1   Self, object, and relationship representations acquired enhanced integrity and coherence.
2   Person representations were increasingly seen in relationship to one another, rather than as isolated figures. Ultimately Mr. A could talk about father and mother as having a marriage in which each parent had a separate mind, with feelings and ideas.

3   Finally, totally new object representations emerged. We may say that
    Mr. A's representational system was restructured so that previously
    isolated, incompatible and unelaborated representations of the mental
    states of self and object ceased to be pathogens.

By creating and elaborating a mental world for his internal objects, these
could change from part objects to whole structures. Understanding the
other in mental state terms requires integrating assumed intentions in a
coherent manner. The initial solution for the child, given the imperative to
arrive at coherent object representations, is to split the representation of the
other into several coherent subsets of intentions (Gergely 1997), primarily
an idealized identity and a persecutory one. Splitting enables the individual
to create mentalized images of others, but these are inaccurate and oversimplified and allow for only an illusion of mentalized interpersonal interchange. Further development of reflective function normally leads to an
integration of these partial representations. The hopelessness of this task in
the face of a deficit in reflective capacity may be seen as the direct cause
of the permanent fragmentation of the internal world of such patients.
The recovery of reflective function, and its active use within the analysis,
enabled Mr. A to integrate his representations, so that his objects could
have conflicted motives and yet retain their coherence.

What brings about representational change?

What aspect of psychoanalysis brings about these changes in representational structure? It is widely recognized that insight is not enough and that
something akin to Loewald's (1960) real object is necessary to explain
change. The primacy of the verbal in psychoanalysis has obscured the
appreciation that representational structures change not only through
insight but also through the experience of the other with the self, whether
the other is speaking or not.

The dichotomy between interpretive insight on the one hand and
relationship-generated change on the other, however, is probably false
(Blatt and Behrends 1987). It is based on a confusion of means and ends.
Verbal communications by the analyst may change representational
structures in the patient's mind, and we may, if we wish, talk of such
changes as insight as long as the term is restricted to the mental states that
are experienced as motivating behavior in self and other. However, as has
become increasingly accepted (Fonagy et al. 1993), the new relationship
with the analyst, as much as interpretations, readily leads to psychic change
via the modification of representational structures. We know from infant
research that, as we observe the behavior of another, even from our earliest
days, we automatically interpret, infer mental states, and restructure and
potentially enrich our representations of how we see self and other

interacting (Gergely and Watson 1996; Stern 1998). By analogy, the patient observing the analyst is not simply unthinkingly internalizing an experience; what patients benefit from are the constant inferences that they make about the analyst's internal world. The perception of the analyst as having empathy (Emde 1990) or healing intentions (Stone 1961) may bring about changes in object representations through the same mechanism of change as interpretations. Thus there is no clear dividing line between interpretation and new relationship as the means by which therapeutic change is achieved.

So our brief answer to the question, is it the relationship or is it the interpretation, would be, "It is both."

What changes in representational change?

Schematic models of therapeutic change (Abrams 1987; Joffe and Sandler 1969; Sandler and Joffe 1969) attribute therapeutic action to changes in long-term memory that underpin the representational system. However, it seems fair to say that, although the aims of psychoanalysis (Sandler and Dreher 1997) have been greatly elaborated since Freud's original model of undoing repression and recovering memory into consciousness (Breuer and Freud 1895), these advances have not brought with them an updating of the role of memory in the therapeutic process.

Solms and Turnbull (2002) have argued that infantile amnesia is a function not of repression but of the immaturity of the neural structures underpinning autobiographical memory before four years of age. But if infants do not have autobiographical memory, does this mean that early experience has no impact on us? There is now overwhelming evidence that there are at least two forms of memory. Relational experiences during the period of infantile amnesia are remembered in an implicit, procedural way.

We have described before (Fonagy 1999) the distinction cognitive science (Cohen 1984; Cohen and Squire 1980) now makes between two memory systems, both of which have important functions in psychoanalytic treatment. *Declarative* or *explicit memory* is involved with the conscious retrieval of information about the past whereas the *procedural* or *implicit* memory system contains the kind of content-independent information that is involved in acquiring general skills like playing the piano or driving. Declarative memory relates to remembering events and information. The aspect of declarative memory that we, as analysts, have been most concerned with is autobiographical memory, high in self-reference and frequently accompanied by personal interpretation (Conway 1996).

Clyman (1991) was perhaps the first to suggest explicitly adopting the distinction between procedural and declarative memory for use within psychoanalytic models of normal and pathological development. He proposed that the procedural, rather than the declarative, memory system may be involved in the transmission of early experience into adult personality.

Even earlier, Crittenden (1990) suggested that Bowlby's notion of internal working models may be best understood in terms of procedural knowledge. More recently, a group of psychoanalysts working in Boston, including Daniel Stern, Ed Tronick, Karlen Lyons-Ruth, Alexander Morgan and Alexie Harrison, have been working intensively to integrate the concept of procedural memory with ideas about the therapeutic process (Stern 1998).

In agreement with these authors, we believe that experiences contributing to internal representations of object relationships are not, by and large, stored in declarative memory. The extent to which episodes of interaction with the caregiver may be remembered (encoded and stored in auto-biographical memory) may be incidental in the development of internal representations of relationships. What lies at the root of interpersonal problems, the transference relationship, and quite possibly all aspects of the personality that we loosely denote with the term unconscious, is a set of procedures or implicit memories of interactional experience. These may be represented as self–other-affect triads, as Otto Kernberg (1988) has suggested, as a network of unconscious expectations, as Bowlby (1988) conceived, or simply as emergent properties of the nervous system that abstract invariant information through the tendency of neurons to survive together if activated together (Edelman 1987; Stern 1994). They are generic memories or scripts (Nelson 1993) where the child's predominant experience of a relationship is retained. Individual experiences that have contributed to this mental model may or may not be stored elsewhere, but in either case, the model is now autonomous, no longer dependent on the experiences that have contributed to it. The models exist noncon-sciously as procedures that organize interpersonal behavior but are not consciously accessible to the individual unless attention is specifically directed to them.

So where is therapeutic action – in procedural (implicit) memory or in declarative (autobiographical) memory? In our view, memories of past experience can no longer be considered relevant to therapeutic action. Psychic change occurs as a function of a shift of emphasis between different mental models of relationship; this change leads to a change in the pro-cedures one uses in living with oneself and with others. Hence, therapeutic action is predominantly in the procedural memory system, rather than in relatively superficial changes in autobiographical memory. The term superficial is used advisedly here because, it is our contention, experiences constructed in autobiographical memory are more likely to be inaccurate than accurate. Undoubtedly, recovered autobiographical memories will contain the essence of a wide range of events, distilled into a configuration represented within that mental model. In that sense, the autobiographical memory is true. It is true to the model of a particular experience-of-being-with (Stern 1994). However, such a model may be profoundly distorted by fantasies and other intrapsychic experiences. The recovered memory is the outcome not of an undoing of repression but rather of a process of active construction.

In other words, analysands work backwards, pulling together elements of early experience consistent with freshly discovered perceptions of themselves in relation to others. It is not surprising, then, that memories from adolescence and latency will dominate a patient's material despite our conviction that earlier experiences were the formative ones. The mental model uncovered by the patient in analysis is likely to have been generated by early experiences that antedate the development of autobiographical memory and therefore will never be retrieved.

Of course, it is also possible that just as procedural memory may activate specific elements within the autobiographical memory system, so might newly found awareness of a particular experience influence the way an individual experiences himself or herself in relation to others. However, the patient's recovery of an autobiographical memory, like the analyst's delivery of a single interpretation, is highly unlikely in itself to be enough to facilitate change without the accompanying context of a reshaping of a way-of-experiencing-the-other. Conversely, given the neurophysiological evidence that the emotional charge associated with experiences stored subcortically cannot change without cortical involvement (LeDoux 1995), bringing such implicit structures of self–other relationships into conscious focus through the exploration of memories, transference dynamics, and interpretations seems not only desirable but arguably a critical component of therapeutic action.

Bringing it all together

We have outlined three modes of psychic change that may occur in psychoanalytic treatment. These three modes may be differentiated on at least four levels (see Table 12.1): (a) their descriptions; (b) the particular mental processes the analyst will aim to engage in each case; (c) the respective impact that each mode will have on symptomatology; and (d) the techniques that are most pertinent to accomplish the analyst's process aims in that phase of treatment.

Initially, in the treatment of personality disordered individuals, we are most likely to encounter intersubjective shifts. Descriptively, these are defensive strategies that enable the patient to establish coherent self-states by externalizing alien parts of the self onto the therapist. From the point of view of infant research, we can recognize these as flaws in the self-structure that result from misattunement, common in all our histories. The therapy offers an opportunity to increase self-coherence by externalization. As a consequence, symptom reduction is likely to result. The analyst must permit such externalizations in order for the therapy to be tolerable to the patient and seek precisely these moments for interpretation, not of the

Table 12.1   The three modes of psychic change

	Intersubjective shifts	*Disinhibition of mental processes*	*Representational change*
Description	Initial defensive strategy of patient	Enhancement of reflective function	Changing the representation of the patient's picture of the mental world of self and object
Process aim	Allow intersubjective shifts to make therapy tolerable for patient	Move away from psychic equivalence	Fuller, more elaborated model of mental states; integrate split-off representations of objects
Impact on symptoms	Improvement	Worsening	Improvement
Techniques	Dual functioning; see patient beyond enactment; human generosity	Coherent approach; focus on mental states; availability of analyst's mind	Exploration of current object relationship; relationship experienced in the transference

externalization but of what the externalization has left behind. These moments may be short windows of time, when the patient is able to hear yet is still convinced of the success of the externalization. The analyst, his mind colonized by alien ideas, must find sufficient reflectiveness to perceive patients as they are, having distanced himself from an alien self-construction.

The second, concurrent, phase entails the disinhibition of mental processes, particularly of reflective capacity – mental processes that have been defensively inhibited as part of an attempt at adaptation to suboptimal internal and external environments. The clinical aim here is a move away from the infantile duality of psychic equivalence and pretend modes of functioning that antedate reflectiveness and toward engagement of the patient's mind in forms of mental activity that have felt dangerous in the past, such as playing with ideas and different points of view. A complicating aspect of this phase is the almost inevitable worsening of the patient's symptoms. The revitalization of mental processes inevitably induces a heightening of conflicts, which bring with them regression and compromise formation. With consistency and coherence of approach, it is possible for patients to build increasingly clear experiences of their own minds, thereby replacing their defensive disruption of their own thinking and the analyst's access to it. Patients experience an intense hunger for understanding the ways that minds function; they learn this not so much from the specific comments of the analyst but rather through the observation of the analyst's developing a coherent model of their minds – through the experience of a mind's having their mind in mind.

Finally, representational change is the reorganization or restructuring of the representational system. With neurotic patients, this may be all that is required. And because therapists tend to come to the profession with reasonably intact minds, we are often tempted to assume that the patient on the couch also requires no more. Knowledge of infant research alerts one to the primitive mechanisms that may be active even in neurotic, and relatively intact, patients. But representational change will all too readily be reversed unless it becomes integrated with changes at the level of implicit memory. Both self- and other representation may need to alter, and this can be done effectively only in the here and now. Changes in the perception of important others will surely follow.

Conclusion

We have described three phases of a prototypical psychoanalytic treatment. These phases, whilst theoretically coherent as presented, may indeed emerge in a different order in particular treatments. The deepest level of a patient's pathology tends to emerge only as the therapeutic relationship intensifies. As early relationship representations are activated in the intensified transference, the patient's capacity to represent self and other as feeling and thinking beings can appear to fail, and an analytic process characterized by representational change comes to be dominated by intersubjective shifts.

Some further qualifications are in order. Permanent symptomatic improvements should be an inevitable consequence of these steps being followed. Yet process–outcome research clearly demonstrates that close associations between observed process and subsequent outcome are by no means inevitable and may be quite rare (Fonagy et al. 1999). These studies are sobering reminders that our understanding of factors relevant to therapeutic benefit remains limited. In this context, we should remember that this model was proposed as a simple heuristic.

Perhaps the only assertion we can make with confidence is that psychoanalysis creates an interpersonal encounter where the psychoanalyst's mentalistic elaborative stance helps the patient to find himself in the therapist's mind and to integrate this image as part of his sense of self. In this process, there will be a gradual but inevitable transformation of a non-reflective mode of experiencing the internal world that forces an equation of internal and external reality to one where the internal world is treated with more circumspection and respect, as separate and qualitatively different from physical reality. This, we believe, is our inheritance from Freud and is what we should cherish in our daily work with our patients.

Notes

1 This chapter is a tribute to Sidney Blatt, who has overseen in a benevolent way the growth of both our scientific careers. We are indebted to him and delight in being able to contribute to this fitting tribute to one of the great clinician scientists. The chapter also owes a great deal to the editorial talents of Dr. Elizabeth Allison, for whom Mr. A. represents as much of a formative experience as to his analyst.
2 The analyst was Peter Fonagy. Throughout this chapter, the case will be discussed in the first person.

References

Abrams, S. (1987) 'The psychoanalytic process: a schematic model', *International Journal of Psycho-Analysis* 68: 441–52.
—— (1990) 'The psychoanalytic process: the developmental and the integrative', *Psychoanalytic Quarterly* 59: 650–77.
Auerbach, J. S. and Blatt, S. J. (1996) 'Self-representation in severe psychopathology: the role of reflexive self-awareness', *Psychoanalytic Psychology* 13: 297–341.
—— and —— (2001) 'Self-reflexivity, intersubjectivity, and therapeutic change', *Psychoanalytic Psychology* 18: 427–50.
Bateman, A. (1998) 'The concept of enactment and "thick-skinned" and "thin-skinned" narcissism', *International Journal of Psycho-Analysis* 79: 13–25.
Bion, W. R. (1962) *Learning from Experience*, London: Heinemann.
—— (1967) 'Notes on memory and desire', *Psychoanalytic Forum* 2: 272–3 and 279–80.
Blatt, S. J., and Auerbach, J. S. (2000) 'Psychoanalytic models of the mind and their contributions to personality research', *European Journal of Personality* 14: 429–47.
—— and Behrends, R. S. (1987) 'Internalization, separation-individuation, and the nature of therapeutic action', *International Journal of Psycho-Analysis* 68: 279–97.
—— and Blass, R. B. (1990) 'Attachment and separateness: a dialectical model of the products and processes of development throughout the life cycle', *Psychoanalytic Study of the Child* 45: 107–27.
Bowlby, J. (1988) *A Secure Base: clinical applications of attachment theory*, London: Routledge.
Breuer, J. and Freud, S. (1895) 'Studies on hysteria', in J. Strachey (ed. and trans.) *The Standard Edition of the Complete Psychological Works of Sigmund Freud*, vol. 2, London: Hogarth Press, pp. 1–305.
Britton, R. (1995) 'Psychic reality and unconscious belief', *International Journal of Psycho-Analysis* 76: 19–23.
—— (1998) *Belief and Imagination*, London: Routledge.
Cavell, M. (1993) *The Psychoanalytic Mind*, Cambridge, MA: Harvard University Press.
Clyman, R. B. (1991) 'The procedural organization of emotions: a contribution

from cognitive science to the psychoanalytic theory of therapeutic action', *Journal of the American Psychoanalytic Association* 39: 349–82.

Cohen, N. (1984) 'Preserved learning capacity in amnesia: evidence for multiple memory systems', in L. R. Squire and N. Butters (eds) *Neuropsychology of Memory*, New York: Guilford, pp. 83–103.

—— and Squire, L. R. (1980) 'Preserved learning and retention of pattern-analyzing skill in amnesia: dissociation of knowing how and knowing that', *Science* 210: 207–9.

Conway, M. A. (1996) 'Autobiographical knowledge and autobiographical memories', in D. C. Rubin (ed.) *Remembering Our Past: studies in autobiographical memory*, New York: Cambridge University Press, pp. 67–93.

Crittenden, P. M. (1990). 'Internal representational models of attachment relationships', *Infant Mental Health Journal* 11: 259–77.

Dennett, D. C. (1978) *Brainstorms: philosophical essays on mind and psychology*, Montgomery, VT: Bradford.

Edelman, G. M. (1987) *Neural Darwinism: the theory of neuronal group selection*, New York: Basic Books.

Emde, R. N. (1990) 'Mobilizing fundamental modes of development: empathic availability and therapeutic action', *Journal of the American Psychoanalytic Association* 38: 881–913.

Fonagy, P. (1995) 'Playing with reality: the development of psychic reality and its malfunction in borderline patients', *International Journal of Psycho-Analysis* 76: 39–44.

—— (1999) 'Memory and therapeutic action (guest editorial)', *International Journal of Psycho-Analysis* 80: 215–23.

—— Gergely, G., Jurist, E. and Target, M. (2002) *Affect Regulation, Mentalization, and the Development of the Self*, New York: Other Press.

—— Kachele, H., Krause, R., Jones, E. and Perron, R. (1999) *An Open Door Review of Outcome Studies in Psychoanalysis*, London: International Psychoanalytical Association.

—— Moran, G. S., Edgcumbe, R., Kennedy, H. and Target, M. (1993) 'The roles of mental representations and mental processes in therapeutic action', *Psychoanalytic Study of the Child* 48: 9–48.

—— and Target, M. (1996) 'Playing with reality: 1. theory of mind and the normal development of psychic reality', *International Journal of Psycho-Analysis* 77: 217–33.

—— and —— (1997) 'Attachment and reflective function: their role in self-organization', *Development and Psychopathology* 9: 679–700.

—— and —— (2003) *Psychoanalytic Theories: perspectives from developmental psychopathology*, London: Whurr.

Gergely, G. (1997) 'Margaret Mahler's developmental theory reconsidered in the light of current empirical research on infant development', paper presented at the Mahler Centennial Conference, Sopron, Hungary.

—— and Watson, J. (1996) 'The social biofeedback model of parental affect-mirroring', *International Journal of Psycho-Analysis* 77: 1181–212.

Goodman, S. (1977) *Psychoanalytic Education and Research: the current situation and future possibilities*, New York: International Universities Press.

Joffe, W. G. and Sandler, J. (1969) 'Comments on the psychoanalytic psychology of adaptation, with special reference to the role of affects and the representational world', *International Journal of Psycho-Analysis* 49: 445–54.

Kennedy, H. and Moran, G. (1991) 'Reflections on the aims of child psychoanalysis', *Psychoanalytic Study of the Child* 46: 181–98.

Kernberg, O. F. (1988) 'Psychic structure and structural change: an ego psychology-object relations theory viewpoint', *Journal of the American Psychoanalytic Association* 36: 315–37.

Kerridge, I., Lowe, M. and Henry, D. (1998) 'Ethics and evidence based medicine', *British Medical Journal* 316: 1151–3.

Kohut, H. (1972) 'Thoughts on narcissism and narcissistic rage', *Psychoanalytic Study of the Child* 27: 360–400.

Koós, O. and Gergely, G. (2001) 'The "flickering switch" hypothesis: a contingency-based approach to the etiology of disorganized attachment in infancy', in J. Allen, P. Fonagy and G. Gergely (eds) *Contingency Perception and Attachment in Infancy: special issue of the Bulletin of the Menninger Clinic*, New York: Guilford, pp. 397–410.

LeDoux, J. E. (1995) 'Emotion: clues from the brain', *Annual Review of Psychology* 46: 209–35.

Levy, K. N. and Blatt, S. J. (1999) 'Attachment theory and psychoanalysis: further differentiation within insecure attachment patterns', *Psychoanalytic Inquiry* 19: 541–75.

—— —— and Shaver, P. R. (1998) 'Attachment styles and parental representations', *Journal of Personality and Social Psychology* 74: 407–19.

Loewald, H. W. (1960) 'On the therapeutic action of psycho-analysis', *International Journal of Psycho-Analysis* 41: 16–33.

—— (1979) 'Reflections on the psychoanalytic process and its therapeutic potential', *Psychoanalytic Study of the Child* 34: 155–67.

Mayes, L. C. and Spence, D. P. (1994) 'Understanding therapeutic action in the analytic situation: a second look at the developmental metaphor', *Journal of the American Psychoanalytic Association* 42: 789–816.

Modell, A. H. (1976) '"The Holding Environment" and the therapeutic action of psychoanalysis', *Journal of the American Psychoanalytic Association* 24: 285–307.

Nelson, K. (1993) 'Explaining the emergence of autobiographical memory in early childhood', in A. Collins, S. E. Gathercole, M. A. Conway and P. E. Morris (eds) *Theories of Memory*, Hove, England: Erlbaum, pp. 355–85.

Rosenfeld, H. (1964) 'On the psychopathology of narcissism: a clinical approach', *International Journal of Psycho-Analysis* 45: 332–7.

Sackett, D. L., Rosenberg, W. M., Gray, J. A. M., Haynes, R. B. and Richardson, W. S. (1996) 'Evidence based medicine: what it is and what it isn't', *British Medical Journal* 312: 71–2.

Sandler, J. and Dreher, A. U. (1997) *What Do Psychoanalysts Want: the problems of aims in psychoanalytic psychotherapy*, London: Routledge.

—— and Joffe, W. G. (1969) 'Towards a basic psychoanalytic model', *International Journal of Psycho-Analysis* 50: 79–90.

Schlessinger, N. and Robbins, F. (1983) *A Developmental View of the Psychoanalytic Process*, New York: International Universities Press.

Solms, M. and Turnbull, O. (2002) *The Brain and the Inner World: an introduction to the neuroscience of subjective experience*, New York: Other Press.

Stern, D. N. (1994) 'One way to build a clinically relevant baby', *Infant Mental Health Journal* 15: 36–54.

—— (1998) 'The process of therapeutic change involving implicit knowledge: some implications of developmental observations for adult psychotherapy', *Infant Mental Health Journal* 19: 300–8.

Stolorow, R. and Lachmann, F. (1978) 'The developmental prestages of defenses: diagnostic and therapeutic implications', *Psychoanalytic Quarterly* 47: 73–102.

Stone, L. (1961) *The Psychoanalytic Situation: an examination of its development and essential nature*, New York: International Universities Press.

Target, M. and Fonagy, P. (1996) 'Playing with reality: 2. the development of psychic reality from a theoretical perspective', *International Journal of Psycho-Analysis* 77: 459–79.

Viederman, M. (1991) 'The impact of the real person of the analyst on the psycho-analytic cure', *Journal of the American Psychoanalytic Association* 39: 451–89.

Wallerstein, R. S. (1965) 'The goals of psychoanalysis: a survey of analytic viewpoints', *Journal of the American Psychoanalytic Association* 13: 748–70.

Chapter 13

How often are relationship narratives told during psychotherapy sessions?

Lester Luborsky, Tomasz Andrusyna, and Louis Diguer

I should begin this chapter with a few words about Sidney Blatt, in whose honor this chapter is written. Sid and I have had a fruitful association for many years. Most of our interchanges have been about psychoanalytic theory, and it is therefore fitting that I share with him and with all of you more about my Core Conflictual Relationship Theme (CCRT) method (Luborsky 1977), a method that pertains to patients' own accounts of important events that they wish to discuss. It was for that reason too that Sid was one of the few analysts whom I invited to attend the award ceremony in 1999 for my American Psychological Foundation Gold Medal for Lifetime Achievement. In the chapter, I discuss research that derives from the CCRT method – specifically, an investigation of the links between the CCRT and the narratives told during psychotherapy.

Many important theorists (e.g., Habermas 1968; Ricoeur 1977; Schafer 1983, 1992; Spence 1982) have proposed that psychoanalysis is essentially a narrative process, that is, a process in which patients come to tell new, more integrated and coherent stories about themselves and their lives. It has even been suggested by Bruner (1986, 1990) that the narrative is a basic cognitive structure, parallel to the computational mode that underlies the intellectual abilities investigated by Piaget (1972). But despite a rich theoretical literature, little attention has been devoted to the empirical study of how narratives actually function in psychotherapy, and therefore no one knows what role or roles stories actually play in psychotherapeutic treatment. To investigate these issues, my colleagues and I have proposed the concept of a *relationship episode* (RE). A relationship episode (RE) is a narrative account of a personally meaningful event in a relationship, either with others or with the self. The recognition of such narratives about other persons in psychotherapy is usually simple: the patient's account names the main other person and then tells a narrative about the interaction of the patient with this main other person. It has become more and more generally recognized since its first use in psychotherapy research by Luborsky (1976, 1977) that relationship narratives are scorable units about episodes in relationships that are regularly told during psychotherapy sessions (Luborsky

1992). In the Penn Psychotherapy Project the usual rate of telling these narratives during psychotherapy was a mean of 4.1 REs per session (Luborsky *et al.* 1988; Luborsky and Crits-Christoph 1998; Crits-Christoph *et al.* 1994).

The main themes in these REs can and should be used by the therapist to formulate the CCRT. The CCRT score of each session turns out to be somewhat like a clinical version of the transference pattern. In terms of the specifics of the method, the thought units in each RE are scored according to the three basic components of the CCRT: wishes, responses from others and responses of self. This coding system can be used as the basis for the therapist's interpretations given during the treatment sessions (Luborsky and Crits-Christoph 1998), and it has been noted by Blatt and colleagues (Blatt, Auerbach and Aryan 1998) that the three components of the CCRT form the skeleton of a narrative.

In this chapter, we will discuss the frequency of REs during sessions and the desirability of their use in interpretations. We will also provide a few impressionistically generated hypotheses about the factors explaining the frequency of these narratives in terms of their rate per session.

Aims of the study

The main aims of the present chapter are (a) to update our knowledge of the frequency of relationship narratives in psychotherapy sessions and (b) to discover more about factors that might explain the frequency of narratives in psychotherapy sessions, such as the gender of the patients, their time in treatment, and the outcome of the treatment.

Method

We reexamined the frequency of telling relationship narratives during psychotherapy in a sample of 41 patients in a treatment study of patients with a DSM-IV (American Psychiatric Association 1994) diagnosis of major depression or of major depression, chronic. We then examined our clinically based explanations about the frequency of relationship narratives in the early sessions and in the late sessions of short-term supportive-expressive (SE) psychotherapy, a form of psychoanalytic psychotherapy that involves the therapist's (a) facilitation of a *supportive* relationship with the patient and (b) understanding of the patient's verbal *expression* of psychological material (Luborsky 2002). The subsample of 31 patients independently diagnosed with major depression were in psychotherapy for a mean of 16 sessions; the 10 patients diagnosed with major depression, chronic, were seen for a mean of 20 sessions. These two subsamples were combined for this report because differences in their outcomes were not statistically significant (Luborsky *et al.* 1996).

Measures

Relationship episodes (REs)

REs are mostly about relationships with people; only a very few are about nonhuman content. Those involving relationships with people were therefore the only ones used in this chapter. Independent judges reliably identified and then reliably CCRT-scored the REs throughout the transcript of each session. The average interjudge agreement results of eight different samples were for Wishes, 87%, for Responses from Others, 97%, and for Responses of Self, 89%; the weighted Kappas for these three components were .60, .68, and .71, respectively (Luborsky and Diguer 1998).

Completeness of the narratives

The relationship episodes were also rated for their completeness on a 5–point scale (Luborsky and Crits-Christoph 1998). Our usual rule, that only those narratives rated 2.5 and above on this scale, was used in the study.

Beck Depression Inventory (BDI)

This is a reliable questionnaire that measures the severity of depression (Beck et al. 1961; Beck et al. 1988). The questionnaire was filled out by the patient at the end of each psychotherapy session. Our outcome measures were twofold: (a) the termination BDI score and (b) the change in BDI score from early to late in treatment.

Results and discussion

The frequency of telling REs during psychotherapy sessions is moderately high

For the 41 patients in SE psychotherapy, the mean frequency of relationship narratives, 5.6 REs per session, was found to be higher than in previous studies. Some of this is reviewed in Luborsky (1984), and as noted previously, the mean frequency of REs per session in the Penn Psychotherapy Study had been 4.1 (Luborsky and Crits-Christoph 1998). But in another study, Crits-Christoph et al. (1999) found a much smaller mean frequency of only 2.4 REs per session. This lower frequency probably reflected the constraints of their reliance on a different method of collecting REs – the presentation for judgment of each narrative in random order and by itself, rather than in the context of an entire session. The latter method, the rating of REs within the context of a session transcript, is the standard approach for identifying narrative units. Nevertheless, the frequency of REs in this sample must then be compared with that in other samples to try to explain why different samples vary in the rate of telling REs in psychotherapy, as in Luborsky, Barber and Diguer (1992).

We were also interested in understanding why telling REs is such a common behavior among psychotherapy patients. We have seen that patients in psychotherapy, in telling each narrative, often conveyed that they have behavioral problems. They report examples, such as the working out of their problem, in their accounts of relationship events. One possibility, among several, is that patients find it adds vividness and veracity to their description of their problems to illustrate them through their narratives of events (Luborsky and Crits-Christoph 1998). Another is that people often come to therapy to resolve specific life incidents or memories – memories that are presented as narratives.

The rate of telling REs in psychotherapy sessions tends to decrease over the course of the sessions in a treatment

Within a treatment, *early* has tended to refer to occurrences within the first 30 per cent of the sessions, and *late* to occurrences within the last 30 per cent of the sessions. There is a drop-off in frequency of REs from the beginning to end of most psychotherapies; that is, REs are more often told early in treatment, and their frequency progressively diminishes as the treatment goes on. The mean of the early REs is 6.8 per session, the mean of the late REs is only 4.5 per session, and the difference is highly significant, $t(40) = 4.60$, $p < .0001$, $r^2 = .41$.

This novel phenomenon of a drop-off in frequency of telling REs has never been written about before, although we have found it is a rather marked phenomenon that is shown by 32 of the 41 patients in our sample. Why this spontaneous drop-off in frequency occurs can be only partly understood by examination of the session. It probably happens largely because the patient must know which narratives have already been told in the earlier sessions, and patients apparently follow a principle not to repeat the same ones again in later sessions, perhaps also because in later sessions the therapist is already familiar with these narratives. Additionally, in later sessions, patients tend to talk more about what is happening in the therapy room between the patient and therapist. However, in many treatments, some of the main REs are reexamined as the treatment goes on, rather than more new ones being told.

There are gender differences over time in the rate of telling REs

An analysis of gender differences (see Table 13.1) showed several clear trends. Men tend to tell far fewer REs than do women, with a mean of 4.2

Table 13.1   Gender differences in frequency of Relationship Episodes

Gender group	Frequency of Relationship Episodes in sessions	
Men (n = 8)	4.2 REs/session	
Women (n = 33)	6.0 REs/session	p = .055
Men early	4.75 REs/session	
Women early	7.24 REs/session	p = .036
Men late	3.6 REs/session	
Women late	4.7 REs/session	n.s.

REs per session throughout treatment, whereas women tell a mean of 6.0 REs per session. The difference is almost significant, with $t(40) = 1.977$, $p = 0.055$, $r^2 = .09$. This finding is consistent with our predictions regarding gender and the telling of relationship narratives. As Blatt (1995; Blatt and Shichman 1983) has noted, women are likely to be relational, rather than self-definitional, in their personality styles, and for men, this pattern is reversed. Thus, it is unsurprising that women tend to tell more REs than do men. Further analysis of the results shows that this difference is mainly in *the early sessions*, where the mean for men is only 4.75 but for women is 7.25, a significant difference with $t(40) = 2.167$, $p = 0.036$, $r^2 = .107$. In late sessions, however, the difference in means is in the same direction but is no longer significant: For men, it is 3.6 at this point, and for women, it is 4.7, with $t(40) = 1.066$, $p = 0.2929$, $r^2 = .028$. Men tell a steady low level of REs throughout treatment, whereas women tell many REs early in treatment but only about the same as men late in treatment. In fact, 21 per cent of the women in our sample were very high in the number of REs told, but none of the men were.

Another finding with regard to gender was that women were significantly more depressed at the beginning of therapy than were men. Women's early BDI was 29.2; men's early BDI was 23.5; $t(40)$ 2.130, $p = 0.04$, $r^2 = .104$. It is possible, therefore, that level of depression is a stronger predictor of telling REs than is gender. We cannot easily sort this out, however, because our sample consists of 33 women but only 8 men, although the findings did nevertheless support our predictions significantly regarding depression and gender.

Frequency of telling REs is typically unrelated to outcome, yet an unusually high frequency is associated with poor treatment outcomes

To examine the relation of the number of REs to the outcomes of the treatment, we first calculated the correlation for these variables within the whole sample of 41 patients. We found the general trend is toward a positive but nonsignificant association of frequency of REs with outcome of treatment, $r(39) = .23$, $p < .13$, but with one major outlier removed, the correlation reaches significance, $r(38) = .44$, $p < .02$.

However, the strong clinical impression about this relationship, even before our statistical analyses were done, was that it does not fit the entire distribution. Our clinical hypothesis at the outset of the study was that the relationship holds mainly at the extremes of the frequencies. We therefore divided the sample of REs per session into three levels of frequency (Table 13.2): (a) very low, (b) typical (the largest group), and (c) very high. To do this, we first calculated the standard deviation of the frequency of REs per session, and then we defined the Low group as comprising those participants whose frequency was more than 1 standard deviation below the mean and the High group as those whose frequency was more than 1 standard deviation above the mean. The frequency for the Low group ($n = 8$) was less than 3.24 REs, and that for the High group ($n = 5$) was greater than 8.04 REs.

We went on to compare by Student's t the means of the three groups on our main outcome measure: the change in Beck Depression Inventory from early to late in treatment. We found almost significant confirmation of our clinical hypotheses. The trend showed that those subjects with the very highest number of REs had the least BDI change (the least decrease in their depression) and that those with the usual number of REs had the largest BDI change (the most decrease in their depression).

When we compared the RE frequency groups with the termination BDI, we found a significant Student's t for the high frequency, as compared with the middle frequency, group, with $t(1) = 2.02$, $p < 0.05$. A separate analysis showed no significant difference among the groups in their initial BDIs; therefore, we see that those patients with the typical frequency of REs per session had a better outcome (mean termination BDI = 11.6) than those with the very high number of REs per session (mean termination BDI = 21.3), even taking initial BDI into account. In conclusion, the telling of very many REs (more than 8 per session) appeared to be associated with factors detrimental to a patient's beneficial outcome of therapy. Those patients who told a very low number of REs were somewhere in between, with a mean termination BDI of 14.3 but with better outcome than those in the high group.

The further understanding of these findings must, for now, rely only on clinical impressions. The patients who fill up much of the session with a

Table 13.2   Frequency of Relationship Episodes (REs) in relation to
psychotherapy outcome

Very low frequency	Middle frequency	Very high frequency
More than one Standard Deviation below mean		More than one Standard Deviation above mean
Less than 3.24 REs	3.24 to 8.04 REs	More than 8.04 REs
(*n* = 8)	(*n* = 28)	(*n* = 5)

$$p = .05$$

Mean termination BDI = 14.3	Mean termination BDI = 11.6	Mean termination BDI = 21.2

very high frequency of REs appear to have interfering attitudes toward their treatment. Such patients may believe the way to get help in psychotherapy is to tell many stories, especially stories that are associated with the problems that the patient wishes to solve. Other patients may have little interest in understanding the REs but much interest in letting the therapist know by the stories how badly he or she has been treated by others. Another less frequent attitude might be the patient's view that allowing for too much exchange with the therapist outside of telling the stories may permit time for the therapist to say things that will make the patient anxious. Another possibility is that these patients do poorly in treatment because they are too disorganized to focus on a few central, defining narratives.

Summary and conclusions

A sample of 41 patients with a diagnosis of either major depression or major depression, chronic, and treated by SE psychotherapy has revealed the frequency and meanings of the rate of telling relationship episodes during psychotherapy sessions. First, the rate of telling of relationship narratives has reconfirmed the usual high frequency of these narratives in each session – a mean of 5.6 REs per session in this sample. Second, it has shown that the patient's rate of telling these relationship episodes tends to decrease over the course of the psychotherapy. Third, there are gender differences in the rate of telling relationship episodes, with women telling significantly more narratives in the early sessions but then coming down in frequency late in psychotherapy to become closer to the lower rate of men. Fourth and finally, the rate of telling these relationship episodes is not significantly related to the outcome of the psychotherapy, *except* for one condition: a *very* high frequency of telling these episodes is significantly associated with poor outcomes of the psychotherapy. We also explored some of the possible explanations for these findings.

References

American Psychiatric Association (1994) *Diagnostic and Statistical Manual of Mental Disorders*, 4th edn, Washington, DC: American Psychiatric Press.

Beck A. T., Steer R. A. and Garbin M. G. (1988) 'Psychometric properties of the Beck Depression Inventory: twenty-five years of evaluation', *Clinical Psychology Review* 8: 77–100.

—— Ward, C., Mendelson, M., Mock, J. and Erbaugh, J. (1961) 'An inventory to measure depression', *Archives of General Psychiatry* 4: 561–71.

Blatt, S. J. (1995) 'Representational structures in psychopathology', in D. Cicchetti and S. Toth (eds) *Representation, Emotion, and Cognition in Developmental Psychopathology*, Rochester, NY: University of Rochester Press, pp. 1–33.

—— and Shichman, S. (1983) 'Two primary configurations of psychopathology', *Psychoanalysis and Contemporary Thought* 6: 187–254.

—— Auerbach, J. S. and Aryan, M. (1998) 'Representational structures and the therapeutic process', in R. F. Bornstein and J. M. Masling (eds) *Empirical Studies of Psychoanalytic Theories, vol. 8: empirical studies of the therapeutic hour*, Washington, DC: Americal Psychological Association.

Bruner, J. S. (1986) *Actual Minds, Possible Worlds*, Cambridge, MA: Harvard University Press.

—— (1990) *Acts of meaning*, Cambridge, MA: Harvard University Press.

Crits-Christoph, P., Connolly, M. B., Shappell, S., Elkin, I., Krupnick, J. and Sotsky, S. (1999) 'Interpersonal narratives in cognitive and interpersonal psychotherapies', *Psychotherapy Research* 9: 22–35.

—— Demorest, A., Muenz, L. and Baranackie, K. (1994) 'Consistency of interpersonal themes for patients in psychotherapy', *Journal of Personality* 62: 499–526.

Habermas, J. (1968) *Knowledge and Human Interests*, J. J. Shapiro (trans.), Boston: Beacon Press, 1971.

Luborsky, L. (1976) 'Helping alliances in psychotherapy: the groundwork for a study of their relationship to its outcome', in J. L. Claghorn (ed.) *Successful Psychotherapy*, New York: Brunner/Mazel, pp. 92–116.

—— (1977) 'Measuring a pervasive psychic structure in psychotherapy: the core conflictual relationship theme', in N. Freedman and S. Grand (eds) *Communicative Structures and Psychic Structures*, New York: Plenum Press, pp. 367–95.

—— (1984) *Principles of Psychoanalytic Psychotherapy: a manual for supportive-expressive treatment*, New York: Basic Books.

—— (1992) 'Does psychotherapy research really offer good ideas for psychotherapists?', *Journal of Psychotherapy Practice and Research* 1: 310–12.

Luborsky, L. (2002) 'Supportive-expressive dynamic psychotherapy: its central principles, procedures, and empirical supports', *Encyclopedia of Psychotherapy* 2: 1–6.

—— Barber, J. P. and Diguer, L. (1992) 'The meanings of narratives told during psychotherapy – the fruits of a new operational unit', *Psychotherapy Research* 2: 277–90.

—— and Crits-Christoph, P. (1998) *Understanding Transference: the core conflictual relationship theme method*, 2nd edn, Washington, DC: American Psychological Association.

—— —— Mintz, J. and Auerbach, A. (1988) *Who Will Benefit from Psychotherapy? predicting therapeutic outcomes*, New York: Basic Books.

—— and Diguer, L. (1998) 'The reliability of the CCRT measure: results from eight samples', in L. Luborsky and P. Crits-Christoph (eds) *Understanding Transference: the core conflictual relationship theme method*, Washington, DC: American Psychological Association, pp. 97–108.

—— —— Barber, J. P., Cacciola, J., Moras, K., Schmidt, K. and DeRubeis, R. (1996) 'Outcomes of short-term dynamic psychotherapy for chronic versus non-chronic major depression', *Journal of Psychotherapy Research and Practice* 5: 152–9.

Piaget, J. (1972) Intellectual evolution from adolescence to adulthood, *Human Development* 15: 1–12.

Ricoeur, P. (1977) 'The question of proof in Freud's psychoanalytic writings', *Journal of the American Psychoanalytic Association* 25: 835–71.

Schafer, R. (1983) *The Analytic Attitude*, New York: Basic Books.

—— (1992) *Retelling a Life: narration and dialogue in psychoanalysis*, New York: Basic Books.

Spence, D. P. (1982) *Narrative Truth and Historical Truth: meaning and interpretation in psychoanalysis*, New York: Norton.

Chapter 14

Research perspectives on the case study

Single-case method

Stanley B. Messer and Laura McCann

The traditional narrative case study or vignette has been the major method of reporting psychoanalytic observations and outcomes since the publication of Freud's cases. There are several advantages to this method. The presenting psychoanalyst is on the scene as the material unfolds and is in a privileged position to know the intricacies of what occurred over a substantial period of time. A case study can summarize large quantities of material and do so in a rich and variegated fashion. Well-written cases allow material to come alive in a compelling way, allowing us to know the unfolding sequence of events, major emergent themes, and the results of the analysis or therapy. By publishing case write-ups, treating therapists permit readers to participate in their sense of discovery and excitement in elaborating new ideas and techniques.

What, then, is wrong with this picture? After all, case study possesses the comforting force of a lengthy and venerable tradition, covers the relevant ground, and allows for the independent scrutiny of others. Advantages notwithstanding, the lens through which we will view the case study – that of normative science – will highlight flaws in this rosy methodological picture. Although the scientific lens that we apply is not flawless, it does possess certain advantages over the traditional case study method, as we shall try to demonstrate in this chapter. We will therefore present an alternative methodology, the single subject approach to psychoanalytic cases. This approach falls within the spirit of Sidney Blatt's work insofar as it reflects his lifelong efforts to apply scientific method to psychoanalytic theory and therapy.

Difficulties with the case report

A major problem with the case report is that it is based on one person's view only. Although it is true that the analyst reporting the data is a highly trained observer, the case material he or she presents is, of necessity, selective. What is not recorded may be technical mistakes that are not remembered or are simply omitted to avoid guilt or shame (Spence 1998).

We cannot assume that accounts readied for publication are veridical because psychoanalysis has taught us that memory is infiltrated by wishes and a confirmatory bias (Spence 2000). We have to rely on the analyst's report because typically we do not have a record of the actual dialogue that transpired between patient and analyst. Such data filtering occurs on at least two levels – what data get reported and the inferences that the analyst draws from them. We can illustrate the problem with examples taken from a recently edited psychoanalytic volume that reports cases of patients seen in psychoanalysis as children and then again as adults. It should be noted that examples could have been chosen as readily from other sources.

In describing the psychoanalytic treatment of Lisa, her 8-year-old patient, Marschke-Tobier (2000: 76) writes:

> there was very little that didn't come quickly into the realm of her sexualized sadomasochistic fantasies and behaviors. Examples of her sadomasochistic mode of relating recurred in varying forms throughout the analysis in her battles over taking things home from the treatment room that began during the first week of treatment. This was followed by her attempts to get me physically involved with her in scary, exciting games; her later use of reading in sessions; her consistent use of the toilet during sessions; and in her ongoing pattern of leaving sessions by bouncing down the stairs on her bottom, which appeared in the first weeks of treatment and remained throughout.

Both the theme and the evidence on which it draws are selected by the treating analyst and by the analyst alone. The evidence is not randomly chosen or systematically sampled but is, we presume, that sample of Lisa's behavior that struck the observer as cohering around the particular theme of sadomasochistic behavior. That is, the material is chosen from a large field of possibilities for its persuasive or rhetorical effect (e.g., Spence 1994) and leaves out other material that may contradict the theme.

Furthermore, the specific inference is made that such behavior is sadomasochistic. Might not an uninvolved observer see these behaviors quite differently, perhaps as evidence of defiant oppositionalism without the added inference of its being sexualized? Alternatively, Lisa may be viewed as trying to master interpersonal fears by recreating a degree of intensity in her relationship to the analyst. There is nothing in the material, such as her reading or her use of the toilet, that in any obvious way speaks to sexual excitement or sadomasochism. Is bouncing down the stairs necessarily sexually gratifying? The interpretation of the behavior – that is, the naming of the theme – seems to derive more from the author's adherence to psychoanalytic drive theory than from anything in the girl's behavior as it is described.

Moreover, if we had a different hypothesis about the meaning of the material – and we have suggested just two possibilities – we would have a hard time supporting or refuting it because we have available only the data that the analyst chooses to present. In this sense, the record is not truly public in the manner that science requires. In a traditional case study, there is no ready way to check either the analyst's or our own hypotheses against the original material. Thus, what we have is an instance of the argument from authority, in which the presenter completely controls access to the information (Spence 1993).

Another case report presented in the same volume by Colarusso (2000) comes closer to the requirement that the data be open to inspection. There are copious vignettes that are partly narrative summaries but also include dialogue between analyst and patient. After reading these brief excerpts, readers are in a better position to arrive at their own interpretation of the material and to draw independent conclusions. Colarusso gives us not only the dialogue but the immediate follow-up to it, and this information also helps readers gauge the effect, or "mini-outcome," of a particular line of interpretation. This moves the case study in the direction of meeting scientific requirements.

Nevertheless, even this presentation falls short of empirical research standards. For one thing, we are not told whether the excerpts, referred to by the author as "clinical vignettes" (Colarusso 2000), are verbatim accounts or summaries reconstructed from the analyst's notes – a matter that affects their evidentiary status. For another, the data supplied are very partial and frequently do not allow for independent confirmation. To illustrate the problem, here is an excerpt from session 37 of his treatment of a 9-year-old patient, Jim, with whom he was involved in play:

> The analyst (A) decided to begin to approach the patient's conflict over his aggression.
>
> *A:* Gee, Jim, what happened, first you were involved in the war and suddenly you say you're bored. You sure didn't seem bored.
>
> *Jim:* Well, I was.
>
> *A:* Maybe, but maybe something else happened. I wonder if you became nervous about how open you were about bombing the houses like that. Like you thought you were too tough. Maybe you were worried about what I would think of you for acting like that.
>
> *Jim:* No.
>
> *A:* Didn't the same thing happen last week? First you were going to fight against me and then suddenly we were brother and sister on the same side. I think you must have had similar feelings then and changed the sides because of them.
>
> Jim denied the interpretation but he had obviously heard it. He began to draw and talk about his fear of doing poorly on some upcoming tests in school.
>
> (Colarusso 2000: 21)

When the analyst says that Jim had obviously heard the interpretation, he seems to infer this from Jim's turning to drawing and talking about his fear of failing school tests. However, neither these behaviors nor Jim's denial makes it obvious to us that the effect of the interpretation was confirmed, nor might it necessarily seem so to others exposed to the same material.

To express the nature of the problem of narrative case report in psychometric terms, what is lacking is evidence of reliability and validity. *Reliability* refers to the ability of two or more observers to rate particular constructs in a similar way. With variables as abstract as those used by psychoanalysts, achieving reliability is no easy task (e.g., Seitz 1966). But without it, we do not have the objectivity our research lens requires. *Validity* refers to the ability of a measure to assess the construct that it claims to assess. In the current example, if the aim is to assess the adequacy of an interpretation, one would want an objective measure of its effect on the subsequent associations or behavior of the patient according to specified criteria like the production of new material or a change in the patient's affective state.

In addition to assessing the effects of within-session interventions, psychoanalysis necessarily needs to be concerned with gauging molar changes over time. Rosenbaum (2000), in another chapter in the same book, describes his narrative evaluation, conducted at the start of treatment and at termination, with subsequent occasional updates either from his patient's parents or from the young patient. From a research perspective, however, what is most desirable in evaluating change is to have the perspective of three parties, namely therapist, patient, and independent interviewer. Psychotherapy research has shown that these perspectives tend to differ but are at least moderately correlated. Each has its advantages and disadvantages. To rely mainly on patients' accounts may be to ignore their transference feelings, which can distort what they report. Therapists, too, have a stake in the outcome and thus can be overly influenced by countertransference reactions. Outside observers do not have the subjective and emotional investment of either the patient or therapist and, in fact, their ratings tend to be less positive than patient or therapist ratings (e.g., Green *et al.* 1975). But patients may reveal their feelings less fully to an outside evaluator who, in addition, lacks the privileged information of the therapist. Although including all three sources of assessment is desirable, it does not resolve the problem of how to interpret lack of agreement among these several sources. Even within an empirical research paradigm, there is no escaping the need for interpretation of the data of personality and change (Messer, Sass and Woolfolk 1988).

An evaluation of change should be conducted at least at initiation, upon termination, and at a follow-up after a minimum of six months to a year. The areas of change that are assessed might include symptoms (e.g.,

Symptom Check List-90-R, Derogatis 1983); conflicts (e.g., Core Conflictual Relationship Theme, Luborsky and Luborsky 1993; Idiographic Conflict Formulation Method, Perry 1994); quality of object relations (e.g., Concept of the Object on the Rorschach scale, Blatt, Brenneis, Schimek and Glick 1976; Object Relations Inventory, Blatt *et al.* 1992; Quality of Object Relations, Piper and Duncan 1999); the increased ability to connect emotional schemas to words (e.g., Referential Activity, Bucci and Miller 1993); degree of complexity and differentiation of object representations (e.g., Thematic Patterning Scale of Object Representations II, Geller *et al.* 1992); and the attainment of insight (e.g., Morgan Insight Rating Scale, Morgan *et al.* 1982). These and other scales allow for an objective assessment of whatever variables are deemed most important to the investigator.

A still larger question is what we are trying to learn from these assessments. If it is to understand the effect of analysis on particular problems, we need to study enough cases with those problems to be able to draw general conclusions. Preferably we would also want to follow an untreated, or differently treated, control group of similar cases – a task that is decidedly difficult to accomplish. For examples of psychoanalytic studies of a large number of patients, see Fonagy and Moran (1990) and Target and Fonagy (1994). Fortunately, there are other methods for arriving at generalizable conclusions, one of which is single-case research, the topic of the remainder of this chapter.

What is single case research?

Single-case research is a type of intrasubject research in which there is an aggregation of data across cases, and the generality of one's findings is established through replication on a case-by-case basis (Hilliard 1993: 373–4). What this means is that in order to determine how we can most usefully understand what does and does not change as a result of an intensive psychoanalytic psychotherapy or analysis, we must first investigate what changed in each particular case and only then look for common threads among them. This may seem obvious, but the more general tendency in empirical research would be to lump the cases together right from the start.

Intrasubject research designs are concerned with the temporal unfolding of variables that are free to vary within individual subjects. Such designs therefore involve the repeated measurement or observation of a variable or variables over time. One process variable of interest might be, let us say, change in the patient's level of emotional experiencing following interpretations. If complete transcripts of sessions were available, we could test the hypothesis that emotional responsiveness to interpretations tends to increase over the course of analysis or therapy.

The problem of generalizability in single-case research

Within a single-case paradigm, generalizability, or external validity, is demonstrated through replication on a case-by-case basis. This approach has been called the N-of-one-at-a-time design. Hilliard (1993), borrowing from the behavioral tradition, distinguishes two types of case-by-case replication – direct replication and systematic replication.

Direct replication "refers to the attempt to replicate the findings in subjects that are similar in terms of the individual-differences variables that are viewed as affecting the phenomenon of interest" (Hilliard 1993: 376). Our hypothetical example or hypothesis above would involve direct replication. The individual-difference variable would be interpretations, and "the phenomenon of interest" their effect on patients' emotional experience.

Systematic replication, on the other hand, "refers to the attempt to show that the findings differ in predictable ways when one selects subjects that differ along the critical individual-difference variables" (Hilliard 1993: 376). To continue with our example, if we studied cases that differed in the quantity, timing, or accuracy of interpretations, we would predict a discernible difference in patients' emotional responses.

Classification of single-case designs

Studies of single cases may be either quantitative or qualitative. Hilliard (1993: 377) classifies single-case designs as case studies, single-case quantitative analyses, or single-case experiments according to three criteria: (a) whether the data are quantitative or qualitative; (b) "whether the independent variables are directly manipulated by the experimenter" (referred to as experimental) or not (passive-observational); and (c) "whether the focus of the study is testing hypotheses that have been formulated a priori" (in a context of justification) "or generating hypotheses to be tested in later research" (in a context of discovery). *Case studies* are based on qualitative data and passive observation whereas *single-case quantitative analyses* use quantitative data and passive observation. Either design may be used to test or generate hypotheses. (*Single-case experiments*, which are seldom used in psychotherapy research, involve quantitative data, direct manipulation of independent variables, and hypothesis testing.) The following sections will discuss qualitative case studies and single-case quantitative analyses in greater detail and will offer examples of psychotherapy research that employ single-case design.

The qualitative case study

Hilliard (1993) reserves the term *case study* for designs based on qualitative data and passive observation. Qualitative case studies are the cornerstones of the study of psychoanalysis. As discussed above, they have come under criticism, both from within and outside psychoanalytic circles, for too often laying the patient on the Procrustean bed of one psychoanalytic theory or another. Edelson (1985) attempted to reclaim scientific status for the case study, that is, to bring it into the context of justification. He set out minimal standards that should be met by case studies claiming to be scientific: Authors should: (a) clearly state their hypothesis about the case and demonstrate how that hypothesis accounts for their observations; (b) separate observation from interpretation and specify what observations would be grounds for rejecting the hypothesis; (c) state the limits of the scope of the hypothesis and refute competing hypotheses; and (d) acknowledge any biases that may have influenced their observations. Fonagy and Moran (1993) set out similar criteria, to which they added that information should be gathered from more than one source – for example, from follow-up interviews with the patient in addition to the therapist's write-up.

Spence (1993) provided another set of guidelines intended to improve case studies in his presentation of the recommendations of the Committee on Scientific Activities of the American Psychoanalytic Association. The Committee and Spence encouraged the adoption of certain conventions in reporting case material: First, the analyst's statements are presented in capital letters; this obviates the need for labeling the speakers in any other way and facilitates a computer search of the transcripts if that is desired. Second, each statement is categorized as either: a noncommunicated thought, shown in parentheses; an approximate wording of spoken discourse, presented without quotation marks; or "exact wording of spoken discourse, marked by quotation marks" (Spence 1993: 45). Third, a series of columns should be used to record later commentaries on the case. The latter is reminiscent of a page of Talmud, where commentaries by different scholars and from different time periods are printed in columns surrounding the original text.

Adopting these conventions would make clinical psychoanalytic material more readily available than it has been in the past, and therefore invite the kind of dialogue that can lead to greater clinical understanding. From an empirical perspective, however, adopting these conventions would not obviate the need for audiotaping or using some other means for obtaining verbatim transcripts of sessions.

In more recent writings, Spence (2001) has emphasized the importance of context and timing in understanding the significance of any clinical happening. Therapists' private awareness of what has proceeded throughout the therapy surely colors their understanding of the material, and this context is not available to the reader. In our own research, described below, we take both context and timing seriously. Spence also points out that within a two-person psychology, the meaning that patients attribute to the therapist's words may be very different from the version described in the case report. Although our research takes account of patients' responses, we did not elicit their or therapists' unvoiced thoughts, as Spence would recommend. This is difficult to achieve but can be partially accomplished in the case study by the therapists' making more of an effort to present patients' thoughts and feelings, as well as their own.

The quantitative analysis of single cases

The quantitative analysis of single cases requires either access to the case as it is occurring (in order to administer questionnaires, and so on) or complete transcripts of the case. Hilliard (1993: 377) proposes the term single-case quantitative analysis for "the situation in which quantitative techniques for analyzing the temporal unfolding of variables . . . are applied to single cases without the direct manipulation of any of the variables studied."

There are many examples of such studies in the literature on psychotherapy process and outcome. First we will review briefly a series of studies based on a single psychoanalysis – the case of Mrs. C. These studies were made possible by the fact that this six-year-long, five-day-a-week analysis was completely audiotaped.

One of the first groups to study Mrs. C. was the Mount Zion Psychotherapy Research Group, led by Joseph Weiss and Harold Sampson. (The publications of this group are too numerous to list here, but see Weiss and Sampson *et al.* [1986], and Silberschatz and Curtis [1993], which include a review of previous research, for a sampling.) Weiss and Sampson used the case of Mrs. C. as the testing ground for their particular psychoanalytic theory, known as control-mastery theory. According to this theory, people are able to assert some control over their unconscious mental lives.

In a therapeutic context, the theory suggests that patients enter psychotherapy with an unconscious plan for testing pathogenic beliefs and working toward certain goals. Weiss and Sampson viewed Mrs. C.'s pathogenic beliefs as centering around her exaggerated sense of responsibility for others and her fear of hurting them, derived from separation guilt and survivor guilt dynamics, which are as universal in Weiss and Sampson's theory as is the Oedipus complex in Freud's. They predicted that she would work to disconfirm her pathogenic beliefs in the analytic relationship by testing the analyst to see if he would be hurt when she disagreed with or criticized him and that the analysis would succeed to the extent that the analyst passed the tests. This series of studies (Weiss and Sampson 1986) used the basic strategy of the *events paradigm*, which asks, "Which specific therapist interventions introduced in which momentary contexts will lead to which immediate and subsequent impacts?" (Stiles, Shapiro and Elliott 1986: 174).

Mrs. C. was later studied by Jones and Windholz (1990), who employed the Psychotherapy Process Q-set (PQS). The PQS has the virtue of being both richly descriptive and amenable to quantitative analysis. For each session, raters sort the 100 items of the PQS into a forced-normal distribution of nine categories, ranging from least characteristic to most characteristic. Items include statements such as "Patient's interpersonal relationships are a major theme," and "Analyst adopts a supportive stance" (Jones and Windholz 1990: 995).

These authors applied PQS to transcripts of 70 sessions chosen in 10-session blocks from the entire course of Mrs. C.'s analysis to examine the pattern of changes that occurred in the analytic process over time. In general, Mrs. C. became more trusting of and dependent on the analyst in the early years of her analysis and at the same time developed a greater capacity for free association and easier access to her emotional life. The middle period was marked by the development of a transference neurosis, with worsening symptoms and heightened resistances. These were resolved in the late phase.

The study demonstrated that "psychoanalytic case material can be studied in a formal systematic manner . . . [that] clinical impressions can be placed on a reliable, verifiable basis, and that clinical knowledge can be documented in a form that potentially allows replication" (Jones and Windholz 1990: 1011). The authors claim that the Q-set method revealed these patterns more clearly than a reading of the transcripts would have done.

Spence, Dahl, and Jones (1993) again chose Mrs. C. as the single subject in their study of the impact of interpretation on associative freedom. They found that the influence of interpretation on associative freedom varied as a function of the phase of treatment. In particular, in the middle and late stages of treatment, when the analyst referred to a defensive style, pointed to a recurrent theme, or discussed Mrs. C.'s dreams or fantasies, she showed an increase in associative freedom. The effect was strongest in the later stages of the analysis, when an interpretation could be shown to exert a positive influence on free association up to three hours after it was offered. When used early in the treatment, however, these interpretations did not appear to affect Mrs. C.'s ability to associate freely. The authors speculate that it is the development of a positive transference that allows interpretations to have their desired effect.

Having briefly considered some of the ways in which a single long-term case may be studied using empirical methods, we will now describe our own project that used research methods to study several brief psychodynamic cases.

A research project on the process of brief psychodynamic therapy

The Rutgers Psychotherapy Research Group set out to study the kinds of therapist interventions that lead to progress in brief psychodynamic therapy. In the present context, this research program can serve to illustrate in some detail single-case research in a format that is applicable to other forms of psychoanalytic therapy as well. In addition to single-case design, an important feature of our approach is the employment of as much context as possible in scoring therapist and patient utterances. That is, the method attempts to place the rater in the same position of privilege as the therapist in having access to the entire stream of material as it unfolds. By doing this we hoped to study psychoanalytic therapy as it is taught and practiced, namely by noting how well the therapist tracks the patient's constantly shifting needs and how patient progress accelerates or stagnates in response (Messer and Holland 1998).

We were interested in two therapist variables: (a) quality of process; and (b) adherence to a focus, and their relationship to one patient variable, degree of progress or stagnation. *Quality of therapist process* includes three aspects: attunement to the patient on a moment to moment basis; therapist competence, which refers to the adequacy or skill with which a therapist applies psychodynamic technique; and interpersonal manner, which refers to the way that the therapist relates to the patient. We constructed a 7-point Likert Scale, the Rutgers Therapist Process Scale, with anchor points defining the meaning of each numerical rating. All therapist interventions, or, in some studies, five-minute blocks of dialogue, were scored for quality of process in the order in which they occurred, thus preserving their meaning in context.

To measure *adherence to a focus*, we chose the Mt. Zion Plan Formulation Method (PFM). In reviewing transcripts – from cases provided by the Mt. Zion group, as well as from our own – we found ourselves in disagreement with the Mt. Zion group on the nature of the central dynamics. Where they saw (in accordance with the tenets of Weiss's theory) instances of survivor and separation guilt that prevented patients from achieving independence, we saw issues of separation anxiety and immature dependency wishes, in accordance with Fairbairn's (1946) object relations theory. That is, they understood these patients as concerned primarily about harming others with whom they were entangled in relationships whereas we perceived them as overly needy of these others.

This suggested a study: Is the Mt. Zion Plan Formulation Method transportable to another setting in which investigators are not wedded to Weissian theory? The Rutgers and Mt. Zion groups each selected a case for study from their archive of audio recorded and transcribed cases. We each created Plan Formulations according to the Mt. Zion fourfold scheme, which includes items pertaining to patient goals, obstructions to these goals (i.e., pathological beliefs), tests that the patient might pose for the therapist, and insights to be acquired (Curtis and Silberschatz 1997). Both groups were able to rate the plan items reliably, but each group endorsed very different plans. That is, the Mt. Zion Plan reflected their cognitive-dynamic theoretical emphasis, and the Rutgers Plan reflected our object relations emphasis (Collins and Messer 1991; Messer 1991). The second therapist variable, adherence to a focus, then became two variables, namely, the extent to which therapist interventions compatible with each Plan were able to predict patient progress. All three scales were found to possess good reliability (Messer *et al.* 1992). Thus, we had three reliable therapist variables – quality of process, and plan compatibility of interventions according to two plans, the Rutgers Plan and the Mt. Zion Plan. Therapist statements were scored on the Plan Compatibility of Intervention Scale (PCIS; Weiss *et al.* 1986).

Turning to the patient variable, our research group created a scale, the Rutgers Psychotherapy Progress and Stagnation Scale, with eight subscales capturing patient progress and stagnation as psychodynamically conceived. The scale included areas such as exploration of significant material, development of insight, focus on the self, and emotional experiencing. The subscales were measured globally by means of a Likert Scale ranging from +3 for progress to –3 for stagnation. We applied the scale to the two cases and achieved satisfactory interrater reliability (Messer *et al.* 1992).

With the four reliable measures in hand, the question we posed was, "Could patient progress/stagnation be predicted from (a) therapist goodness of process and (b) compatibility of therapist interventions with a plan?" For the moment, we will refer to the Rutgers Plan, but we will return to its comparison with the Mt. Zion Plan below.

We found modest but significant correlations between both therapist variables and progress as measured over the therapy as a whole and for many of the individual sessions. However, we noticed that the significant correlations tended to cluster in the middle sessions. We then examined the correlations by phase of therapy – beginning, middle, and termination phase – because this is often how brief dynamic therapy is conceptualized. The results (Messer *et al.* 1992) were that, for both cases, therapist adherence to the Rutgers Plan correlated significantly with patient progress in the early and middle phases and that quality of therapist process correlated with progress in the middle phase. The correlations for the termination phase were not significant. What we understood from these results was that defining and working on the focus or plan was most important in the early and middle phases and the quality of therapist interventions mattered most when therapist and patient were in the thick of working on the focus in the middle phase.

We then compared the correlations between plan compatibility – based on Fairbairn's object relations theory or on Mt. Zion's cognitive-dynamic theory – and patient progress in these three phases. The pattern of correlations across the three phases was quite clear: The Rutgers PCIS correlated positively in five of the six instances (three phases for each of two patients), whereas the Mt. Zion PCIS correlated negatively in five of the six instances, three of them significantly (Tishby and Messer 1995). That is, compatibility with the object relations plan was associated with patient progress, but compatibility of interventions with the Mt. Zion cognitive-dynamic plan predicted stagnation.

This line of research has implications for the practice of brief psychodynamic therapy. It suggests that therapist adherence to a focus is salutary for patient progress with those suitable for this form of treatment, at least in the early and middle phases of therapy. Furthermore, not any focus will do; the results point to there being more and less useful ways of formulating a focus in specific cases. Of course, we do not know just how widely these findings might generalize. Neither do we know whether a specific outlook, such as Fairbairn's object relations theory, is generally more fitting than other approaches, such as Weiss and Sampson's cognitive-dynamic theory, or if, as we suspect, it depends on the nature of the specific case.

The Rutgers Psychotherapy Progress Scale subsequently was refined so that all eight aspects could be measured separately. Studies have been conducted that demonstrate good reliability and validity (Holland, Roberts and Messer 1998). Our hope is that this line of research will continue to allow for the scientific study of the process of psychoanalytic therapy and for the comparison of different theoretical approaches within it.

Advantages and disadvantages of single-case research

In the conflict between a hermeneutic or narrative approach and a positivistic or scientific one, the study of single cases presents an attractive middle way for the researcher interested in studying psychotherapy, including psychoanalysis. More and more, psychotherapy researchers are becoming aware of the importance of context in determining the meaning of events in psychotherapy. The modest findings of traditional group comparison designs in their efforts to identify relationships between process and outcome variables have been widely noted. Perhaps this failure is due to the inability of such designs to capture the subtle processes of psychotherapy. The study of single cases holds more promise in this area because it allows the kind of fine-grained analysis and sensitivity to context that are necessary for a sophisticated understanding of psychotherapy processes.

Although in this chapter we present single-case research as an example of "normative science," we should point out that the study of single cases has long been regarded with suspicion by practitioners of experimental science. The study of single cases has only recently begun to regain some respectability within scientific circles (e.g., Kazdin 1998; Yin 1994). Normative science values large-N studies above all others, and to the extent that it is desirable to generate results that may be immediately applied to a large number of people or situations, the single-case design is at a disadvantage. Replication on a case-by-case basis is a time-consuming, albeit worthy, endeavor.

However, in an effort to improve psychotherapy outcomes, one new line of clinical research blends a single-case emphasis with large scale samples. It monitors individuals, rather than groups of patients (Lambert 2001), but then compares the progress of these individuals to that of a reference group that is similar along the dimensions of interest. It draws on new and sophisticated techniques like probit analysis, survival analysis, and hierarchical linear modeling to effect this comparison. A variant of this model is what Fishman (1999) refers to as the pragmatic case study. It is the effort to create a data base of cases with an emphasis on contextual detail and the unique life circumstances of the individual. The goal is to collect relevant process and outcome data from each case in a systematic manner and to use the cumulative data base to guide treatment of future cases. (But see Messer [2000] for the difficulties involved in this approach from a psychoanalytic perspective.)

Another new research endeavor is known as hermeneutic single-case efficacy design: it uses a "mixture of quantitative and qualitative information to create a rich case record that provides both positive and negative evidence for the causal influence of therapy on client outcome" (Elliott 2001: 317). What is particularly admirable about this method is that it searches for negative evidence to rule out competing explanations as to how nontherapy events might have caused client improvement. A related approach is "multiple case depth research" (Schneider 1999), which combines both case-study methodology and depth-experiential therapeutic principles. It stresses converging lines of multiple sources of evidence for its standard of validation, posing three questions (Schneider 1999: 1532): (a) are the data plausibly linked to theory; (b) is the theory plausibly generalizable; and (c) is the conclusion plausibly disconfirmable? Its advantage over single-case design is that it allows for cross-case comparisons and greater generalizability.

Innovations like these will add to the attractiveness of single-subject case studies. From the point of view of a hermeneutic or narrative approach, on the other hand, any empirical treatment of a subject as complex as that of psychoanalysis or psychotherapy must inevitably fall short of capturing its richness and variety, its complexity, and its many layers of meaning. In this view, the qualitative case study is the method best suited to study the subject matter of psychoanalysis. As we have seen, however, not all case studies have measured up to the task, and we stress the importance of improving the presentation of narrative material in the qualitative case study, as well as of expanding the availability of recorded psychoanalytic therapies for further single-case quantitative studies.

References

Blatt, S. J., Bers, S. A. and Schaffer, C. E. (1992) The assessment of self, unpublished research manual, Yale University, New Haven, CT.

Blatt, S. J., Brenneis, C. B., Schimek, J. G. and Glick, M. (1976) 'Normal development and psychopathological impairment of the concept of the object on the Rorschach', *Journal of Abnormal Psychology* 85: 364–73.

Bucci, W. and Miller, N. E. (1993) 'Primary process analogue: the referential activity (RA) measure', in N. E. Miller, L. Luborsky, J. P. Barber and J. P. Docherty (eds) *Psychodynamic Treatment Research: a handbook for clinical practice*, New York: Basic Books, pp. 387–406.

Colarusso, C. A. (2000) 'The analysis of a neurotic boy', in J. Cohen and B. J. Cohler (eds) *The Psychoanalytic Study of Lives over Time*, New York: Academic Press, pp. 17–48.

Collins, W. D. and Messer, S. B. (1991) 'Extending the plan formulation method to an object relations perspective: reliability, stability, and adaptability', *Psychological Assessment* 3: 75–81.

Curtis, J. T. and Silberschatz, G. (1997) 'The plan formulation method', in T. D. Eells (ed.) *Handbook of Psychotherapy Case Formulation*, New York: Guilford Press, pp. 116–36.

Derogatis, L. R. (1983) *SCL-90-R: administration, scoring and procedural manual II*, Baltimore, MD: Clinical Psychometric Research.

Edelson, M. (1985) 'The hermeneutic turn and the single case study in psychoanalysis', *Psychoanalysis and Contemporary Thought* 8: 567–614.

Elliott, R. (2001) 'Hermeneutic single-case efficacy design: an overview', in K. J. Schneider, J. F. T. Bugental and J. F. Pierson (eds) *The Handbook of Humanistic Psychology*, Thousand Oaks, CA: Sage, pp. 315–26.

Fairbairn, W. R. D. (1946) 'Object relations and dynamic structure', in W. R. D. Fairbairn (1954) *An Object Relations Theory of the Personality*, New York: Basic Books, pp.137–51.

Fishman, D. B. (1999) *The Case for Pragmatic Psychology*, New York: New York University Press.

Fonagy, P. and Moran, G. S. (1990) 'Studies on the efficacy of child psychoanalysis', *Journal of Consulting and Clinical Psychology* 58: 684–95.

—— and Moran, G. S. (1993) 'Selecting single case research designs for clinicians', in N. E. Miller, L. Luborsky, J. P. Barber and J. P. Docherty (eds) *Psychodynamic Treatment Research: a handbook for clinical practice*, New York: Basic Books, pp. 37–52.

Geller, J. D., Hartley, D., Behrends, R., Farber, B., Andrews, C., Marciano, P., Bender, D. and Brownlow, A. (1992) *Thematic Patterning Scale of Object Representations II*, unpublished manuscript, Department of Psychology, Yale University, New Haven, CT.

Green, B. L., Gleser, G. C., Stone, W. N. and Seifert, R. F. (1975) 'Relationships among diverse measures of psychotherapy outcome', *Journal of Consulting and Clinical Psychology* 43: 689–99.

Gruen, R. J. and Blatt, S. J. (1990) 'Changes in self and object representation during long-term dynamically oriented treatment', *Psychoanalytic Psychology* 7: 399–422.

Hilliard, R. B. (1993) 'Single-case methodology in psychotherapy process and outcome research', *Journal of Consulting and Clinical Psychology* 61: 373–80.

Holland, S., Roberts, N. E. and Messer, S. B. (1998) 'Reliability and validity of the Rutgers Psychotherapy Progress Scale', *Psychotherapy Research* 8: 104–10.

Jones, E. E. and Windholz, M. (1990) 'The psychoanalytic case study: toward a method for systematic inquiry', *Journal of the American Psychoanalytic Association* 38: 985–1015.

Kazdin, A. E. (1998) *Research Designs in Clinical Psychology* (3rd edn), Needham Heights, MA: Allyn and Bacon.

Lambert, M. J. (2001) 'Psychotherapy outcome and quality improvement: introduction to the Special Series on patient-focused research', *Journal of Consulting and Clinical Psychology* 69: 147–49.

Luborsky, L. and Luborsky, E. (1993) 'The era of measures of transference: the CCRT and other measures', in T. Shapiro and R. N. Emde (eds) *Research in Psychoanalysis: process, development, outcome*, Madison, CT: International Universities Press, pp. 329–51.

Marschke-Tobier, K. (2000) 'The case of Lisa: from the "baddest girl in the class" to feeling sad and lonely: reflections on the analysis of an 8–year-old girl', in J. Cohen and B. J. Cohler (eds) *The Psychoanalytic Study of Lives over Time*, New York: Academic Press, pp. 67–94.

McCullough, L. (1993) 'Standard and individualized psychotherapy outcome measures: a core battery', in N. E. Miller, L. Luborsky, J. P. Barber and J. P. Docherty (eds) *Psychodynamic Treatment Research: a handbook for clinical practice*, New York: Basic Books, pp. 469–96.

Messer, S. B. (1991) 'The case formulation approach: issues of reliability and validity', *American Psychologist* 46: 1348–50.

—— (2000) 'A psychodynamic clinician responds to Fishman's case study proposal', *Prevention and Treatment*, 3(9), posted 3 May 2000. Online. Available <http://journals.apa.org/prevention/volume3/pre0030009c.html>.

—— and Holland, S. J. (1998) 'Therapist interventions and patient progress in brief psychodynamic therapy: single-case design', in R. F. Bornstein and J. M. Masling (eds) *Empirical Studies of Psychoanalytic Theories, vol. 8, empirical studies of the therapeutic hour*, Washington, DC: American Psychological Association Press, pp. 229–57.

—— Sass, L. A. and Woolfolk, R. L. (eds) (1988) *Hermeneutics and Psychological Theory*, New Brunswick, NJ: Rutgers University Press.

—— Tishby, O. and Spillman, A. (1992) 'Taking context seriously in psychotherapy research: relating therapist interventions to patient progress in brief psychodynamic therapy', *Journal of Consulting and Clinical Psychology* 60: 678–88.

Morgan, R. W., Luborsky, L., Crits-Christoph, P., Curtis, H. and Solomon, J. (1982) 'Predicting the outcomes of psychotherapy using the Penn Helping Alliance rating method', *Archives of General Psychiatry* 39: 397–402.

Perry, J. C. (1994) 'Assessing psychodynamic patterns using the idiographic conflict formulation method', *Psychotherapy Research* 4: 239–52.

Piper, W. E. and Duncan, S. C. (1999) 'Object relations theory and short-term dynamic psychotherapy: findings from the Quality of Object Relations Scale', *Clinical Psychology Review* 19: 669–86.

Rosenbaum, A. L. (2000) 'The case of Charlie: the analysis of a child', in J. Cohen and B. J. Cohler (eds) *The Psychoanalytic Study of Lives over Time*, New York: Academic Press, pp. 125–44.

Schneider, K. J. (1999) 'Multiple-case research: bringing experience-near closer', *Journal of Clinical Psychology* 55: 1531–40.

Seitz, P. (1966) 'The consensus problem in psychoanalytic research', in L. Gottschalk and A. Auerbach (eds) *Methods in Research in Psychotherapy*, New York: Appleton-Century-Crofts, pp. 209–25.

Silberschatz, G. and Curtis, J. T. (1993) 'Measuring the therapist's impact on the patient's therapeutic progress', *Journal of Consulting and Clinical Psychology* 61: 403–11.

Spence, D. P. (1993) 'Traditional case studies and prescriptions for improving them', in N. E. Miller, L. Luborsky, J. P. Barber and J. P. Docherty (eds) *Psychodynamic Treatment Research: a handbook for clinical practice*, New York: Basic Books, pp. 37–52.

—— (1994) *The Rhetorical Voice of Psychoanalysis: displacement of evidence by theory*, Cambridge, MA: Harvard University Press.

—— (1998) 'Rain forest or mud field: guest editorial', *International Journal of Psychoanalysis* 79: 643–7.

—— (2000) 'Remembrances of things past', *Journal of Clinical Psychoanalysis* 9: 149–62.

—— (2001) 'Case reports in a two-person world', *Psychoanalytic Psychology* 18: 451–67.

—— Dahl, H. and Jones, E. E. (1993) 'Impact of interpretation on associative freedom', *Journal of Consulting and Clinical Psychology* 61: 395–402.

Stiles, W. B., Shapiro, D. A. and Elliott, R. (1986) 'Are all psychotherapies equivalent?', *American Psychologist* 41: 165–80.

Target, M. and Fonagy, P. (1994) 'Efficacy of psychoanalysis for children with emotional disorders', *Journal of the American Academy of Child and Adolescent Psychiatry* 33: 361–71.

Tishby, O. and Messer, S. B. (1995) 'The relationship between plan compatibility of therapist interventions and patient progress: a comparison of two plan formulations', *Psychotherapy Research* 5: 76–88.

Weiss, J., Sampson, H. and the Mount Zion Psychotherapy Research Group (eds) (1986) *The Psychoanalytic Process: theory, clinical observation, and empirical research*, New York: Guilford Press.

Yin, R. K. (1994) *Case Study Research: design and methods* (2nd edn), Thousand Oaks, CA: Sage.

Part V

Applied psychoanalysis

Greed as an individual and social phenomenon

An application of the two-configurations model[1]

Paul L. Wachtel

Sidney Blatt was a mentor to me in many different ways. When I arrived at Yale as a young first year graduate student, I was more in need of a mentor than I realized. Still quite naive, and relatively unfamiliar with the field of psychology after having majored in physics as an undergraduate, I was far from ready for prime time. But I had the extraordinary stroke of luck of being assigned to Sid as a research assistant in connection with my National Institute of Mental Health fellowship. For a young student who did not yet even know about the tensions so prevalent in our field between hard-headed research and sensitive, intuitive clinical engagement, being assigned to Sid was a blessing. Sid was, and is, one of the rare individuals in our field who stands out in both realms, and having the opportunity to work so closely with him at the start of my graduate school career helped me not to have to choose between the two sides of my own nature either.

By the time I was applying for internships, Sid had moved the center of his participation at Yale from the psychology department to the role of chief psychologist at the Yale Psychiatric Institute (YPI). Thus, when I interned at YPI, I got to have Sid as a mentor in a second way. Now working closely with him in the clinical realm, I had the opportunity to immerse myself in *his* ability to immerse *himself* in the experiences of others. Whether it was going over a Rorschach protocol or a therapy session, working with Sid meant appreciating what the words "depth" and "sensitivity" really meant.

Finally, when it came time to do my dissertation, it will not surprise you that I chose Sid to be my mentor in still one more way. I recall beginning a project that, for various logistical reasons, did not work out and finding myself, in September of the year I hoped to graduate from Yale, starting from scratch sans proposal, sans data, sans idea. Nine months later, I had my Ph.D. in hand. I suspect that most of you, looking back on your own experience writing your dissertations, might wonder if I signed a pact with the devil to get myself out of New Haven so quickly. Quite the opposite. The pact I signed, as it were, was with the most extraordinarily helpful, facilitative, dedicated mentor one could possibly hope for – Sid.

Now it is true that by some odd omission Sid did not introduce me to my wife. I still wonder how he could have been so derelict in his seeming commitment to take care of virtually every aspect of my life during my years as a graduate student. But fortunately, someone else I knew at Yale introduced me to Ellen just after I had left New Haven. And because that has worked out very, very well, I think Sid can be forgiven for this one lacuna (a word I learned from Sid). I am delighted to be able to offer at least a down payment here on the enormous debt I owe to Sid in so many ways.

Blatt's two-configurations model

Over the past 25 years, Sid Blatt's two-configurations model (e.g., 1974, 1995; Blatt and Shichman 1983) has been one of the most innovative and important contributions to our understanding of personality dynamics and development. The model stresses the development of personality along two key dimensions – the establishment of mature, satisfying interpersonal relationships and the formation of a cohesive, effective self or identity. In much of his writings, Sid has termed the first line of development *anaclitic* or *relational*, and he has referred to the second line as *introjective* or *self-definitional*. The model has been particularly prominent in research on psychopathology in general and depression in particular. But the two-configurations model is rooted as well in a still broader vision. It explores and elaborates on a tension that has been noted by thinkers about human nature throughout the centuries. Humans are both part of nature and apart from nature – separate, differentiated beings and a part of a larger whole that is absolutely essential for their survival. We suffer from our knowledge of our separate existence and from our awareness of the future – and hence of death. At the same time, this awareness is our essential defining quality as human and the foundation of all that is unique to our species.

Much as with nature, society too is both the context that makes our lives possible and the womb from which we struggle throughout life to emerge. The warm nurturing waters of human contact and social connection in which we swim and from which we derive our social and psychological nutrients are also waters that threaten to engulf and drown us. Anxiety is almost inevitable in negotiating this Janus-faced dilemma that is quintessential to our species. If we secure too strongly our connection with nature and with society, we are in danger of losing our uniqueness, our identity, indeed our very sense of selfhood or being. But if we dedicate ourselves too single-mindedly to creating a self, even to being true to our perceived inner yearnings and perceptions, we run an equally terrifying risk – losing touch with the very ground of our being, our intimate connection, indeed our inseparability from, the larger context of nature and of society.

Different cultures pull for a resolution of this tension in one direction or the other – the distinction between individualistic and collectivist cultures is a widely applied one in cross-cultural research (Triandis 1995) – but in fact people in *every* culture experience these competing pulls. The proportions and the modal behaviors or values may differ, but the need to deal with the fundamental conflict is common to all.

One particularly important feature of the two-configurations model, setting it apart from almost all of the other approaches to this core dilemma in human life, is its grounding in the traditions both of psychoanalysis and of empirical psychological research. On the one hand, in contrast to more speculative or anecdotally rooted understandings, the two-configurations model has been put repeatedly to the test of systematic controlled research. On the other hand, however, unlike formulations about personality that are derived rather exclusively from factor analyses of questionnaires or some other simplifying methodology that purchases seeming precision at a high cost, the two-configurations model is rooted as well in the complex vision of personality development that derives from psychoanalysis. Thus, like all psychoanalytic conceptualizations, it is dynamic, rather than categorical. The two configurations are not alternative categories into which people are put. They are not even "percentages of variance," with people conceptualized as showing a little of this, a little of that. Rather, they are inclinations or orientations *in tension*. As is true of all psychoanalytic formulations, at the center of this model is conflict, paradox, and an ongoing need to come to terms with powerful and competing inclinations.

People do differ in the degree to which they manifest anaclitic or introjective tendencies, and it is true that an extreme overweighting in either direction is likely to be associated with pathology. But health is not measured by the degree to which the person achieves a fifty-fifty balance. Balance is indeed important, but it is a *dialectical* balance, a balance that reflects the ongoing dynamic effort to reconcile conflicting needs and proclivities. The optimal balance for any particular person is a reflection of that person's genetic inheritance, early developmental experience, later developmental experiences, and, very importantly, the interpersonal and societal context in which the person's behavior and experience are manifested. This means not only that the social and relational context in which the person's orientation *developed* is crucial but also that the context in which it is *presently* manifested can elicit, in differing configurations and proportions, quite different facets of the complex whole that is the person. The same individual who is especially concerned with separation, competency, and self-definition in one context may well be more concerned with a sense of belonging or being nurtured and cared for in another. This is not an inconsistency but a reflection of the inherently contextual nature of personality or, as I have discussed it elsewhere, of the specificity of human experience (Wachtel 2000).

Introjective and anaclitic orientations as bound opposites

Although the concept of introjective and anaclitic lines of development points to a fundamental tension in almost all of us, it does not imply two separate "types" of people. Not only are the two orientations woven together empirically, in the readily observed variability and contextuality of their manifestations; they are not even *conceptually* independent. By this I do not mean that they are not distinct or that they are not clearly delineated conceptually. Rather, what I mean is that they are conceptualized in a way that illuminates their quality of being not simply opposites but *bound* opposites, opposites in a kind of intrinsic tension, such that each inclination is powerfully and fundamentally shaped by the other. It is out of the very way that we attempt to merge, attach, root ourselves in the other or in society that our need for separation, boundaries, or self-definition emerges and is heightened. And it is in our very efforts to define ourselves as separate and self-sufficient that our need for connection is fueled. One side cannot be achieved without, as a very feature of achieving it, the other being introduced anew. We cannot resolve the tension by choosing one or the other but only by continually and creatively weaving them together in the fabric of our lives.

In this conceptualization, the two-configurations model resembles Piaget's complementary processes of assimilation and accommodation. Here too, each process cannot be adequately understood, cannot even really be defined, without reference to the other. Consider, for example, what happens when a child who has developed an initial schema of *dog* comes into contact with a kind of dog that he has not seen before, say a Chihuahua or a Great Dane. When the child learns to include either of these new experiences in his schema of dog, he is clearly assimilating them to that schema. But in the very effort to do this, the child is also accommodating the schema to take them in. It is no longer the same schema, simply because it is now a schema that includes these new outliers that previously were not part of the child's vision of what the category dog included. It is the very act of assimilation that produces the accommodation and the very act of accommodation that enables the assimilation. Neither could proceed without the other.

Social implications of the model: bound opposites and the phenomena of greed

The understanding of the two-configurations model in terms of bound opposites, of dynamic rather than categorical distinctions, has important implications not only for how we view personality development and psychopathology but also for how we understand many phenomena that are central to the operation of our society as a whole. Any society, and especially one as complex as ours, has as one of its central challenges reconciling these two essential features of human psychology. A society that fails to make room for what might be called the anaclitic side of life, for our continuing need for relatedness and our continuing dependence on each other throughout life, breeds alienation and leaves people enormously vulnerable to the vagaries of nature, markets, or other sources of potential disaster. Even the hardest of hard-right ultra-individualistic ideologues (or at least those who have any hope of being electable) acknowledge that we need some kind of safety net for those who are in need. Reliance on individual responsibility alone is a recipe for disaster, both socially and individually.

At the same time, if a society makes insufficient space for self-definition, if the need for boundaries, relative autonomy, or the development of the unique aims and values that create a distinct identity are persistently thwarted, the result is likely to be stultifying conformity and an absence of initiative and motivation. The now-defunct Soviet Union might be thought of as an example of such a society.

The task of a society is to create a way of life in which these two strands of human nature interact in a dynamic and creative way, with neither predominating to a degree that it crowds out the other. As with individuals, distortions and hypertrophies can develop in societies too, but as with individuals, these hypertrophies always have a price and are inherently unstable. Ideologues may, in one sense, almost be defined by their failure to appreciate the dialectical nature of human needs and motivations. Perhaps a primer of Blatt's two-configurations theory should be required reading for anyone running for office!

Greed as a social phenomenon

In this chapter, I wish to focus on one particular realm in which the social and the psychological converge and in which the two-configurations model provides potential illumination – the phenomenon of greed. I choose greed as my focus both because it is a topic I have recently begun to explore in my own research and because it is especially central to the dynamics of our society. At least since the time of Adam Smith, it has been clear that greed can be a powerful engine of economic growth and productivity. As Smith (1776, Book I, Chapter II: 2) put it, in a widely quoted passage, "It is not from the benevolence of the butcher, the brewer, or the baker that we expect our dinner, but from their regard to their self-interest."

To be sure, greed and self-interest are not necessarily the same thing. And a strong case can be made that Smith used the latter term (that is, *self-interest*) precisely because he meant that, rather than greed. But Smith's thinking has been retrofitted, one might say, by an ideological strain that has become in many respects the dominant one in our society. The constant stimulation of desire for more and more material goods in all of us and the single-minded pursuit of that experienced need for more and more by each individual in the society is seen by leading voices in our nation's academic and political life as the fuel that ignites our economy and makes us a strong and prosperous nation.

It can be said that the economic side of life dominates so much in American society because economists have been so successful in persuading people that it is the only side of life that need be considered. In the ideology that – through the rhetorical magic of mathematical equations – passes for economic "science," explicit concern with the feelings and needs of others, except insofar as those feelings and needs are important to discern for the purposes of marketing and product development, is not only unnecessary but misguided. Attention to the needs of the community as a whole or to its least privileged members impairs the remarkable alchemy through which the invisible hand of the market most effectively turns the base metal of individual greed into social gold.

Interestingly, if we turn to Adam Smith himself, we see that from the outset he understood that the wish for more for oneself must be pursued both in tension with and, from a broader perspective, in concert with – or in the term I introduced earlier, in *bound opposition to* – another equally crucial set of human motivations and inclinations. Smith discussed this second crucial dimension under the rubrics of natural sympathy and moral sentiments. A good society – indeed, even a society that functions well economically – depends on a degree of trust and trustworthiness that enables people to count on the honesty, integrity, and good will of those with whom they interact and without which even the capacity to engage effectively in hard-nosed negotiation breaks down. When greed alone prevails, greed itself is thwarted; when each person has no inhibition in maximizing profit by providing cheap, damaged, or dangerous goods, none can engage intelligently in trade.

Importantly, however, Smith's vision of a good society goes beyond simply the modicum of honesty required for the pursuit of self-interest to be reasonably enlightened. As he put it in *The Theory of Moral Sentiments*:

> All the members of human society stand in need of each other's assistance . . . . Where the necessary assistance is reciprocally afforded from love, from gratitude, from friendship and esteem, the society flourishes and is happy. All the different members of it are bound together by the agreeable bonds of love and affection . . . . Society . . . cannot subsist among those who are at all times ready to hurt and injure one another.
>
> (Smith 1753: 124–5)

In a contemporary context, writers like the political scientist Robert Putnam have made similar points about our own society and the challenges it faces.

In essence, then, the dynamics of greed in a well-functioning society must be dialectically balanced, as must the anaclitic and introjective tendencies in a healthy personality. Putting together Sid Blatt and Adam Smith, we may say, combining both conceptual frameworks, that ambition, striving for success, and seeking to stand out are essential components of a vital society and economy but only when balanced by a corresponding element of caring, concern, solidarity, or fellow feeling for others. When the first is lacking, interdependence regresses to dependency, and one may perhaps depict the society itself as problematically anaclitic, lacking dynamism, productivity, innovation, or willingness to take risks or to lead. When the second is lacking, one may think of the society as problematically introjective, the alienated, competitive struggle among hostile and isolated monads described by social critics from Hobbes (1651) to Marx (1964) to Fromm (1941, 1955).

Insatiability and heedlessness

Given its importance both in individual lives and in our society as a whole, greed has been a rather neglected topic in the psychological literature. Among psychoanalytic discussions of the topic, a Kleinian perspective has been particularly prominent (e.g., Boris 1986; Emery 1992; Klein 1957). These writings, although at times suggestive, have tended to be breath-takingly speculative. They have also given enormous emphasis (perhaps, one might say at the risk of a bad pun, overweening emphasis) to the experience of the infant at the breast. Consequently, they offer few paths toward understanding the ways in which variations in greed among individuals and societies are related to larger social phenomena.

In part, the neglect of the concept of greed – both in the psychoanalytic literature and in the larger literature of psychology in general – reflects the origins of the concept of greed not in the empirical tradition of psycho-logical research but in the judgmental tradition of moral exhortation. It reflects as well the considerable ambiguity and imprecision in our usage of the terms *greed* and *greedy*. If one, for example, looks through the literally thousands of references to greed in the Lexis-Nexis index of newspapers, magazines, and other news and media sources, it is readily apparent that the variations in tone, nuance, and both connotative and denotative refer-ence point are enormous. In thinking about these varied uses and meanings of the term, I have provisionally, in my own research, attempted to introduce some order by distinguishing between two broad classes of usage – greed as *insatiability* and greed as *heedlessness*.

In some ways, the former may be seen as pointing to how greedy individuals hurt (or at least frustrate) themselves, and the latter to how, through their greed, they hurt others. The distinction, like almost all distinctions in the psychological realm, is by no means hard and fast. Thus, for example, King Midas might well serve as a poster child for the insatiability dimension. As rich as he was, it was simply not enough. And ultimately, the story of Midas is clearly a story of how greed brings ruin to the greedy person himself. But we can certainly agree that things do not go well for Midas's daughter either. And indeed, the insatiability of the greedy person has almost inevitable impact on others.

Similarly, if we consider who might be the poster child for the second meaning of greed, heedlessness, a good candidate might be Gordon Gekko, the character in the film *Wall Street* (Pressman and Stone 1987). Gekko's signature statement, "Greed is good," comes from the mouth of a man who is amorally indifferent to the impact of his actions on others. He wants his, and the devil take the hindmost. Yet at the same time, two things are worth noticing. First, Gekko hardly seems like a genuinely happy or fulfilled man. His greed has an impact on him as well. Second, one important sign of his discomfort with his total indifference is his need to rationalize it. This rationalization, "Greed is good" is the mantra of our entire system, a claim that, ultimately, selfish behavior not only does not hurt others but is essential to everyone's welfare. Remember Adam Smith on the butcher and the baker (leaving out, of course, Smith's insights about the moral sentiments).

Greed and the two-configurations model

Can the two-configurations formulation shed any further light on the distinction I have been discussing thus far? Perhaps we might speculate that the insatiability dimension has some relationship to the anaclitic line of development and the heedlessness dimension to the introjective. Might we, for example, see a disguised or altered expression of what Blatt has called anaclitic in the greedy person's insatiable hunger, in feelings of emptiness and lack of support and nurturance that fuel a relentless sense of needing more? Similarly, in greed marked more by the dimension of heedlessness, are we observing a pathology of drivenness and self-definition, an inability to integrate the needs and feelings of others into one's own aims either because the boundaries of the self, perceived at one level as too permeable, are defensively bolstered and hardened or because driving voices from within drown out the voices of other people's needs and experiences?

To be sure, insatiability can derive from an unquenchable desire for achievement or at least for signs of achievement. And, conversely, what I am calling heedlessness can at times derive from a sense of entitlement that comes from feeling, "I have never received the love and protection I desire from others." So there is not a simple one-to-one correspondence, and this, of course, is not surprising because the two configurations Blatt has studied do not reduce simply to greed, nor does greed reduce to those two configurations. They are potentially related but by no means equivalent concepts.

Nonetheless, exploring the ways in which greed, materialism, and consumerism do and do not map onto the two-configurations model can add illuminating dimensionality to our understanding of the social and motivational implications of greedy behavior. At times, we may note, an overly materialistic orientation is a means toward independence from other people, toward a substitution of *things* for people. But at other times, it can be almost the opposite. In one patient I saw a number of years back, for example, who had a seemingly insatiable desire for material things, those material things were clearly in the service of ingratiating himself with others or of making himself attractive to them, a sadly ineffective effort to connect with other people, rather than to be independent.

Stimulated by the two-configurations model, one might suggest that, in contrast to the distinction between insatiability and heedlessness (though partially overlapping with that distinction), the various manifestations of greed might also be usefully categorized according to whether the primary aim is one of *filling* up the self with good stuff or one of *shoring* up the self with signs of achievement and success. Although the (anaclitic) fear of being a hungry self (or a lonely self) and the (introjective) fear of being a weak self are by no means totally independent, they do represent different loadings or emphases that, as in other arenas in which roughly the same distinction has been applied, can have quite significant implications.

From the vantage point of the two-configurations model, we may ask about greedy behavior whether it supports primarily the sense of belonging, being connected, being taken care of or, in contrast, of being masterful and bounded, to use for this latter orientation the terminology emphasized by Cushman (1990) in another application of psychological perspectives to the analysis of social issues. And one thing that immediately becomes clearer from this vantage point, and quite interesting as well, is that although one might think of greed as something that disrupts social ties, and of the greedy person as unpopular as a result of greed, we may also see that certain forms of greed (and of the related phenomena of materialism and consumerism) are largely designed to make oneself more desirable or attractive to others. These efforts may not succeed (as many neurotic tendencies do not succeed), but that is at times their aim, and whether we are considering the implications for treating an individual in psychotherapy or of working to change problematic social trends, it is useful to understand the distinctive motivational configurations that underlie the pattern with which we are concerned. When someone wants lots of money, expensive clothes, a big house, all the signs of success, sometimes it is to enhance the sense of self-efficacy and independence, but at other times it is a way of winning people over. The two-configurations model helps us to see more clearly a distinction between kinds of greed or motives for greed that may not be immediately evident in the morphology of the behavior itself.

Put differently, people who are particularly driven by feelings (conscious or unconscious) of dependency, neediness, or emptiness, who need to be filled up by others, who manifest inclinations toward more hysterical forms of personality organization, may well be more inclined, when greedy, to be hungry, to feel they need more and more simply because they do not have enough. At the same time, because their greed is anaclitically rooted, they may be wary of alienating others, may be hesitant to offend by *actually* taking more than their fair share, even as their *desires* feel endless and their capacity to feel they have enough is limited. As the two-configurations model helps us to understand, greed of this sort may be characterized more by resentfulness than by actual accumulation; such people feel perpetually unsatisfied but also perpetually prevented from acting to take or get what they think they need.

In contrast, people more focused on self-definition, on the maintenance of clear boundaries between self and other, or on struggling with feelings of inadequacy or insufficient power or independence, may be more likely, when greedy, to be characterized by the dimension I have called heedlessness. Their greed is, one might say, less pathetic and more aggressive. That is, they are struggling less with feelings of needing to be filled up and more with feelings of needing to be strong and dominant. Fine tuning themselves to the needs of others in order to elicit protection and nurturance from them is of less concern than making sure that others are not dominating or disdaining them. The need for more and more is, one might say figuratively, to display the musculature of the body's surface, rather than to fill its empty interior. Thus, the heedlessness dimension of greed may be expected to bear some relationship to the introjective dimension of Blatt's two-configurations model, with its emphasis on boundaries, separation, and self-definition.

Greed, the anaclitic-introjective distinction, and Horney's tripartite model of moving toward, away, and against

The distinctions that I have been discussing thus far overlap in interesting ways with Horney's (1945) conceptualization of the moving-toward and the moving-against neurotic trends, with an additional and more complex relation to what she refers to as the moving-away trend. Like the two-configurations model, Horney's conceptualization is often mistakenly viewed as a typology when it is in fact a depiction of inclinations in tension, competing inclinations of the same individual, even if, as with the anaclitic-introjective distinction, individuals may be identifiable as occupying different ends of the continuum with regard to their relative emphasis on one or the other of these inclinations.

It is perhaps easiest to see how the anaclitic or dependent dimension corresponds to the moving-toward trend in Horney's scheme. In both, there is an experience (sometimes conscious, sometimes mostly unconscious) of intense neediness and of turning to others for support and nurturance. If greed is characterized by an overtone of either of these tendencies, it will be greed of the insatiably hungry variety, and although the *expression* of this hunger or the resentment or despair it generates may alienate others, the strongest underlying *aim* is to cement the ties to them, to prevent the feared occurrence of abandonment, to maintain a sense of safety or well-being through being protected, cared for, loved.

The introjective or self-differentiation dimension also maps usefully onto Horney's theoretical scheme, but in this instance, it seems to partake of both the moving-against trend and the moving-away. The distinctions between the moving-against and the moving-away trends are manifold and fundamental, but in the present context perhaps what is most important is that in the former category (the moving-against), one is still very closely tied to others and needs them, even if that need is less evident because the need is expressed through dominance. But whereas one cannot be dominant or dominating without the presence and participation of others, one can be independent, or at the very least can strive for independence and experience oneself as independent, quite apart from any connection to others. In the sense that the self-definition dimension is one in which the firmness of the *boundaries* of the self is at issue, with a desire for more sharply defined boundaries or a fear that the boundaries are dangerously permeable, it is a dimension of experience that overlaps quite extensively with what is implied in Horney's moving-away trend. If we view this motivational configuration from the vantage point of greed and materialism, the function of a vast cache of material goods is to substitute for people and to diminish the need for them because one *has* (in the most literal sense) whatever one needs.

However, in the sense that the introjective dimension refers to being self-critical around themes of adequacy, success, admirability, etc., it overlaps significantly as well with the moving-against trend, in which anxiety is warded off through what might be called – seemingly paradoxically but actually quite straightforwardly – a "desperate" show of strength. Indeed, some of the vulnerability of the individual who is plagued by negative or depressive feelings along the introjective dimension may be usefully understood in terms of the failure of the moving-against strategy really to liberate the person from the "taint" of needing others – that is, with the persistence, as Horney describes, of neediness beneath the bravado or, more accurately, with the persistence of conflict between wanting to dominate and wanting to be taken care of.

Thus, from the vantage point of the two-configurations theory, the moving-away trend may be seen as occupying a position further along the self-definition dimension, a position even more radically dedicated to eliminating or erasing the vulnerability that inheres in needing people (or in *acknowledging* one's need for people).

In future empirical investigations of both the Blatt and the Horney conceptualizations, it would be of considerable interest to explore where people's experience and behavior sort into a tripartite model (corresponding to the dimensions of toward, against, and away) and where they sort into a bipolar model, as implied in the related but nonetheless distinct two-configurations model. In the pursuit of greater understanding of the psychological dynamics of greed, similar attention to parsing out where a two-configurations model captures most of the variance and where a tripartite model is preferable would be a useful issue to explore.

Concluding comments

For all of the difficulties and ambiguities in the concept of greed, I have chosen to make it a focus of this chapter – and an important element in the work I am currently pursuing beyond this chapter – because it seems to me a key nexus between some of our most pressing social problems and the more private discontents that plague many individually in our society. Psychoanalytic discourse and analysis often has paid insufficient attention to the impact of the values, institutions, pressures, assumptions, and messages of the larger social system on people's sense of well-being or of distress and unhappiness. Although the larger agenda of psychoanalysis has always included a concern with how the values, habits, and institutions of society seep into (as they are also shaped by) the psychological depths of the individual, the carrying out of this agenda has often been hampered by a priori assumptions about the inordinate impact of early familial experiences. These assumptions tend to render society but a distant shadow or ghostly epiphenomenon, simply the elaboration of patterns that have already been well set before the child begins elementary school.

If psychoanalytic social criticism is to be vital, it must take seriously the impact of real social and economic forces without reducing them simply to manifestations of the intimate sphere writ large. At the same time, the strength of a psychoanalytic analysis lies in highlighting the ways in which the impact of those larger social forces is complicated by and intertwined with unconscious emotional pulls and attitudes, conflict and the struggle to keep certain experiences out of awareness, and the anxiety and vulnerability that neither riches nor power can quell. One key to illuminating this enormously complex set of interconnecting force fields lies in the elaboration of both the phenomenology and the motivational underpinnings of whatever psychological phenomena are being investigated.

In pursuing better understanding of the phenomenon of greed, the distinctions that Sid Blatt has explored for more than a quarter century and articulated in the evolving two-configurations model seem to me of great utility. The suggestions offered in this chapter are speculative, one provisional way of applying the model that is based on both my recent immersion in the study of greed as a psychological phenomenon and extrapolations stimulated by the two-configurations theory. In emphasizing the conceptualization of bound opposites in the two-configurations theory, I have tried to highlight the dynamic nature of a framework that is sometimes misunderstood to be merely categorical and to show how this dynamic understanding of a key dialectic in human development has applications and potentials well beyond its original areas of application. Much as Sid's way of thinking inspired me as his student at the very beginning of my career, I find that, after more years than either Sid or I would probably like to admit to, my own thinking continues to be nourished by his ideas.

Note

1 The author is pleased to acknowledge the support of PSC-CUNY grant number 63674 00 32 "The Psychological Study of Greed".

References

Blatt, S. J. (1974) 'Levels of object representation in anaclitic and introjective depression', *Psychoanalytic Study of the Child* 29: 107–57.
—— (1995) 'Interpersonal relatedness and self-definition: two personality configurations and their implications for psychopathology and psychotherapy', in J. L. Singer (ed.) *Repression and Dissociation: implications for personality theory, psychopathology, and health*, Chicago: University of Chicago Press, pp. 299–335.
—— and Shichman, S. (1983) 'Two primary configurations of psychopathology', *Psychoanalysis and Contemporary Thought* 6: 187–254.
Boris, H. (1986) 'The "other" breast: greed, envy, spite and revenge', *Contemporary Psychoanalysis* 22: 45–59.
Cushman, P. (1990) 'Why the self is empty: toward a historically situated psychology', *American Psychologist* 45: 599–611.
Emery, E. (1992) 'The envious eye: concerning some aspects of envy from Wilfred Bion to Harold Boris', *Melanie Klein and Object Relations* 10: 19–29.
Fromm, E. (1941) *Escape from Freedom*, New York: Holt, Rinehart & Winston.
—— (1955) *The Sane Society*, New York: Holt, Rinehart & Winston.
Hobbes, T. (1651) *Leviathan*, ed. C. B. MacPherson, Harmondsworth, England: Penguin, 1968.
Horney, K. (1945) *Our Inner Conflicts*, New York: Norton.
Klein, M. (1957) *Envy and Gratitude*, London: Tavistock.
Marx, K. (1964) *The Economic and Philosophic Manuscripts of 1844*, ed. D. J. Struik and trans. M. Milligan, New York: International Publishers.

Pressman, E. R. (Producer) and Stone, O. (Director) (1987) *Wall Street* [motion picture], United States: Twentieth Century Fox.

Putnam, R. D. (2000) *Bowling Alone: the collapse and revival of American community*, New York: Simon & Schuster.

Smith, A. (1753) *The Theory of Moral Sentiments*, Oxford, England: Clarendon Press, 1976.

—— (1776) *An Inquiry into the Nature and Causes of the Wealth of Nations*, Oxford, England: Clarendon Press, 1976.

Triandis, H. (1995) *Individualism and Collectivism*, Boulder, CO: Westview Press.

Wachtel, P. L. (2000) 'Specificity and the future of psychotherapy integration', paper presented at the Annual Meeting of the Society for the Exploration of Psychotherapy Integration, Washington, DC, May 8, 2000.

Chapter 16

Narcissism as a clinical and social phenomenon

Diana Diamond

This chapter is rooted in a dialogue that I had with Sidney Blatt over 15 years ago, when he read an earlier draft of it that I submitted as part of my application for a postdoctoral fellowship at Yale Medical School. In my interview for the position, Sid told me right off the bat that he liked the paper very much and even wished he had written it himself. He then gave me a paper (Blatt 1983) that he had written, "Narcissism and Egocentrism as Concepts in Individual and Cultural Development," that illuminated some of the problematic areas of my own paper, and that enabled me finally to finish it. In that first dialogue I was introduced to the spirit of generosity and generativity that characterizes Sid's role as a mentor. The two lines of development, relatedness and self-definition, that have been so fundamental to his theoretical and research investigations have also guided his relationships with the many students and colleagues whom he has mentored over the years. It is with gratitude for all the ways in which my relationship with Sid has enhanced my own capacity for relatedness and self-definition that I offer this chapter.

The age of narcissism

It is a truism that we live in a narcissistic age. The narcissistic personality of our time is said to possess a grandiose but enfeebled self whose precarious integration depends on others' constant, admiring regard and on a barrage of external stimuli from an increasingly complex, bureaucratized social order. Disorders of narcissism cripple a growing mass of isolated, self-obsessed and rootless individuals who wander through our society substituting shimmering surfaces for sustained creativity or commitments, blind adherence to the imperatives of political and bureaucratic organizations for individual morality, and shallow encounters for the prolonged exploration of the interiority of the other that we used to define as intimacy. The rise of narcissism is thought to account for a range of social phenomena from fundamentalism to corporate greed. Recently, a *New York Times* columnist (Race 29 July 2002: 2) observed that CEOs who put self-image and self-promotion before the health of their companies or public good were "lost in a narcissistic fog" and attributed their false sense of power and invincibility to "the ecosystem of narcissism" that pervades corporate life.

How did this kind of person become the characteristic, if not the dominant, figure of our society? Critical social theorists attribute the trend toward narcissism to a variety of changes in our society and culture. These include changes in family structure and the process of socialization; the spread of bureaucracy that reaches its tentacles into the sphere of private life, strangling individual initiative and self-sufficiency; the obsession with consumption or the tendency to commodify everything, including human experience; and the array of media images that substitutes stereotyped reflections for a genuine mirroring of individual complexities (Adorno 1968; Horkheimer and Adorno 1944; Lasch 1978). Psychoanalytic theorists, on the other hand, have focused on the clinical extremes of this general social trend, documenting through case studies and theoretical writings the early developmental fixations and distortions that have led to the emergence of narcissistic disorders (Kernberg 1975, 1980, 1984; Kohut 1971, 1977, 1984).

Psychoanalysts and critical social theorists each address only one aspect of the social totality in which narcissism and its disorders is embedded. The central tenet of this chapter is that social and psychological perspectives on narcissism are mutually interpenetrating, although ultimately distinct and irreducible. In this regard, the chapter is inspired by the work of critical social theorists who hold that society reaches into the individual to shape him or her in its own image and for its own requirements while, within the individual, social processes are transformed into intrapsychic structures, governed by their own language and laws (Adorno 1967, 1968; Horkheimer and Adorno 1944). The tools of social theory can help us to understand how society constitutes the individual, producing social character types, but it is the tools of psychoanalysis that enable us to decode the highly variable ways, pathological as well as nonpathological, in which social sedimentation settles within the individual psyche.

Since its inception, psychoanalysis has been concerned with the interconnections between individual psyche and social trends, normal character structure and its pathological formations. The idea of a continuum between psychic health and abnormality, first formulated by Freud (1940), has found new centrality within psychoanalytic thought with the emergence of narcissism as a clinical concept and a social phenomenon.[1] Narcissism, which encompasses normative strivings for perfection, mastery, and wholeness as well as pathological distortions of these strivings, is thought to be a fundamental aspect of human experience that both shapes history and culture and in turn is shaped by them (Alford 1988). Despite the interpenetration of psychoanalysis and social thought around the issues of narcissism, it is important to emphasize that psychoanalytic and social perspectives on narcissism are distinct, if complementary. From the traditional psychoanalytic point of view, narcissism refers to the trans-historical, universal human tendency to invest libido in the self, and is characterized by two positions: (a) a primary one, occurring before the boundary between self and other has been established, in which there is libidinal investment in a rudimentary, undifferentiated self; and (b) a secondary one, in which the libido reverts to the self after self–other differentiation has taken place (Freud 1940). It should be noted that in Freud's (1914) original formulations of these concepts, the stage of primary narcissism involved libidinal investment in the self-representation that was differentiated from representation of objects. This theory dovetails with recent findings from infant research suggesting that infants are born with the perceptual and cognitive apparatus to differentiate between self and object from birth on, findings that lead some theorists to reject the notion of a stage of primary narcissism involving indifference to objects or lack of early self–other differentation (see Auerbach [1993] for a comprehensive discussion of these issues). However, as Green (1993: 72) has pointed out, Freud's concept of primary narcissism, whether it describes an actual developmental stage or not, retains value as an explanatory concept to account for the "blurring of mental frontier that occurs even in normal persons . . . and the return to an undifferentiated infantile state of mind, characterized by an 'oceanic feeling'."

From the psychoanalytic point of view, then, narcissism and its disorders are conceptualized in terms of the vicissitudes of the formation of the self and its relation to objects. By contrast, narcissism as a social phenomenon refers to the trend towards the apotheosis of the self in every sphere of social and cultural existence. This chapter attempts to advance our under-standing of narcissism as a social and a psychological phenomenon by integrating psychoanalytic and critical social perspectives on the topic. The first part of the chapter reviews theories of narcissism and its disorders in the work of the two psychoanalytic object relations theorists most influential in their development – Otto Kernberg and Heinz Kohut – with particular attention to these theorists' attempts to provide a social dimension to their clinical thought. The second section traces the concept of narcissism in the work of several critical social theorists who have sought to use psychoanalytic concepts in social analysis. This chapter identifies two perspectives on narcissism that have emerged in both psychoanalytic and critical social thought.

The concept of narcissism in psychoanalytic theory

Kohut and Kernberg have done for narcissism what the novelist Charles Dickens did for poverty in the nineteenth century (James 1973). Just as Dickens illuminated both the social roots and individual idiosyncrasies of poverty through his fiction, Kernberg and Kohut, through case studies and theoretical writings, have sketched the by now familiar clinical portrait of the narcissistic personality. Both Kohut and Kernberg agree that the narcissistic personality is characterized by a pathological grandiose self – a self-formation that may present the appearance of smooth and effective social functioning, with few manifest symptoms, but that obscures, at best, a tenuous and attenuated sense of self and chronic fluctuations of self-regard and, at worst, severe estrangement from self and others. Over time, however, narcissistic personalities reveal a certain superficiality in work and intimate relationships. Such individuals lack the well-integrated and cohesive set of internalized self (and object) images that provide depth and continuity to experience. Both Kernberg and Kohut recognize that the grandiose self of the narcissistic personality may meet the requirements of an advanced, industrial, bureaucratic society because it is stable enough to fit into the routinized, performance-oriented structure of work yet, lacking an integrated core, is easily manipulable by the mass media and bureaucratic institutions.

The clinical writings of Kernberg and Kohut have provided us with an opportunity to examine a general social phenomenon under the illuminating, if circumscribed, lens of the clinical microscope. There are significant differences in the work of the two theorists that have established two major perspectives on narcissism and its disorders within psychoanalysis. Kernberg has developed a conceptualization of narcissistic personality disorders that remains within the mainstream of traditional psychoanalytic thought, in that he integrates his conceptualizations of narcissism and its disorders with drive theory, although drives in Kernberg's (1990) view are bound up in a complex mesh of affectively-charged early experiences with objects. For example, Kernberg (1984: 189) writes, "The development of normal and pathological narcissism always involves the relationship of self representation to object representation and external objects as well as instinctual conflicts involving both libido and aggression." For Kohut, by contrast, an understanding of narcissism and its disorders necessitated a revision of psychoanalytic metapsychology, a repudiation of drive theory, and a refashioning of its basic assumptions along the lines of a self psychology that from its inception was hailed as a paradigm shift within psychoanalytic thought (Ornstein 1978).

The two theorists hold divergent views over the nature and etiology of the grandiose self. Kernberg (1975) defines the grandiose self of the narcissistic personality as a severely pathological structure that involves a condensation in the course of early preoedipal development of the real self (special qualities of the child), the ideal self (fantasies of the self's perfection and power), and the ideal object (fantasies of the parent as all giving and all loving) and that lead to distortions in both ego and superego formation. Kohut (1984), in contrast, conceptualizes narcissistic disturbance as arising from an arrest at one of three normative phases of infantile narcissism: (a) the grandiose self, in which a parental selfobject is engaged to mirror and confirm the infant's feelings of omnipotence and perfection; (b) the alter ego or twinship, in which a parental selfobject provides the child with the experience of essential alikeness; or (c) the idealized parent imago, in which the child projects his or her sense of global omnipotent perfection onto an idealized parental selfobject with whom he or she seeks to merge. Positing a line of development for such narcissistic structures separate from that of object relations, Kohut hypothesizes that, through a process of transmuting internalization, these archaic selfobject relationships will be transformed into adult self-structures, the grandiose self into realistic and stable forms of self-esteem and ambitions, the alter ego and twinship into skills or talents that serve to integrate ambitions and ideals, and the idealized parent imago into mature goals and values that form the basis for intrapsychic structures such as the ego ideal and the superego. If the original needs for mirroring, twinship, and idealizing experiences were frustrated by unempathic responses of the selfobjects, archaic residues of unmodulated grandiosity, need for alikeness, and idealization will persist in the adult personality and will lead to narcissistic pathology.

If one contrasts these views, one finds that Kohut's original bifurcation of early development into narcissistic and object-instinctual lines leads him to reify the narcissistic moment in relationships. Kohut posits a radical disjunction between object relations of the narcissistic and object-related types. Kernberg, on the other hand, in keeping with his position that no single developmental line can be supraordinated to others in understanding normal and pathological development, conceptualizes object relations as a complex admixture of narcissistic and object-oriented strivings and identifications. He points out that in intimate relationships the object is always loved for both its unique otherness *and* its capacity to enhance the self, such that "the investment of objects and the investment of the self in the gratifying relations with such objects go hand in hand" (Kernberg 1975: 323).

At the crux of the debate between the two theorists is the fate of the oedipus complex. Kohut (1977, 1984) reconceptualized the oedipal stage as a way station in the process of self-formation that may be unattainable by those with narcissistic deficits. According to Kohut (1977: 277) "unless the child sees himself as a delimited, abiding, independent center of initiative, he is unable to experience the object-instinctual desires that lead to the conflicts and secondary adaptations of the Oedipal period." Kernberg (1975, 1976) by contrast maintains that the oedipus complex is the funda- mental drama of early development that profoundly affects preoedipal or narcissistic, as well as oedipal, pathology.

Two portraits of narcissistic disorders emerge from Kohut's and Kernberg's conceptualizations of oedipal and preoedipal development. In keeping with his view of narcissistic disorders as involving severe pathology of self and object relations, Kernberg emphasizes the unbridled grandiosity of these patients, their ruthless exploitation of others, and their emotional coldness and shallowness. Kohut, in keeping with his focus on narcissistic disorders as arrests at normative developmental processes, emphasizes not only the overt grandiosity but also the painful timidity and the preoccupation with secret grandiose fantasies, not only the self-aggrandizement but also the submission to others perceived as powerful and omnipotent of these patients. Subsequent psychoanalytic investigations, both clinical and empirical, have confirmed such a spectrum of narcissism and its disorders, ranging from the self-aggrandizing, overt type to the self-effacing, covert type (Cooper 1998; Gabbard 1986; Wink 1991).

Kohut, Kernberg, and psychoanalytic trends

Both Kohut's and Kernberg's reconceptualizations of the theory and treatment of narcissistic personality disorders signal a trend within psychoanalytic thought both to emphasize and to depathologize concepts of narcissism and the self. Kernberg (1980) defines the self as a specific structure within the psychic apparatus that is synonymous with internalized self-representations and is not separate from the ego. In contrast, Kohut (1977) defines the self as a bipolar psychic configuration that develops as an independent structure unto itself. Because of his almost mystical conception of the self as an independent and enduring psychic configuration that emerges out of specific types of self–object relationships distinct from object-instinctual object relationships, Kohut assigns the self an importance and autonomy within the intrapsychic apparatus that is unprecedented within psychoanalytic thought. In evaluating the contributions of Kohut and Kernberg, more classically oriented analysts like Spruiell (1974) and Loewald (1979) have described the increasing emphases on ego instead of id, self instead of ego, and narcissistic instead of oedipal transferences and dynamics.

More productive, however, than such interminable debates within psychoanalytic thought about the hegemony of drives versus object relations, primary narcissism versus primary attachments, or the prevalence of disorders of the self versus oedipally based disorders are recent attempts by Blatt (Blatt and Shichman 1983; Westen 1990) and others to understand narcissistic disorders within the framework of a broader theory of normal and pathological personality development that synthesizes clinical observations with empirical research. The investigations of Kohut and Kernberg and subsequent theorists suggest that narcissistic disorders fall on a continuum that parallels the two major developmental configurations identified by Blatt: an anaclitic line of relatedness and an introjective line of self-definition, each of which represents distinct moments in an ongoing developmental spiral of normal personality development and pathological formations (Blatt and Shichman 1983). The unbridled grandiosity of the overt narcissist represents a distortion of the strivings for uniqueness, mastery, and perfection that are characteristic of the introjective line of self-definition while the idealization of and surrender to omnipotent others of the covert narcissist represents a distortion of anaclitic strivings for relatedness.

Kohut, Kernberg, and cultural trends

The emergence of narcissism and self-formation as central, pivotal foci within the work of Kohut and Kernberg must be understood not only in terms of current trends within psychoanalytic thought but also in terms of the broader cultural context that may influence the direction of psycho-analytic theory and technique. Kohut attributes the increase in narcissistic disorders to our society's inability to afford the same legitimacy to our healthy narcissistic strivings, which he defines as "our ambitions, our wish to dominate, our wish to shine, and our yearning to merge into omnipotent figures" (Kohut 1971: 365), that it affords to object-instinctual strivings. Commenting on the hypocritical attitudes towards narcissism in our society, which he compares to Victorian hypocrisy towards sex, Kohut (1971: 365) writes, "Officially the existence of the social manifestations emanating from the grandiose self and the omnipotent self-object are denied, yet their split-off dominance everywhere is obvious."

Kohut's self psychology may signal the creation of an ideology of the self at a point in history when true individuality is on the wane, and the subject is said to be disappearing (Adorno 1968). A self-less age breeds preoccu-pation with selves. One analyst, puzzling over why his patients take so high an interest in the self, surmises that it is because "they cannot take themselves – their selves for granted; they constantly need to confirm themselves" (Bursten 1977: 110). The question must be posed to what extent this trend in psychoanalytic thought toward a focus on disorders of narcissism and the self is itself a reflection, on the theoretical level, of cultural processes and patterns that have been designated by Lasch (1978) as the culture of narcissism.

Kohut and Kernberg provide somewhat divergent opinions on the extent to which social determinants have contributed to psychoanalytic trends. Although he rejects any direct correspondence between social alienation and the narcissistic personality's subjective experience of emptiness and self-estrangement, Kernberg actually provides a compelling argument for continuity between narcissistic personality disorders and narcissism as a social trend in his astute observation that the narcissistic individual may not only be asymptomatic but may indeed embody those traits that guarantee success in contemporary bureaucratic structures. According to Kernberg (1975: 308), it is precisely the narcissistic personality's emptiness, lack of emotional depth, and curious lack of involvement with others that cause him or her to function optimally in certain "political and bureaucratic organizations in which lack of commitment means survival and access to the top." Kernberg (1975) hypothesizes that social alienation alone cannot in itself foster the self-estrangement and inner deterioration of object relations experienced by the narcissistic individual because object relations refer not to actual interpersonal interactions but to the intrapsychic structures, formed through the experience of early familial relationships, that constitute the basis for such interactions. At other points, however, he does allow that, over several generations, social trends like family uprootedness, social disorganization, the bureaucratization of work, and the ubiquitous stereotyped images offered by the mass media might eventually permeate the immediate relational world of the child, catalyzing changes in intrapsychic structure (Kernberg 1975). As a case in point, Kernberg (1989) has explored the ways in which mass culture, with its array of banal and stereotyped images, both reflects and reinforces the psychological characteristics of latency, including conventional thinking and simplistic morality, the tendency to seek an individual identity in group norms, and the seeking of substitute gratification for sexuality and aggression through cultural conformity and consumption.

In contrast to Kernberg, who conceives of a dialectical process whereby social processes and psychological development might mutually reinforce or resist each other, Kohut (1977) hypothesizes that the narcissistic personality, with his or her shifting and tenuous sense of self, is a direct reflection of the characteristic psychological predicament of our age. As evidence, he notes the prevalence of themes and images of self-cohesion and self-fragmentation in the contemporary arts. Kohut (1977) specifically attributes the rise of narcissistic disorders to changes in the family and to concomitant changes in the early relational experience of the child. According to Kohut, the nineteenth-century middle-class family, with its clutch of extended family, servants, and nurses offered its members a rich and varied constellation of object relationships, that, when internalized, provided depth and continuity to the personality. Indeed, the chief problem for the child in such an emotionally dense familial environment was an excess of parental warmth and closeness, bordering on seductiveness. In contrast, the twenty-first century middle-class family, isolated from extended kin and community and often disrupted by divorce and social mobility, may predispose children to narcissistic personality disorders by providing an impoverished emotional atmosphere and a dearth of object relationships.

Kohut (1977: 271) also surmises that the severing of the public sphere of work from family life has deprived the child of the opportunity to "participate emotionally . . . via concrete, understandable imagery, in the parents' competence and in their pride in the work situation where their selves are most profoundly engaged." The encapsulation of parent–child relations within the isolated and shrunken nuclear family unit lends a shadowy and insubstantial quality to parent–child interactions that contributes to the narcissistic individual's shifting and tenuous sense of self and reality.

The thwarted narcissistic strivings and attenuated self formation that are the legacy of the contemporary family have implications for ego and superego development that affect group as well as individual psychology. Kohut (1977: 365) warns that the failure of early mirroring and idealizing self–object relationships may precipitate the "unrestrained pursuit of grandiose aims and resistenceless merger with omnipotent self-objects." The population's submission to an idealized Führer in Nazi Germany is cited as an historical example of such collective eruption of frustrated archaic narcissistic needs and aspirations, as is the surrender of rational judgment and individual autonomy to religious cults and fundamentalist groups.

In sum, both Kohut and Kernberg, to varying degrees, offer intriguing formulations about the connections between narcissistic pathology and the way the self is constructed in our society. For a more comprehensive understanding of the ways in which a narcissistic society reaches into the individual to create the self-estrangement and self-attenuation noted in narcissistic personality disorders, we must turn to the work of the social theorists.

The concept of narcissism in critical social theory

Although they draw heavily on psychoanalytic conceptualizations of narcissism, which they described as one of Freud's "most magnificent discoveries," (Adorno 1968: 88), critical social theorists of the Frankfurt School understand narcissistic pathology as representing the crystallizations within the psyche of certain social processes. According to the critical theorists, every society organizes the instinctual strivings and relational needs that form the basis of individual personality and identity into those characteristic patterns that come to constitute the predominant character types. In keeping with the psychoanalytic notion of a continuum between psychic health and abnormality, critical social theorists have identified prevailing forms of psychopathology as exaggerations of such predominant character types. For critical social theorists, the pattern of the ego's conflicts and regressions is determined not only by interpersonal or intrapsychic factors but by objective aspects of the social world, including economic structure, characteristic familial forms, and political organization of a society (Adorno 1967, 1968; Alford 1988; Lasch 1978; Marcuse 1955).

Critical social theorists have developed two positions on the social meaning of narcissism that parallel those delineated by Kohut and Kernberg in psychoanalytic thought. Most notably Horkheimer (1936),

Adorno (1967, 1968), and Lasch (1978) see the prevalence of narcissistic personality disorders as an ominous indication that the underlying character structure in our society is enfeebled and fragmented, unbuttressed by strong identifications and parental introjects, and thus increasingly susceptible to direct social manipulation. In their understanding of the social meaning of narcissism, the work of Horkheimer, Adorno, and Lasch parallels that of Kernberg, who connects the narcissistic personality's emotional shallowness, inner emptiness, and passive orientation to reality to the demands of contemporary bureaucratic and political organizations for a malleable and unreflective citizenry.

A less prominent but nonetheless clearly discernible strain within critical theory, developed originally by Marcuse (1955) and elaborated by Aronowitz (1980), emphasizes the potentially emancipatory aspects of narcissism. Critical theorists in this tradition insist that narcissism, which involves erotic connection with the self and the world, represents a potential empowerment of the self and a subversive withdrawal from a repressive reality. This elevation of narcissism to the archetype of another existential relation to reality, the historical moment of which has arrived, parallels the emergence of Kohut's self psychology. Each of these perspectives on narcissism will be reviewed and critiqued in turn.

Narcissism as the enfeeblement of the self: the work of Horkheimer, Adorno, and Lasch

Horkheimer, Adorno, and Lasch trace the emergence of narcissism as a dominant character trait and the prevalence of narcissistic personality disorders as prevailing forms of psychopathology to the collapse of paternal authority and the dilution of maternal nurturance as families and the processes of economic production have changed. The usurpation of the parental functions by the media, the schools, and the apparatus of social welfare have diluted parental authority and interfered with the capacity of children to form strong psychological identifications with parents. The authority and autonomy of the father is increasingly undermined by the trivialization of his role in production while the efficacy and nurturance of the mother are vitiated by the increasing professionalization of childrearing and by the lack of social validation for her role as guardian of those qualities (i.e. love, tenderness, reciprocity) antithetical to the reduction of human beings to mere appendages of the production process.

In the view of Horkheimer, Adorno, and Lasch, the decline of parental (and particularly paternal) authority interferes with processes of internalization, both oedipal and preoedipal. The oedipus complex is valorized by these theorists as the vehicle not only for the internalization of the father's authority but also as the basis for moral autonomy that might serve as a locus of social resistance. They surmise that many individuals in our society are deprived of a strong figure for identification by virtue of the father's absence from the home and his powerlessness in the social world, and consequently, the individual no longer develops a strong ego through protracted struggles with a loved and revered, if feared, father. Lasch (1978) points out that the failure of internalization leaves the individual prone to primitive fantasies about the father of an unnecessarily harsh and punitive nature, with the result that the superego remains primitive, personified, and prone to be projected onto the social world, in turn perceived as dangerous and irrational. Although Benjamin (1978) and others have criticized the Frankfurt School for ignoring the extent to which firm internalizations are based on gratifying preoedipal experiences with the mother, Horkheimer and Adorno observe that the decline in paternal authority also deforms the relationship between mother and child, setting the stage for the inadequate separation between self and other that is the hallmark of narcissistic pathology.

A further psychological consequence of the collapse of parental authority within the family involves the transformation in the individual's relationship to external authority. Adorno (1968) notes a tendency among individuals in mass society to form merger-like identifications of a preoedipal or narcissistic nature with idealized leaders, who are experienced as enlargements of the subject's own personality. Such poorly differentiated, enfeebled selves, who regress to early incorporative forms of identification and primitive defenses like excessive idealization, were described as narcissistic by Horkheimer and Adorno (1944). In their view, narcissism replaces internalization as the dominant psychological mode of our time.

The inflation of narcissism in the personality coincides with the "triumph of society over the individual" (Adorno 1968: 95). Denied channels of mastery and individuation, the ego turns back on itself. The inflation of narcissism within the ego, which results from this regression, represents only one moment before its total dissolution as an autonomous force. Horkheimer and Adorno surmise that the increase of narcissistic personality disorders signals a transformation in the nature of human subjectivity. It entails the end of the individual with a rich, complex, and autonomous inner life and the truncation of the capacity for active mastery, rather than passive submission to reality.

In their tendency to emphasize the pathological aspects of the trend toward narcissism, the work of Horkheimer and Adorno corresponds primarily to that of Kernberg within psychoanalytic thought. The trend toward ego weakness and the failure of differentiation, the decline of the oedipus complex and the stunted ego and superego development, and the tendency toward merger-like identifications and slavish submission to irrational authority that they observe in the general nonclinical population all have their counterparts in the clinical picture of the narcissistic personality developed by Kernberg.

Narcissism as empowerment of the self: the work of Marcuse and Aronowitz

Kohut's benevolent view of narcissism as a normal developmental line that under optimal conditions fosters the individual's quest for blissful perfection and expansion of self has its parallel in critical social thought in Marcuse's and Aronowitz's conception of narcissism as an orientation to reality that is progressive as well as regressive, self-enhancing rather than self-depleting. Like Kohut (1971, 1977), Marcuse deplores the pervasive Western bias against narcissism and reinterprets narcissistic modes of being and relating as not only desirable but also as historically viable, insisting that "narcissism may contain the germ of a new reality principle" (Marcuse 1955: 169). Marcuse (1955) maintains that advances in technology have created the conditions for reconciliation between the pleasure principle, which in advanced capitalist societies has been deformed through a process that he termed "repressive desublimation," in which sexual pleasure is channeled into mindless consumption, and the reality principle. According to Marcuse (1955: 198), such a reconciliation would "reactivate early stages of the libido, which were surpassed in the development of the reality ego." These stages are termed narcissistic by Marcuse; they entail deeply gratifying, if archaic, modes of relating and being involving play, polymorphous sexuality, and merger experiences between self and other, self and world.

Like Kohut, Marcuse seeks support for his reconceptualization of narcissism in a particular interpretation of Freud's theory of primary narcissism. He insists that primary narcissism not only represents a phase in the development of the libido in which ego and external objects are unified but also symbolizes the archetype of another existential relation to reality. Primary narcissism implies not an impoverishment or shrinking of the self but an enlargement of the self's boundaries to include the external world. As evidence for this position, Marcuse quotes Freud's statement that primary narcissistic states persist in the mature psyche as the oceanic feeling of limitless extension and 'oneness with the universe' (Freud 1930: 72).

Aronowitz (1980) expands on the emancipatory potential in the empowerment or overvaluation of self inherent in narcissistic states. For Aronowitz, as for Marcuse, narcissism represents the ascendance of a preoedipal or polymorphous form of eros, one that is inherently disruptive of the process of inscription of the social order on the individual that occurs during the oedipal stage. Narcissism, as a negative moment of refusal against a repressive social order, is indicative, for Aronowitz (1980: 67), of the potential "surfacing of desire as a social force." In sum, Marcuse and Aronowitz elevate narcissism, with its potential for self–other dedifferentiation, to the prototype for the eradication of stultifying boundaries between public and private, individual and society, heterosexual and homosexual, play and labor, personal and political.

Marcuse's (and Aronowitz's) reinterpretation of narcissism corresponds to that of Kohut in several respects.[2] Marcuse's elevation of narcissism to an archetype of a less anguished and compartmentalized relation to reality corresponds to Kohut's (1966: 265) conception of cosmic narcissism as a "new expanded transformed narcissism . . . which transcends the bounds of the individual." Perhaps most important, both theorists emphasize the empowering aspects for the self of narcissistic ego states and downplay its pathological distortions. Within critical social theory, then, Marcuse's reconceptualization of narcissism represents a parallel trend to Kohut's normalization of narcissism – the acceptance and even inflation of its importance for the personality – within psychoanalytic thought.

Critique and conclusion

The correspondences in the work of the psychoanalytic and critical social theorists suggest that a continuum exists between narcissism as a psychological phenomenon and narcissism as a social trend. On the principle, shared by psychoanalytic and critical theorists alike, that abnormal character structure represents the hidden truth of the normal, we can seek clues in the narcissistic personality to the characteristic personality of our time. The narcissistic personality is plagued with chronic feelings of unreality and emptiness but a sense of futility, meaninglessness, and self-doubt is evident in the general population as well. The grandiose self of the narcissistic personality maintains its precarious equilibrium through the constant admiring reflection of others, but a tendency to define the self in terms of external reflection and a widespread admiration of narcissistic figures are characteristic of our age. The narcissistic personality cultivates a protective emotional shallowness and is incapable of object relationships of depth, but the search of the general population for new sensations and experiences militates against the cultivation of deeply intimate bonds over time.

Although there is clearly a correspondence between narcissistic pathology and social trends termed narcissistic, neither psychoanalytic nor critical theorists have adequately explored the complexities of such a continuum – its discontinuities as well as its continuities. In their search to distill the social meaning from individual personality types, the critical social theorists may have overly obscured the boundary between the normal and the pathological. Their quest to discern the contours of the normal in the magnifying mirror of the abnormal leads the critical social theorists to eradicate the polarity maintained within psychoanalytic thought, between normal and pathological narcissism.

In the line of critical social thought spawned by Horkheimer, Adorno, and Lasch, the concept of narcissism loses its psychoanalytic specificity as a form of individual psychopathology involving early developmental distortions as it becomes conflated with every social and cultural trend these theorists deplore. These theorists portray the culture of narcissism as a social tapestry that inevitably weaves the narcissistic personality into existence. The strands of the culture of narcissism are spun from different aspects of the society – from the bureaucratization of work, the breakdown of the family, the hegemony of the media, and the clutch of consumption – but the end result is a totalizing fabric from which there is no escape and against which there is no possibility of resistance.

Just as for Horkheimer and Adorno, the normal becomes a mere diluted reflection of the abnormal, for Marcuse and Aronowitz the normal pole of the continuum of narcissism is mythologized and idealized while the pathological pole is dismissed as ideological distortion and denied a real existence altogether. Both Marcuse and Aronowitz hypothesize that early narcissistic states characterized by the blurring of boundaries between self and other can continue to coexist with a mature reality-oriented ego to the enrichment of the self. But they fail to distinguish between regression to archaic narcissistic states that are fundamentally pathological in nature and those that are potentially self-enhancing. Regardless of which position on the social meaning of narcissism is emphasized – narcissism as regression and fragmentation of self, or narcissism as empowerment and transcendence of self – the eradication of the polarities between normal and pathological narcissism sets the stage for the transformation of narcissism into a totalizing concept with limited utility for social analysis.

Psychoanalysts, on the other hand, in their intensive and prolonged exploration of the intrapsychic sphere in a dyadic situation are in a position to understand the highly variable ways, pathological as well as nonpathological, in which the social is encoded in the deepest recesses of the individual psyche. However, psychoanalytic theorists fail to comprehend the ways in which their own theories reflect the characteristic distortions of the culture of narcissism. Kohut's self psychology is indeed the perfect theoretical complement to the culture of narcissism, for it elevates narcissism not only into a new paradigm for psychoanalysis but also into a worldview. Rather than conceptualizing human development as an inter-subjective process with the strand of narcissism or self-regard as merely one moment in this process, as do, for example Kernberg and others, Kohut magnifies the narcissistic moment in development, focusing inordinately on the development of self-structure to the exclusion of object relations. The positioning of a fundamental cleavage in the developmental process, which separates the consolidation of self-structure from the vicissitudes of object relations, may represent a reification of the narcissistic moment in development. Kohut may hypothesize the existence of two separate and independent developmental axes not because such a separation exists in any absolute or universal sense, as he claims, but because he is led to perceive such a cleavage as a result of certain social processes. This is not to say that the phenomena defined by Kohut and others as narcissistic do not exist.

Indeed, the question is irrelevant. Instead, it seems important to explore the complex dialectic between the phenomena we observe as clinicians, the theories that enable us to perceive and understand them, and the social climate that allows those theories to flourish.

In sum, neither psychoanalytic nor critical social theorists have adequately explored the connections between social narcissism, or the trend toward shallow self-absorption, rootless pleasure seeking, and lack of continuity and depth in object relations in the general, nonclinical population, on the one hand, and narcissistic personality disorders as a specific pathological structuring of the personality on the other. Future investigations in both psychoanalytic and critical social thought should explore the extent to which persons may embody social trends that are now being termed narcissistic without suffering from narcissistic personality disorders as they are defined in the psychoanalytic literature.

Blatt (1983) is one of the few theorists who offers a dialectical view of the relationship between normal and pathological narcissism, between social trends and individual personality development, that avoids the pitfall of narcissism as a totalizing concept. Blatt distinguishes between narcissism, which he refers to as pathological developmental processes of self formation with limited applicability to normative individual or cultural development, from the Piagetian concept of egocentrism, a stage of normative development that is far more useful for linking individual development to social and cultural change. Narcissism, in Blatt's view, characterizes an enfeebled self in defensive retreat from object relations via introjective or anaclitic mechanisms while egocentrism involves a cognitive process through which the individual confounds his or her views and actions with those of others and that is gradually overcome through a process of decentration.[3] Blatt, like Lasch and Adorno, affirms that a highly mobile, technological society may in fact heighten egocentrism by offering the individual an expanded range of choices and opportunities, even while it disrupts extended kin networks and interpersonal ties, but he suggests that it would be a mistake to view these developments only through the distorting pathogenic prism of narcissism and its disorders. Instead he affirms that the rise of narcissism in contemporary society in fact represents only one moment of heightened egocentrism that hearkens new levels and opportunities for decentration in cultural development involving the recognition and integration of multiple, diverse perspectives.

Indeed, Blatt (1983: 301) affirms that the culture of narcissism may in fact "involve our struggles to decenter from a level of egocentrism – from a conception of nature and society based on cultural absolutism to a new level of integration and synthesis based on individual and cultural relativism." The destruction of cultural absolutes in the form of family structure, values, and dominant cultural forms has the potential in the view of Blatt and others to afford disenfranchised individuals and social groups greater recognition and integration into our cultural reality. Hence Blatt's analysis poses the postmodern question about whether the rise of narcissism in individual pathology and social discourse heralds the death throes of the autonomous individual or the birth pangs of new sources of autonomy in the self's strivings for perfection, mastery, and recognition.

Notes

1 It should be noted that Freud introduced the concept of narcissism as distinct from object love, without the assumption that this was a psychological aspect of modernity or that there was a social dimension to narcissism.

2 It should be noted that, in contrast to Kohut, who abandoned drive theory in his later formulations, Marcuse, like the majority of the critical social theorists, holds fast to Freud's libido theory, seeing in the notion of drives and the conflicts within the personality that they entail a source of resistance to the social order. Additionally, Marcuse is closer to Kernberg in his commitment to the drives and in his recognition of the ubiquitous threat of aggression.

3 From a Piagetian perspective, development is conceptualized as a process of decentration in which the individual not only gradually learns to distinguish his or her own perspective and experience of reality from that of others, and increasingly recognizes the independence of his or her cognitive processes from those of others, but also recognizes that he or she is responsible for the construction of reality and the meaning ascribed to it. Piaget's formulations constitute a genetic epistemology that provides explanatory constructs for cultural, as well as individual, development.

References

Adorno, T. W. (1967) 'Sociology and psychology', *New Left Review* 46: 67–80.
—— (1968) 'Sociology and psychology', *New Left Review* 47: 79–95.
—— (1978) 'Freudian theory and the patter of fascist propaganda', in A. Arato and E. Gebbardt (eds) *The Essential Frankfurt School Reader*, Oxford: Basil Blackwell.
—— Frenkel-Brunswik, E., Levinson, D. and Sanford, N. (1950) *The Authoritarian Personality*, New York: Harper.
Alford, F. C. (1988) *Narcissism: Socrates, the Frankfurt School, and psychoanalytic theory*, London and New Haven, CT: Yale University Press.
Aronowitz, S. (1980) 'On narcissism', *Telos:* 44: 65–74.
Auerbach, J. S. (1993) 'The origins of narcissism and narcissistic personality disorder: a theoretical and empirical reformulation', in J. M. Masling and R. F. Bornstein (eds) *Empirical Studies of Psychoanalytic Theories, vol. 4: psychoanalytic perspectives on psychopathology*, Washington, DC: American Psychological Association.
Benjamin, J. (1978) 'Authority and the family revisited: or a world without fathers?', *New German Critique* 13: 35–57.
Blatt, S. J. (1983) 'Narcissism and egocentrism as concepts in individual and cultural development', *Psychoanalysis and Contemporary Thought* 6: 291–303.

Blatt, S. J. and Shichman, S. (1983) 'Two primary configurations of psychopathology', *Psychoanalysis and Contemporary Thought* 6: 187–254.

Bursten, B. (1977) 'The narcissistic course', in M. C. Nelson (ed.) *The Narcissistic Condition: a fact of our lives and times*, New York: Human Sciences Press,.

Cooper, A. M. (1998) 'Further developments in the clinical diagnosis of narcissistic personality disorder', in E. F. Ronningstam (ed.) *Disorders of Narcissism: diagnostic, clinical and empirical implications*, Washington, DC: American Psychiatric Press.

Freud, S. (1914) 'On narcissism: an introduction', in J. Strachey (ed. and trans.) *The Standard Edition of the Complete Psychological Works of Sigmund Freud*, vol. 14, London: Hogarth Press, pp. 69–102.

—— (1930) 'Civilization and its discontents', in J. Strachey (ed. and trans.) *The Standard Edition of the Complete Psychological Works of Sigmund Freud*, vol. 21, London: Hogarth Press, pp. 59–145.

—— (1940) 'An outline of psychoanalysis', in J. Strachey (ed. and trans.) *The Standard Edition of the Complete Psychological Works of Sigmund Freud*, vol. 23, London: Hogarth Press, pp. 144–207.

Gabbard, G. O. (1986) 'Two subtypes of narcissistic personality disorder, *Bulletin of the Menninger Clinic* 53: 527–37.

Green, A. (1993) *On Private Madness*, Madison, CT: International Universities Press.

Horkheimer, M. (1936) 'Authority and the family', in *Critical Theory*, trans. M. J. O'Connell *et al.*, New York: Seabury Press, pp. 47–128.

—— and Adorno, T. W. (1944), *Dialectic of Enlightenment*, trans. John Cumming, New York: Herder and Herder 1972.

James, M. (1973) '*The Analysis of the Self: a systematic approach to the psychological treatment of narcissistic personality disorders*', book review, *International Journal of Psycho-Analysis* 54: 363–8.

Jay, M. (1973) *The Dialectical Imagination: a history of the Frankfurt School and the Institute of Social Research, 1923–1950*, Boston: Little Brown.

Kernberg, O. F. (1975) *Borderline Conditions and Pathological Narcissism*, New York: Aronson.

—— (1980) *Internal World and External Reality: object relations theory applied*, New York: Aronson.

—— (1984) *Severe Personality Disorders*, New Haven, CT: Yale University Press.

—— (1989) 'The temptations of conventionality', *International Review of Psychoanalysis* 16: 191–205.

—— (1990) 'New perspectives in psychoanalytic affect theory', in R. Plutchik and H. Kellerman (eds) *Emotion: theory, research and experience*, New York: Academic Press, pp. 115–130.

Kohut, H. (1966) 'Forms and transformations of narcissism', *Journal of the American Psychoanalytic Association* 14: 243–72.

—— (1971) *The Analysis of the Self*, New York: International Universities Press.

—— (1977) *The Restoration of the Self*, NewYork: International Universities Press.

—— (1984) *How Does Analysis Cure?*, Chicago: University of Chicago Press.

Lasch, C. (1978) *The Culture of Narcissism: American life in an age of diminishing expectations*, New York: Norton.

Loewald, H. W. (1979) 'The waning of the Oedipus complex', *Journal of the American Psychoanalytic Association* 27: 751–75.

Marcuse, H. (1955) *Eros and Civilization: a philosophical inquiry into Freud*, Boston, MA: Beacon Press.

Ornstein, P. (ed.) (1978) *The Search for the Self: selected writings of Heinz Kohut, 1950–1978*, vol. 2, New York: International Universities Press.

Race, T. (2002, 29 July) 'Executives are smitten, and undone, by their own images'. *New York Times*. Online. Available HTTP: <http://www.newyorktimes.com> (accessed 29 July, 2002).

Spruiell, V. (1974) 'Theories of the treatment of narcissistic personalities', *Journal of the American Psychoanalytic Association* 22: 268–78.

Westen, D. (1990) 'The relations among narcissism, egocentricism, self-concept, and self-esteem: experimental, clinical, and theoretical considerations', *Psychoanalysis and Contemporary Thought* 13: 183–239.

Wink, P. (1991) 'Two faces of narcissism', *Journal of Personality and Social Psychology* 61: 590–7.

Chapter 17

Attachment and separateness and the psychoanalytic understanding of the act of faith

Rachel B. Blass

The psychoanalytic literature on religion points to a major shift in recent years in the analytic understanding of the act of faith. The shift is from Freud's negative assessment of it as an unrealistic act based on infantile needs and wishes to Winnicottian assessments of it as a potentially positive act of relatedness within the realm of transitional phenomena. In the present chapter, I will explore the act of faith and this shift in understanding in the light of a psychoanalytic developmental model that has been evolved by Sidney Blatt and some of his collaborators in the course of the past two decades. This model, which considers the maturation process throughout the life cycle in terms of a dialectical relationship between two developmental lines, that of attachment (relatedness) and that of separateness (self-definition), helps elucidate central psychological dimensions of the act of faith and points to the ways in which these dimensions are overlooked in the shift from Freudian to Winnicottian understandings of this act. In turn, this clarification and the complex interaction between attachment and separateness that is revealed in the act of faith help refine the developmental model and the distinction between its different facets.

The attachment and separateness developmental model

During the 1980s, Sidney Blatt, together with some of his colleagues (myself included), formulated a model of personality development that described two central developmental lines that were, in effect, finding expression in various psychoanalytic theories – a line of attachment or relatedness and a line of separateness or self-definition (Blatt and Shichman 1983; Blatt and Blass 1990, 1992, 1996; Blass and Blatt 1992, 1996). Development in the attachment line is concerned with the quality of the individual's relationships – the capacity to form and maintain stable relationships and to integrate them into a sense of self in relation to an other. Development in the separateness line, in contrast, is concerned with the individual as a self-contained and independent unit. Individuation, differentiation, and autonomy are developmental achievements that lead to a stable sense of self as separate, guided by clear conceptions of goals and values. Although personality theories tend to consider to some degree both of these dimensions, most theories usually emphasize primarily one or the other. Within psychoanalytic theory, an emphasis on attachment may be seen most clearly in the works of British object relations theorists, who focus on the development of interpersonal relationships and themes of dependency, care, affection, mutuality, reciprocity, and intimacy (e.g., Balint 1952; Fairbairn 1952; Guntrip 1969; Winnicott 1958, 1971). And an emphasis on separateness is best exemplified by the contributions of those who define development in terms of separation and individuation (e.g., Blos 1979; A. Freud 1974; Mahler 1974). The developmental model proposed by Blatt and his colleagues was aimed at formally conceptualizing the relationship between these two lines and the dialectic that exists between them throughout the life cycle. The model, based on a revision of Erikson's eight-stage formulation of psychosocial development (Erikson 1959, 1982), provided a framework for such a conceptualization that has proved valuable to the understanding of development, personality theory, pathology, the therapeutic process, and various experiential states (Blass and Blatt 1992, 1996; Blatt and Blass 1992, 1996).

Attachment and separateness and the act of faith

In this chapter, I present an application of the attachment and separateness model to the understanding of the act of faith. The focus here will be specifically on the kinds of psychological functions, capacities, or states that come into play as the individual manifests belief in a transcendent God – that is, as he or she asserts the existence of such a transcendent reality. Several points and distinctions are important here. Defining the issue in this way, faith is considered in terms of the moment of the act. What is central are the kinds of events that are taking place in the course of the act itself, rather than on the believer's ongoing stable capacities. This allows for the possibility that, in the act of faith, processes take place that are not necessarily consistent with the individual's general capacities. A parallel would be an examination of the kinds of processes that occur in the act of love, rather than of the kind of personality that is capable of love.

This definition of the issue to be studied also stresses the relational nature of the act of faith. Faith is a belief *in* God. Moreover, because God is regarded here as a transcendent being, a special kind of relationship is supposed to be involved. For believers, God is real and yet not part of the natural order of things. God is not another object in the world (Leavy 1990). Without taking into account this aspect of the relationship, it would not be possible to speak of the act of faith in the traditional and common sense of the term. But this definition of the issue does not make any theological assumptions regarding the existence of God, nor would it be within the legitimate realm of the present psychoanalytic exploration to do so. Rather, it stresses that what will be examined are the kinds of psychological functions or capacities that are involved in the act of faith as it is described by traditional religious and theological accounts, independent of the objective validity of these accounts. As I shall argue, examination of this issue points to an interesting interplay between the two developmental lines that is relevant beyond the specific question of faith.

In what follows, I will outline some of the main processes involved in the act of faith in terms of the attachment and then the separateness developmental lines and will do so in a way that will allow us to then address the meaning and consequences of the contemporary shift within psychoanalysis towards a Winnicottian understanding of faith.

Faith and the attachment line

The involvement of attachment capacities and functions in the act of faith seems rather clear. Although the very fact that faith entails a relationship to God does not immediately point to its attachment nature, the relational capacities that specifically belong to the attachment line are rather striking in this context. Most notable here is the involvement of trust. It may be seen that the act of faith requires trust on two different levels: There is trust in the knowledge and experience of other believers or the community of belief, and there is trust in God. But these two kinds of trust are less simple than they seem when one takes into account their relationship to processes determined by the separateness developmental line and when the uniqueness of the religious context in which they find expression is taken into account. Trusting the faith of one's community and trusting God are different from trusting that one's friend is telling the truth or that things will work out for the best.

The trust in others that is involved in the act of faith rests neither on an assessment of the credibility of these others nor on the very likelihood of what they have to say. To take a Biblical example, in the book of Exodus, God commands Moses to go to the people of Israel and tell them of His existence and plan of salvation for them. Moses is reluctant, fearing the people's disbelief, and consequently God equips him with a set of miracles and Aaron as a spokesman. But the people do believe. And it seems that it was the words, not the miracles, that were most effective: "And the people believed, and when they *heard* that the Lord had visited the people of Israel and that he had seen their affliction, they bowed their heads and worshipped" (Exodus 4: 31, English Standard Version, italics added). It is suggested here that through listening, the people came to accept as truth the reality spoken of, and then entered their own relationship to God. It is not merely that they understood that Moses was trustworthy and describing a probable course of history and thus provisionally accepted his message. Nor was their response an expression of a general sense of trust. Moses did not trust that they would believe him, but they did, despite the lack of trustfulness that he ascribed them. Thus the act of faith here described exemplifies a kind of trust of others – a trust that leads to a certainty regarding the truth of something that is beyond comprehension. As the medieval mystic St. John of the Cross (1973: 110) writes: "Faith is not knowledge derived from the senses, but an assent of the soul to what enters through hearing."

The example from Exodus focuses on the trust in a single unique individual, the prophet, the leader. But many have emphasized that what characterizes faith is the trust of the believer in the community of believers. As Tillich (1957: 118) writes: "There is no life of faith, even in mystical solitude, which is not life in the community of faith." Throughout the generations, theologians and philosophers of religion have offered various formulations of the nature of this reliance on community and its role in the act of faith. Here too it is not merely that the group supports the faith of individuals, but rather that, as in the encounter with the prophet, the experience of the truth of that to which individuals assent in their faith comes in part through the community. As Meissner (1984: 178) explains, "The believer's faith does not spring from a vacuum but comes to life within a context of belief." Here it is often stressed that the relationship to the community is one in which the individual's faith is confirmed through participation in the broader body of believers. It were as though the individual act of assent of the believer is experienced as just one part of the more general assent of the community. The individual's reliance on the authoritative teachings of the community and its representatives may be better understood in the light of this kind of communal trust.

In this description of the trust of others that is involved in the act of faith, the second kind of trust, trust in God, already finds expression. The relationship with others within the community is typically described as providing an opening to the relationship with God, and it is through this opening that faith comes to fruition. If the trust in the testimony or faith of other believers is not followed or accompanied by a trust in God, then there may be appreciation of faith, a belief in the faith of others, but there is not a real act of faith per se (Marcel 1973). As Tillich (1957: 99) states, "Every act of faith presupposes participation in that toward which it is directed."

This participation entails openness to and trust in the presence of a transcendent God. And although this presence has certain specific qualities depending upon the religion (e.g., love, grandeur, demands, etc.), what is unique and different from all other kinds of relationship is the object's transcendent Godlike nature. It is that God is considered to be an object beyond all the specific qualities that are attributed to other objects, that God is considered to be supernatural and the source of being and not just another being, that makes this relationship unique. There is an inevitable distance or gap in the relationship. Thus, by definition, God can never be fully grasped or comprehended. Although theologians and philosophers have attempted to prove *that* God exists, those same theologians assert that the knowledge of God's nature attained in the act of faith is beyond any rational demonstration (Burrell 1986). To have faith is to have a relationship of trust in another whose very existence does not have the same material certainty of everything else encountered in life. Thus, although faith posits an intimate participation, it is a participation fused with an inevitable separation. Accordingly, after stating that, "every act of faith presupposes participation," Tillich goes on to remark that "there is no faith without separation" (1957: 99–100). He further states: "He who has faith is separated from the object of his faith. Otherwise he would possess it. It would be a matter of immediate certainty and not of faith" (Tillich 1957: 100).

Both in the relationship to the community of faith, and in relationship to God, the sense of trust that is manifested is an openness to the presence of the other, a response to, and total reliance upon him or her, an acceptance and intimacy that is beyond any rational explanation. These are all qualities and capacities associated with the attachment line, as well as with Erikson's stage of trust versus mistrust, which has been posited as belonging to it (Blatt and Blass 1990). Indeed it may be suggested that because of the unique characteristics of the act of faith, its transcendent and ultimate nature, the trust that it manifests is most complete or extreme. Erikson himself at one point seems to suggest this. He maintains that religion is a kind of institution that "throughout man's history has striven to verify basic trust" (1968: 106). When "the glory of childhood . . . survives in adult life . . . [t]rust, then, becomes the capacity for *faith*" (Erikson 1968: 106). Within this framework, the opposite of such trust would be mistrust, a lack of openness, responsiveness, reliance, participation, etc.

It should be noted that there are analytic thinkers who have looked negatively on this kind of trust solely because of the sort of processes it involves. It has been argued that the act of faith that I have been describing here reflects a dangerous form of submission or acceptance of authority. Fromm (1942) most clearly gives voice to this view. He distinguishes between rational and irrational faith – the former being based on one's own experience, thought, or feeling, the latter on submission and acceptance of authority. The act of faith as portrayed here would fall into the latter category. Although it may have an experiential component, it is not rationally grounded and does indeed involve submission and the acceptance of authority. Fromm evaluates this negatively because he sees in it a denial of the self and its positive productive powers. Consequently, he maintains that in the religious realm only those forms of religion "that emphasized man's own power to love, his likeness to God, have preserved and cultivated the attitude of rational faith" and perforce such faith cannot be towards a transcendent object: "Since rational faith is based upon our own productive experience, nothing can be its object which *transcends* human experience" (Fromm 1947: 209–10). The evaluation that the submission involved in the act of faith is based on a kind of misuse of authority and misguided denial of self continues in later analytic writings as well (Balter 1993; Symington 1994, 1999). In such remarks, one can see an instance of the overly strong emphasis on the value of what has been termed the separateness developmental line. Anything that comes at the expense of the autonomous self and its productive powers is regarded very negatively. From this perspective, nothing can be more wrong for a human being than submission. Moreover, these remarks posit an inherent relationship between submission and self-denial. But it may be seen that such a relationship need not be assumed when the self is conceptualized in terms of a dialectical relationship between the two developmental lines because this conceptualization allows for extreme states of relatedness on the one line simultaneously with states of self-assertion on the other.

Faith and the separateness line

On the separateness line of development, there are also two main kinds of capacities that come into play in the act of faith. One of these capacities is again trust, but a trust of a different kind than that of the attachment line. Here this capacity takes the form of trust in oneself, a reliance on one's experience and understanding, a decision to proceed with what one believes (or from the believer's perspective, knows) to be true, even if one can never convince others of its truth. It is a kind of embracing of oneself as an adequate source of knowledge. Interestingly, here the opposite of the capacity for trust is not mistrust, as it is on the attachment line, but doubt. Overcome by self-doubt, the full-hearted embrace of what one on another level believes to be true is forever impeded. New questions and alternative explanations constantly arise. Again it is the transcendent nature of the concept of God, God's existence as a supernatural being, that gives this trust (and doubt) special significance. It is because God is posited as inherently separated, beyond full grasp and comprehension, that trust in oneself is here pushed to the extreme. Reason, as it is commonly understood and so commonly applied in the manifestation of capacities along the separateness line (Blatt and Blass 1992), cannot in itself support or confirm the trust in one's understanding and experience that here comes to the fore.

Kierkegaard refers most clearly to the necessary expression of self-trust in the act of faith. He writes, "Faith is the objective uncertainty with the repulsion of the absurd, held fast in the passion of inwardness, which is the relation of inwardness intensified to its highest" (Kierkegaard 1846: 611). Inwardness is at its highest in the act of faith because "objectively . . . [the believer] then has only uncertainty, but this is precisely what intensifies the infinite passion of inwardness, and truth is precisely the daring venture of choosing the objective uncertainty with the passion of the infinite" (Kierkegaard 1846: 203). As Meissner (1987: 97) explains: "Faith implies an act of the will, a fundamental choice in which man not only radically expresses his subjectivity, but also posits himself in his choosing to will the infinite" (see also Buber 1961).

In making this choice, the doubts are recognized, not ignored. The risk of error is acknowledged but transcended in the choice. Thus some religious writers have focused on the courage that necessarily accompanies the self-determination in the act of faith. Courage is that "element in faith which is related to the risk of faith" (Tillich 1957: 103; see also Tillich 1952). This courage "does not deny that there is doubt, but takes the doubt into itself as an expression of its own finitude and affirms the content of an ultimate concern" (Tillich 1957: 101).

It may be seen here that the trust that is involved in the act of faith from the perspective of the separateness line is based on a positive evaluation of the self. It is an expression of affirmation, of courage, heightened self-determination, and inwardness. But there is another dimension that characterizes the act of faith along this line that is of a very different quality. This is the recognition of self-limitation. In one sense, the limitation of the self may be a product of the involvement of the attachment line, which aims towards the development of self-in-relation, rather than toward a strong autonomous self. But the recognition of limits may come also from *within* the separateness line. And in fact, it may be suggested that the recognition of the limits of the self is what allows for and furthers true attachment. In the act of faith, the recognition of self-limitation that is expressed along the separateness line emerges from a process of self-reflection. In the course of the reflective process, the believer comes to the view that one's experiences (hopes, fears, desires, etc.) point to the existence of a transcendent being beyond oneself and that the self and its potential depends on the existence of that being. That is, the believer is convinced that, to make sense out of his or her experiences, for the course his or her life has taken to have any meaning and any meaningful future, for the believer to be who he or she truly is, the presence of God must be posited. God becomes not only an essential component of the believer's self-understanding but also a component that is needed for the completion of the self. Although the act of completion may be viewed as part of the attachment line, the recognition that precedes this is clearly a separateness process, focused as it is on contemplation and reasoning regarding the self as separate and autonomous.

The description of this reflective process has taken different forms and the manner in which God is perceived through it has differed in essential ways. But common to the process in its different forms and ways is the recognition of the insufficiency of the self in and of itself. For example, Rahner (1978) speaks of the believer's pre-apprehension of the infinity of reality, which becomes known to him or her through a certain kind of experience of freedom and responsibility for one's own life. In this experience the believer "cannot understand himself as subject in the sense of an *absolute* subject, but only in the sense of one who receives being" (Rahner 1978: 34). He continues, "A finite system as such can experience itself as finite only if in its origins it has its own existence by the fact that, as this conscious subject, it comes from something else which is not itself and which is not just an individual system, but is the original unity" (Rahner 1978: 34). Such contemplation of self-experience when truly lived, rather than merely thought through, leads the believer to maintain that one's very being depends on God and comes from God.

Kierkegaard's (1849) well-known psychological and philosophical essay on the experience of despair, *Sickness unto Death*, arrives at a similar conclusion from a somewhat different direction. Kierkegaard's analysis of the experience intends to show how, were it not for dependence of the fullness of our existence on the presence of a creating God that is transcendent to us, the feeling of despair, in the sense of despair "to will to be oneself," would not really be possible. This kind of despair, which one often tries to avoid in various ways, reflects that the self is constituted by a relationship to God and can be itself only within that relationship. Kierkegaard (1849: 14) writes, "The formula that describes the state of the self when despair is completely rooted out is this: in relating itself to itself and in willing to be itself, the self rests transparently in the power that established it." The person cannot be himself or herself without God.

There is no real contradiction that Rahner, Kierkegaard, and other religious thinkers who describe this recognition of limitation also stress personhood, individuality, and inwardness as essential to the act of faith and as strengthened through it. As Kierkegaard (1849: 21) explains, "to have a self, to be a self, is the greatest concession, an infinite concession given to man, but it is also eternity's claim upon him." In other words, it is suggested here that indeed being a self is of infinite value, but to be this self is to recognize that this self is dependent, created, given within a relationship to a transcendent God. The self in itself is always lacking. From this perspective, the fact that the person is completed through a relationship to God and can, although finite, reach out to and participate in God, is viewed as a source of human greatness. In turn, the fact that without God one cannot be oneself and that God remains forever beyond full grasp is viewed as the source of self-limitation.

The capacity to recognize such self-limitation has been described in terms of the quality of humility. When self-trust is dominant in the absence of such humility and without recognition of doubt, then the opposite quality, arrogance, finds expression. Arrogance, a common vice in religious literature, may be seen from a psychological perspective to express a limitation of the act of faith in relation not only to the separateness line, but also to the attachment line. Because in the context of the act of faith, arrogance may be understood as a kind of "identification with God" (Rizzuto 1979: 187), it would also foreclose the possibility of a participation with God.

The value of the attachment and separateness model for the understanding of the act of faith and the new psychoanalytic perspectives on religion

This examination of the act of faith in the light of the attachment and separateness model has highlighted dimensions of self and relationship that this act involves and points to their developmental sources. Psychologically, the act of faith was seen to comprise a complex integration of processes along both the attachment and separateness lines and to be determined in part by the uniqueness of the object of these processes for the believer – God.

In turn, the examination of these capacities in the context of the act of faith refines our understanding of them. For example, the act of faith brings to the fore the distinction between trust in *others*, which is a basic form of relatedness opposed to the state of mistrust, and trust in *oneself*, which is a form of self-affirmation leaning towards autonomy and opposed to the state of doubt. The interactions between these different notions of trust, and the related states of self-loss and self-doubt, arrogance and submission, affirmation and limitation, etc., are useful for the exploration and under-standing of other relational and developmental processes.

There is another way in which the examination of the act of faith in terms of attachment and separateness is of particular significance. This is in its contribution to the understanding of the nature of the shift that has taken place in the past twenty years in psychoanalysis' evaluation of religious belief. This shift clearly may be seen to result from the influence of Winni-cott's thought in the realm of transitional objects and space (Winnicott 1953). Although Winnicott (1963, 1971) himself directly addressed the topic of religious belief on only a few occasions, his views nevertheless have had a profound impact, with later theoreticians taking up his ideas on religion and further developing them in many important ways (Jones 1991; Kakar 1991; Meissner 1984; Rizzuto 1979). Prior to this shift, psychoanalytic understandings of religion were strongly influenced by Freud's views on this topic. Freud said many things about religion, some more positive than others, but what has been retained as the heart of the Freudian position on religion is that belief is an illusion – an idea strongly motivated by wish fulfillment and, in this case more specifically, by wishes for a protective father who would fulfill our dependent needs (Freud 1927) and overcome our feelings of guilt about our being independent (Freud 1913). According to this view, Freud acknowledged that wishes and reality may at times coincide, but he did not think that this was what in fact happened when it came to the issue of belief in God. Rather, because of their early psychic needs, believers posit a transcendent reality that, as a matter of fact, does not exist. There may be certain advantages and disadvantages to the believer's act in this regard, but in any case it entails a mistaken relationship to reality.

Winnicott and his followers did not reject Freud's view of religious belief as illusion but rather elaborated the notion of illusion and ascribed it positive value in this context. Through the notion of transitional objects and space, they maintained that illusion belongs to the intermediate area between reality and fantasy that evolves early in life in the child's inter-actions with his mother and that continues and should continue in certain forms to play an important role throughout life. Illusion is, in Winnicott's words, "an area of *experiencing*, to which inner reality and external life both contribute. It is an area that is not challenged" (1971: 3). Winnicott (1971: 13–14) further states, "The mother's adaptation to the infant's needs, when good enough, gives the infant the *illusion* that there is an external reality that corresponds to the infant's own capacity to create." The illusion is not challenged; the question whether what is perceived was created by the infant or presented from without is not raised. Religious belief is a mature expression of such illusory experiencing. It involves the spreading of the original transitional relationship to the cultural field, as the original relationship naturally dissolves. Winnicott (1971) may be under-stood here to be saying that cultural phenomena are given, not fully created by the individual, but the individual meets these phenomena, finds them anew, and in this sense experiences them as his or her creation. Thus, as long as there is no demand of others that they recognize the objective truth of the belief, illusion provides the believer with an area of relief from the ongoing strain of relating inner and outer reality, an area that may be pleasurably shared with other believers.

This new view of religion as existing in a transitional space, as a legitimate mature illusion, makes irrelevant the question of whether the belief entails a denial of objective reality and lends positive meaning to it. Rather than being an expression of infantile needs that comes at the expense of acknowl-edgement of reality, as it was for Freud, religion may now be regarded as an acceptable form of ongoing relatedness that serves the individual's well-being (Kakar 1991; Jones 1991). Moreover, viewing religious experience in terms of transitional phenomena and illusion provides a good explanatory context for many aspects of this experience (Meissner 1984; Rizzuto 1979).

But the analysis of the act of faith in the light of the attachment and separateness model raises questions whether in certain other respects this apparently positive shift provides an adequate psychological understanding of this religious phenomenon. Others have already raised the question whether viewing religious experience in terms of transitional phenomena leaves room for a transcendent reality of God that is not reducible to imaginary objects (Leavy 1988; Richardson 1992; Spezzano 1994; Wallace 1991), to a kind of "Cosmic Teddy Bear" (Leavy 1988: 155). And some analysts who have conceptualized religious experience in transitional terms have noted the limitations of such psychological terms in describing the transcendent nature of God (Meissner 1990; Rizzuto 1991).

The present examination has shown that integral to the understanding of the processes and capacities of the two developmental lines that come into play in the act of faith is the believer's affirmation of the veridicality of the transcendent. Although the psychological investigator must bracket the question of the veridicality, to bracket the *believer's affirmation* of this veridicality may not only misrepresent the believer but also limit the psychological investigation of important and exclusive dimensions of the act of faith. The transitional and illusory view of religious experience shifts the focus away from this unique affirmation, emphasizing instead the inter-action between personal need and creation on the one hand and environ-mental and cultural givens on the other that is common to a whole range of experience. Instead of focusing on the believer's affirmation of the reality of God, this view focuses on the reality of community, tradition, and culture, as they meet the believer's subjectivity. In contrast, the present examination suggests that although indeed the act of faith entails a meeting between a given cultural context and individual subjectivity, the processes that are unique to the act of faith are drawn forth because of the believer's specific involvement with what he or she considers to be a transcendent reality that is not illusory, albeit lying beyond demonstration. As I have argued, it is this involvement that influences the believer's special relationship of trust with community and God (on the attachment line) and that requires of the believer special self-trust and yet awareness of limitation (on the separateness line).

With the shift to the Winnicottian perspective, the special nature of these processes is, as a rule, put aside in favor of processes more familiar from other experiential domains. The unique nature of trust in relation to community and to God that is required of the believer is often described from this new perspective in terms of more general feelings of trust (Meissner 1987). Emphasis is placed on the "capacity to believe," rather than on belief in God per se (Hopkins 1997: 489). The community is described as a realm for shared experiencing, rather than a vehicle through which truth is conveyed (Symington 1999). Moreover, because the objective existence of God within the believer's experience is bracketed, the scope of the attachment dimension of the act of faith is limited. Whereas one's mother is regarded as having a real presence, God is viewed more as a creation of the believer, a means for the expression of transitional relatedness, than as a potentially real object or initiator of a relationship (Winnicott 1971). Thus a shift towards the subjectivity of the believer and his or her position along the separateness line tends to occur (although it is not a necessary move and clearly not the intention of all those who have furthered the Winnicottian perspective). This shift, however, is not to the issues of trust of self versus doubt in the face of absence and limitations that were earlier shown to be central to the act of faith along the separateness line, for these are not possible without positing the potential reality of God for the believer. Instead what predominates from the perspective of the separateness line is the self's capacity for experiencing, creating, and finding, all with positive affective tones (Jones 1991).

In sum, the present analysis of the act of faith in terms of the attachment and separateness development model not only clarifies and refines the natures of the act and the model of development but also points to the limitations of the contemporary shift to the Winnicottian perspective on religious experience. Because this perspective tends to put aside the reality for the believer of the transcendent object of God, it does not provide an adequate account of many of the unique psychological processes that are required for the act of faith along both developmental lines, and the relational kind of attachment processes that seem to be involved in this act become mainly self-oriented.

It may be seen that this shift from attachment to separateness in the context of the act of faith, when taken to an extreme, can result in a kind of psychology of self-deification. When the *experience* of transcendence cannot be denied and yet the *existence* for the experiencer of a real transcendent object is not acknowledged, it is the self as a psychological entity that comes to be regarded as transcendent. The "act of faith" is then used to describe the individual's relationship to his or her unknown inner personal truth and creativity (Eigen 1981, 1985), and "sacred" is applied to an object in the anticipation of its serving as a means to enhance self-experience (Bollas 1987); it is viewed as immanent, "found in the depths of our inner world" (Jones 1991: 124). Although conceptualized in terms of relationship to the world, to others, and to holiness, transcendence in these formulations remains within the individual's own natural experiencing self. This view is best expressed by Jones (1991) in his examination of religion in the light of contemporary psychoanalytic perspectives. He writes: "The experience of the sacred has a transcendental numinous quality not because the sacred is a wholly other object but because such experiences resonate with the primal originating depths of selfhood" (Jones 1991: 125).

It is in this context that the attachment and separateness developmental model, with its demand for distinction between forms of relatedness to the self and to the object and for the involvement of both forms throughout life, provides a safeguard against such slippage from relationship to narcissism.

References

Balint, M. (1934) *Primary Love and Psychoanalytic Technique*, London: Hogarth Press, 1952.

Balter, L. (1993) 'Review of *Psychoanalysis and Religion: psychiatry and the humanities, vol. 11*', *Psychoanalytic Quarterly* 62: 481–6.

Blass, R. B. and Blatt, S. J. (1992) 'Attachment and separateness: a context for the integration of self psychology with object relations theory', *Psychoanalytic Study of the Child* 47: 189–203.

—— and —— (1996) 'Attachment and separateness in the experience of symbiotic relatedness', *Psychoanalytic Quarterly* 65: 711–46.

Blatt, S. J. and Blass, R. B. (1990) 'Attachment and separateness: a dialectic model of the products and processes of development throughout the life-cycle', *Psychoanalytic Study of the Child* 45: 107–27.

—— and —— (1992) 'Relatedness and self-definition: two primary dimensions in personality development, psychopathology, and psychotherapy', in J. Baron, M. Eagle and D. Wolitsky (eds) *Interface of Psychoanalysis and Psychology*, Washington, DC: American Psychological Association, pp. 399–428.

—— and —— (1996) 'Relatedness and self-definition: a dialectic model of personality development and disturbance', in G. Noam and K. Fischer (eds) *Development and Vulnerability in Relationship*, Hillsdale, NJ: Erlbaum, pp. 309–38.

—— and Shichman, S. (1983) 'Two primary configurations of psychopathology', *Psychoanalysis and Contemporary Thought* 6: 187–254.

Blos, P. (1979) *The Adolescent Passage*, New York: International Universities Press.

Bollas, C. (1987) *The Shadow of the Object*, New York: Columbia University Press.

Buber, M. (1961) *Two Types of Faith*, New York: Harper and Row.

Burrell, D. B. (1986) *Knowing the Unknowable God: Ibn Sina, Maimonides, Aquinas*, Notre Dame: University of Notre Dame Press.

Eigen, M. (1981) 'The area of faith in Winnicott, Lacan and Bion', *International Journal of Psycho-Analysis* 62: 413–33.

—— (1985) 'Toward Bion's starting point: between catastrophe and faith', *International Journal of Psycho-Analysis* 66: 321–30.

Erikson, E. H. (1959) *Identity and the Life Cycle*, New York: International Universities Press.

—— (1968) *Identity: youth and crisis*, New York: Norton.

—— (1982) *The Life Cycle Completed*, New York: Norton.

Fairbairn, W. R. D. (1952) *Psychoanalytic Studies of the Personality*, London: Routledge.

Freud, A. (1974) 'A psychoanalytic view of developmental psychopathology', in A. Freud (ed.) *The Writings of Anna Freud*, vol. 8. New York: International Universities Press, pp. 57–74.

Freud, S. (1913) 'Totem and Taboo', in J. S. Strachey (ed. and trans.) *The Standard Edition of the Complete Psychological Works of Sigmund Freud*, vol. 13, London: Hogarth Press, 1955, pp. 1–161.

—— (1927) 'The Future of an Illusion', in J. S. Strachey (ed. and trans.) *The Standard Edition of the Complete Psychological Works of Sigmund Freud*, vol. 21, London: Hogarth Press, 1961, pp. 5–56.

Fromm, E. (1942) 'Faith as a character trait', *Psychiatry* 5: 307–19.

—— (1947) *Man for Himself*, New York: Holt.

Guntrip, H. (1969) *Schizoid Phenomena, Object Relations and the Self*, New York: International Universities Press.

Hopkins, B. (1997) 'Winnicott and the capacity to believe', *International Journal of Psycho-Analysis* 78: 485–97.

John of the Cross (1973) *Collected Works of St. John of the Cross*, trans. K. Kavanaugh and O. Rodriguez, Washington, DC: Institute of Carmelite Studies.

Jones, J. W. (1991) *Contemporary Psychoanalysis and Religion*. New Haven, CT: Yale University Press.

Kakar, S. (1991) *The Analyst and the Mystic*, Chicago: University of Chicago Press.

Kierkegaard, S. (1846) *Concluding Unscientific Postscript to Philosophical Fragments*, ed. and trans. H. V. Hong and E. H. Hong, Princeton, NJ: Princeton University Press, 1992.

—— (1849) *The Sickness Unto Death*, ed. and trans. H. V. Hong and E. H. Hong, Princeton, NJ: Princeton University Press, 1980.

Leavy, S. (1988) *In the Image of God*, New Haven, CT: Yale University Press.

—— (1990) 'Reality in religion and psychoanalysis', in J. H. Smith and S. Handelman (eds) *Psychoanalysis and Religion*, Baltimore, MD: Johns Hopkins University Press, pp. 43–59.

Mahler, M. S. (1974) *Selected Papers of Margaret S. Mahler*, New York: Aronson.

Marcel, G. (1973) *Tragic Wisdom and Beyond*, Evanston, IL: Northwestern University Press.

Meissner, W. W. (1984) *Psychoanalysis and Religious Experience*, New Haven, CT: Yale University Press.

—— (1987) *Life and Faith: psychological perspectives on religious experience*, Washington, DC: Georgetown University Press.

—— (1990) 'The role of transitional conceptualization in religious thought', in J. H. Smith and S. Handelman (eds) *Psychoanalysis and Religion*, Baltimore, MD: Johns Hopkins University Press, pp. 95–116.

Rahner, K. (1978) *Foundations of Christian Faith*, New York: Crossroad.

Richardson, W. (1992) 'Love and the beginning: psychoanalysis and religion', *Contemporary Psychoanalysis* 28: 423–41.

Rizzuto, A. M. (1979) *The Birth of the Living God*, Chicago: University of Chicago Press.

—— (1991) 'Review of *Psychoanalysis and Religion*', *International Review of Psycho-Analysis* 18: 576–80.

Spezzano, C. (1994) 'Illusion, faith, and knowledge: commentary on Sorenson's "Ongoing change in psychoanalytic theory"', *Psychoanalytic Dialogues* 4: 661–5.

Symington, N. (1994) *Emotion and Spirit*, London: Cassell.

—— (1999) 'Religion and science in psychoanalysis', in S. M. Stein (ed.) *Beyond Belief: psychotherapy and religion*, London: Karnac, pp. 162–78.

Tillich, P. (1952) *The Courage to Be*, New Haven, CT: Yale University Press.

—— (1957) *The Dynamics of Faith*, New York: Harper and Row.

Wallace, E. (1991) 'Psychoanalytic perspectives on religion', *International Review of Psycho-Analysis* 18: 265–78.

Winnicott, D. W. (1953) 'Transitional objects and transitional phenomena', in

Collected Papers: through paediatrics to psycho-analysis, London: Tavistock Publications, 1958, pp. 229–42.

Winnicott, D. W. (1958) *Collected Papers: through paediatrics to psycho-analysis*, London: Tavistock Publications.

—— (1963) 'Morals and education', in *The Maturational Processes and the Facilitating Environment*, London: Hogarth Press and Institute of Psychoanalysis, 1965, pp. 93–105.

—— (1971) *Playing and Reality*, New York: Basic Books.

Chapter 18

The menace of postmodernism to a psychoanalytic psychology

Robert R. Holt

Over a long career, Sidney Blatt has not hesitated to confront subtle psychological topics concerning subjective, even evanescent and often unconscious phenomena. His work on psychological representations and self-definition, for example, proceeds boldly into such territory. One of the many reasons I have such respect for my old friend Sid is that he has never succumbed to the temptation to try to finesse the vexing problems of developing reliable methods for studying them, so that his work can be replicated by others. All too many of our colleagues, psychologists and psychoanalysts alike, invoke instead the trendy cliches of postmodernism, claiming that a new – and not incidentally, a far less demanding – methodology is needed to replace that of the true scientific tradition. It is then, I hope, fitting to help celebrate Sid's many contributions by taking a hard and sustained look at postmodernism, and some of the ways it has had unfortunate effects on our field, psychoanalysis in particular.

Some definitions

A recent book (Fishman 1999; see also Holt 2000) asserts that post-modernism includes hermeneutics, social constructivism, pragmatism, and relativism.

> A core idea in postmodernism is that we are always interpreting our experienced reality through a pair of conceptual glasses—glasses based on such factors as our present goals in this particular situation, our past experiences, our values and attitudes, our body of knowledge, the nature of language, present trends in contemporary culture, and so forth. It is never possible to take the glasses off altogether and view the world as it "really is," with pure objectivity.
>
> (Fishman 1999: 5)

This passage contains some themes that come up again and again in postmodern literature: an attack on "objectivism," portrayed as the notion that it is possible to view the world as it really is, and an espousal of relativism, the doctrine that all knowing is contingent, influenced by a range of determining frameworks.

Sokal and Bricmont (1998) provide a more succinct but narrower definition: Postmodernism is

> an intellectual current characterized by the more-or-less explicit rejection of the rationalist tradition of the Enlightenment, by theoretical discourses disconnected from any empirical test, and by a cognitive and cultural relativism that regards science as nothing more than a 'narration,' a 'myth' or a social construction among many others.
>
> (Sokal and Bricmont, 1998: 1)

It appears that we are talking about a rather general intellectual/cultural phenomenon, reactive and rebellious in its origins, rejecting what was seen as a preceding dogmatic, established tradition, and embracing some form of relativism. But its literature generally lacks clear and explicit definitions, to the point of self-contradiction. It is, moreover, diffuse, vague, and beset with internal contradictions. Richard Rorty, looked up to by many postmodernists as a philosophical guru, has remarked about postmodernism, "It would be nice to get rid of it. It isn't exactly an idea; it's a word that pretends to stand for an idea" ("Think Tank" 1997). And in an irresponsible attack on Harvard generally and the late Henry A. Murray in particular, Alston Chase (2000) construes "positivism" to include moral relativism!

If postmodernism is a reaction against it, what, then, is meant by modernism? Fishman first defines it as "the natural-science-centered worldview deriving from the Enlightenment," calling it "a seductively attractive belief system in its promise of clear, absolute, 'objective' answers in a complex, ambiguous, troubled world" (Fishman 1999: 3). Very shortly, he begins referring to it as positivism, a term one encounters a good deal in postmodern literature, though characteristically it is rarely given an explicit definition, and usually seems to lack much similarity to what philosophers mean by the term. Others, however, define modernism much more broadly, as encompassing many aspects of our contemporary civilization and culture that came to a full flowering in the nineteenth century. I believe that, in many usages, postmodernism implies a rebellion against modernism in this larger sense, in which the culture and social institutions of industrial capitalism play central roles. That is the way I shall use it.

The origins of postmodernism

The modern era emerged during the "Great Transformation" of the sixteenth through nineteenth centuries from a culture permeated by traditionalism. Modern science began shortly before the Enlightenment, a time when established, traditional institutions, dogmas, and doctrines – notably religious ones – were questioned in the name of reason and empiricism. Rapid developments of technology and the factory system of production led to the Industrial Revolution, which very quickly replaced guilds and cottage industries with industrial capitalism. At about the same time, demographic and political revolutions took place also: population in the developed countries increased rapidly, its locus shifting from rural to urban, while monarchies were overthrown in the name of liberty, popular sovereignty, and representative government. Small and interactive communities gave way to cooler, more impersonal and institutional forms of association, the extended family being replaced by the nuclear family. With less social cohesion and more competitiveness came alienation and anomie, poverty, and growing economic inequality. Mass society emerged, with mass production and consumption, universalism, and pressures for conformity. Yet standards of living rose generally, with an extended life span.

This "modern" mode of economic production and distribution is now widespread in the "developed world." That economic system in turn required a new kind of human being (Inkeles 1983), produced in part by universal education. Its schools supply skills needed for the work force and teach the ideologies of capitalism and democracy (or fascism). As compared to the preceding traditionalist culture, modernism demands less relaxed attitudes towards time and obligations. In a similar way, personal relationships have become pervaded by impersonal, legally regulated controls; the gain in efficiency was offset by a loss of emotional gratifications and support.

If the free-market capitalist system is to work well, society should be stable, not subject to frequent political upheavals. That implies political conservatism, the freezing in place of whatever arrangements of power and privilege may exist, however unjust they may be. Capitalism is inherently expansive, working best when there is continuous economic growth. Its workers must be paid enough to survive and become consumers, with constantly expanding desires for the system's outputs. So there must be a way to inculcate a system of materialist values – the belief that happiness is achieved by wealth and the concrete goods and services that it can buy. Advertising and entertainment industries become increasingly predominant means of education. The schools must also, however, produce people who have the technical know-how to plan and build the productive machinery and to invent new types of goods and services. Those engineers and technologists in turn must be fed new information by scientists. Indeed, many students believe that the basic motor of change and expansion in the modern system is provided by science and its practical application, technology.

A major consequence of this last aspect of the modern world is rationalism, not only the techniques of logical and realistic thinking but a set of values that push aside tradition, respect for one's elders and their ways, in favor of demonstrably more efficient and effective ways of matching means to ends. Modernism implies that we should replace our old habits of respecting nonrational traditions and values like those of religion by esteeming science as the ideal realization of rationality and efficiency. This value system includes awe and even fear of scientists because so much of what science consists of is difficult to understand and because it has brought us unimaginable powers of destruction along with its good products.

The tumultuous events of the nineteenth century were accompanied by a gradual questioning of many traditional certainties. Under the influence of Romanticism in the early part of the century, Europeans began to appreciate the exotic, and travelers' tales of the strange customs of foreign peoples became popular reading. For intellectuals, the simple dichotomy of civilized (us) vs. savage or primitive (them) would no longer do; Chinese civilization, for example, was ancient and highly developed, yet unlike that of the West in countless fascinating ways. Its religions and morality commanded respect despite their divergence. It was a short step to moral relativism, the proposal that one ethical system could not be proved to be better than another, simply different. A sharper challenge to orthodoxy's comfortable assumption that "our way is of course the best" could hardly be imagined.

Various other eventful discoveries of the nineteenth century brought similar challenges to ethnocentric dogmatism. The development of non-Euclidean geometries made it evident that any geometry was one member of a large group of formal systems, none of which had the absolute, eternal verity that had long been assumed for Euclid's. Darwin's revolution shook many basic assumptions of contemporary thought, eventually including the presumption that European man was the ultimate goal toward which all biological evolution had been heading. Freud, too, played an important role in showing how various forms of presumably rational thought could be influenced by wishes, fears, and defenses, especially unconscious ones. The developing discipline of hermeneutics turned away from its earlier search for ways to establish the true meaning of a text, an enterprise now declared impossible, for all attributed meanings were relative to the interpreter's purposes, conditions, presuppositions, and other contingencies.

Such influences undermined simple, comfortably egocentric world views and dogmatic systems. Philosophers had long realized that underlying most beliefs are more general ones, their foundations. If this kind of inquiry is pushed far enough, we come to first principles or metaphysics, basic assumptions on which a philosophy or other belief system rests (Pepper

1942). No set of facts, nor any rational analysis, can be found to compel anyone to choose one such set of metaphysical foundations over another. Hence the awkward postmodernist term, antifoundationalism, meaning that "there is no ultimate, provable foundation for any value or idea" (Holland 1999: 153) – that is, none that is provably superior to others. These changes disturb those who, nourished on fundamentalism or the naïve reliance on received wisdom, want to believe in absolutes and therefore feel disillusioned, unanchored, and despairing at the prospect of having only approximate Truth.

One consequence of the relativistic demise of dogmatic fundamentalism was a new metaphysical system, pragmatism. At the heart of its epistemology was a skeptical rejection of Truth as an aim of human inquiry; at best, one could establish that a proposition was found useful in some particular context by a community. All of the versions of postmodernism that I am familiar with seem to have their metaphysical basis in pragmatism.

The obvious drawbacks of modernism have led to various other revolts against it. The socialist and communist movements incorporated numerous aspects of modernism while rejecting capitalism. The 1960s saw a diffuse but powerful rebelliousness against modernism's excesses, with a questioning of many values, ideologies, and institutions. The feminist revolution has brought continuing pressure against patriarchy and male domination. Other oppressed groups, like Americans of African and Asian descent, rebelled against racism, homosexuals against discrimination and for gay rights, while liberally educated youth turned away from dogmatic religious fundamentalism.

But not just the flaws of modernism may be responsible for the current crisis. Consider the growing split between science and humanism, which so worried Henry Adams (1918), and more recently, C. P. Snow (1993). Both of them noted, with some alarm, the emergence of a new class of intellectuals, highly adept in mathematics and hard science and relatively untutored in the humanities but feeling little inner need for them. Each group developed its own jargon, making communication increasingly difficult across the emerging divide, which the Gymnasium-educated gentleman-scientists of earlier centuries had easily bridged. Worse, from the humanists' viewpoint, was the arrogance of the scientifically learned technologists, who cockily implied that they had all the answers. No wonder academic teachers of the arts and literature felt defensive as such parts of their realm as natural philosophy became the preserve of people trained in rigorous disciplines poets did not understand.

It must be conceded that the new intellectuals of the laboratories were often allied with the most aggressive and exploitative masters of modernity. Mumford (1970) has called our attention to the fact that first kings and later merchant princes held the purse strings and were quick to see how their power and privileges could be protected and extended by funding scientists. The latter, being human beings, could hardly fail to do the kind of work their patrons demanded. It was all too easy, therefore, to see the destructiveness unleashed by applications of science, ranging from the machine gun through dynamite to nuclear bombs, as somehow intrinsic to an approach that excludes heart and soul, overlooking the fact that the new technologies produced great advances in many of the positive sides of life. I find it an attractive hypothesis, then, that postmodernism arose in part from real flaws in modernism, in part from defensiveness that turned many nonscientists into antiscientists.

In literary criticism during the three middle decades of the twentieth century, modernism took the form of trends calling themselves formalism and structuralism. In them, critics treated works of literature "as stand-alone, solid, even monumental, things-in-themselves, to be studied and analyzed in and for themselves without much reference to their surroundings" (Holland 1999: 153). The linguistics of de Saussure was of this type. For "structuralist thinkers like Claude Levi-Strauss and Jacques Lacan . . . linguistic structure became . . . an absolute to replace earlier absolutes" (Holland 1999: 154). This extreme position led to an exaggerated backlash in which the importance of context was overemphasized.

In reacting against this new absolutism, Derrida started the post-structuralist movement, and in 1966, founded deconstruction. He took the inherent ambiguity of language to an extreme in which meaning could never be deciphered. In an attempt to expose and overcome the ambiguities and traps of language, he adopted a style of writing that was difficult to the point of impenetrability, partly in hopes that he could get past the binary oppositions implicit in familiar words by means of an arcane vocabulary. This unfortunate and ultimately self-defeating device was taken up and widely imitated by a growing postmodern school of scholars.

According to Holland (1999: 159), "deconstruction says it is not possible for literature or anything else to develop beliefs about the nature of the world and of human experience that are not grounded in political or social history." Moreover, Lyotard (1989, as paraphrased by Holland) asserts that "the 'grand narratives' [of psychoanalysis and Marxism] are no more than language games, each governed by its own rules, and therefore incommensurate with the others." Thus postmodern writers easily fall victim to the pervasive danger of reductionism, although their writings contain more subtle and insightful substance than this brief treatment seems to imply. Notice that postmodernism has had many roots, but almost none in the natural sciences. As a consequence, members of the movement tend to have poor understanding of and little if any first-hand knowledge about the methods and everyday work of scientists.

Some parallels between history and personal development

In reviewing the above bit of history, I was struck by some parallels with another kind of development: the stages of growth of individual personalities. During the past few decades, developmental psychology has extended its range of concern from childhood and adolescence to the adult years. I will focus on the scheme put forward by William Perry (1970), in a book summarizing several years of research at Harvard and Radcliffe.

His procedure should satisfy almost any enthusiast for hermeneutics. In a most nondirective kind of way, he interviewed samples of students from several successive classes after each of their four undergraduate years. Reading through the texts of these recorded conversations, he began to notice a main line of development. Students tended to enter college with what he calls "Basic Dualism," the outlook developed by a child who is constantly corrected and shown the right way, what "we in this family and the authorities" believe in. It contrasts starkly with what's wrong, bad, and stupid – the ways of our enemies. This position is sharply challenged by the encounter with multiplicity as students enter college and find among their peers, as well as in the faculty, many obviously intelligent and decent people with quite different ways and points of view.

To the dismay of many freshmen, the faculty do not offer a set of the right answers to all questions, an array of unquestioned truths. Instead, they constantly challenge students to question assumptions and to realize that issues may be approached from various positions. A common way of coping with the challenge without wholly giving up Basic Dualism is to adopt the formula, "All people are entitled to their own opinions." Bewildered by the difficulty of finding out what their teachers want of them and the path to getting good grades by supplying that, the student usually "transmutes the simple pluralism of Multiplicity into contextual Relativism" (Perry 1970: 57). We need not go into the various forms it takes, with partial or full attempts at retreat or escape.

In the best case, the student realizes that, even though there is no simple, authority-given solution to the problem, living and acting in the real world does require making up your mind. Such choices, at first tentative, help firm up a sense of identity, often aided by identification with wise (as opposed to dogmatic) authorities, and the student moves into the final stage, accepting the necessity of personal Commitment. Though this mature stance differs from relativism through the affirmation of a specific set of values and goals, superficially resembling the initial certainties of Basic Dualism and perhaps including some of the same content, it is actively chosen after a full awareness of other possible options, not passively inherited. I believe that Perry's scheme may be useful by helping us see a way out of the dilemmas of relativism. I hope that you understand, however, that I am not suggesting that all relativists are stalled at a late-adolescent stage of development or any other such easy reductionism.

Why we should be concerned about postmodernism

One major reason to consider postmodernism more mischievous than helpful, despite the fact that it does incorporate some genuine insights and is a step toward a useful sophistication, is that – like most other reactions against a preceding system – it is often carried too far. Perhaps its single most pernicious exaggeration is to reject rationality as part of an outmoded crude modernism. Because modern corporate capitalism tends to be short-sighted and incorporates many injustices, it is easy to reject the ethos of modernism too sweepingly. For example, some postmodern feminists assimilate reason and logic to the male-dominated world of modernism, claiming that women think in different (and often, in superior) ways. To be sure, those hard-nosed extremists who hold up as an ideal a form of rational thinking completely purged of emotion are more often male than female, but it is not difficult to show them, following their own basic procedures, that truly effective thinking must incorporate emotion along with logic (Damasio 1994).

American political thinkers on the left, such as Noam Chomsky and Michael Albert, have vigorously opposed postmodernist thought, as expressed by self-described leftist intellectuals, on the grounds that its rejection of rationality is self-defeating. As part of his contribution to a symposium on postmodern thought, pro and con, Chomsky said:

> many scientists, not too long ago, took an active part in the lively working class culture of the day, seeking to compensate for the class character of the cultural institutions through programs of workers' education, or by writing books on mathematics, science, and other topics for the general public. Nor have left intellectuals been alone in such work, by any means. It strikes me as remarkable that their left counterparts today should seek to deprive oppressed people not only of the joys of understanding and insight, but also of tools of emanci-pation, informing us that the "project of the Enlightenment" is dead, that we must abandon the "illusions" of science and rationality – a message that will gladden the hearts of the powerful, delighted to monopolize these instruments for their own use. They will be no less delighted to hear that science . . . is intrinsically a "knowledge system that legitimates the authority of the boss," so that any challenge to such authority is a violation of rationality itself – radical change from the days when workers' education was considered a means of emancipation and liberation.
>
> (Chomsky 2000)

Chomsky also pointed out the dilemma of anyone who wanted to discuss attacks on the usual procedures of rational discussion: either one had to make arguments using those canons, which in effect presumed the validity of what was under discussion, or else follow an alternative set of procedures that postmodernists never specify. It is indeed striking how those who try to persuade others to abandon the rational heritage of the Enlightenment are intelligible only when they follow the very procedures they attack.

Much of the time, however, the postmodernist literature is expressed in such deliberately obscure language as to be impenetrable. One might think that writing of that type would be so counterproductive that it would be quickly abandoned. Yet that overlooks the sad fact that many people are intimidated and impressed by others who spout learned-sounding technical language, even if it makes no sense when carefully examined. That is true of journal editors and book publishers, too, I am sorry to say. The most lamentable errors of reasoning, confident misstatements of fact, and unintelligible writing may be found in print, and their perpetrators often have great reputations.

Let me turn to the effects of postmodernism on science generally before considering psychology and psychoanalysis. Occasionally these days one sees the phrase, "the science wars," referring to the frontal attack some postmodern writers have mounted against science generally. Most of it has come from a new discipline, called Science Studies (see, for example, the journal *Science as Culture*). Its exponents are joined by a group of armchair intellectuals from university departments of humanities and social studies. With the naïve assumption that others must be just like themselves, they claim that scientists, too, are playing "language games," making up "narratives" that merit no "privileged" status. Some of them seem recently to have discovered that ideas are malleable to the influences of their authors' personal foibles, gender, histories, and predilections and also to such standard "forces" as the material conditions and social ambience of their production. They assume, therefore, that anyone who tries to discover what is reliably valid about the world must have a naïve belief that absolute truth is directly available and needs a lesson in relativity and contingency.

The branch of psychology that studies how we perceive the real world is one of the most rigorous (and thus, for postmodern critics, most "positivistic" and " scientistic"). Yet we owe our detailed understanding of just how various kinds of personal, social, cultural, and other influences bias and shape our perceptions to this discipline (see, e.g., Boring 1957; Klein 1970). Ironically, it is only because those workers understood and used objective scientific method – and assumed the existence of a stubborn external reality – that they were able to do more than make plausible arguments: They actually demonstrated by replicable procedures the biases that interfere with our everyday ability to know nature directly and simply.

Part of the postmodernists' error is that they overgeneralize some of their valid insights, mistakenly upgrading empirical points to metaphysical status. As Sokal and Bricmont (1998: 189) put it, "*Specific skepticism should not be confused with radical skepticism*" (their italics). In addition, much of the most ambitious postmodernist writings by some of the most famous authors suffers from the less forgivable faults of poor scholarship and slanted or reductionistic intellectual history.

Not all postmodernists approach science to attack; many try to borrow its prestige, and act as if the obscurity of their writing is attributable to their arcane scientific knowledge. Sokal and Bricmont (1998) have written a scrupulously fair but deliciously merciless exposé of eight writers of this kind who have great prestige in postmodern circles (especially in Europe). All of them write as if they had intimate familiarity with various of the most difficult branches of mathematics or physics, but all make numerous elementary blunders in talking about these matters, betraying their virtually complete failure of understanding. Happily, Sokal and Bricmont have the easy mastery of the relevant disciplines that most readers lack and can see through all the pretenses. Sokal (1996) is the physicist who perpetrated a brilliant hoax on the editors of the postmodern journal, *Social Text*. He submitted and they printed a paper deliberately designed to make no sense whatsoever while touching all modish postmodern bases. It is noteworthy, I think, that the people who attack scientific method as blind to its own biases do not even uphold decent standards of humanistic scholarship.

Stephen J. Gould, president of the American Association for the Advancement of Science (AAAS) for 1999–2000, considered the "science wars" important enough to attack. He warned against the press picture of science studies as a

> public and scholarly analysis . . . with this supposed struggle depicted as a harsh conflict pitting realists engaged in the practice of science (and seeking an absolute external truth progressively reachable by universal and unbiased methods of observation and reason) against relativists pursuing the social analysis of science (and believing that all claims about external truth can only represent social constructions subject to constant change and unrelated to any movement toward genuine factual knowledge) . . . . But I have never met a pure scientific realist who views social context as entirely irrelevant, or only as an enemy to be expunged by the twin lights of universal reason and incontrovertible observation. And surely, no working scientist can espouse pure relativism at the other pole of the dichotomy. . . . If all science arises as pure social construction, one might as well reside in an armchair and think great thoughts . . . .
>
> The true, insightful, and fundamental statement that science, as a quintessentially human activity, must reflect a surrounding social

context does not imply either that no accessible external reality exists, or that science, as a socially embedded and constructed institution, cannot achieve progressively more adequate understanding of nature's facts and mechanisms.

(Gould 2000: 259–60)

Many scientific statesmen have been directing attention to the diminishing proportion of our brightest young people who are enrolling in scientific courses in universities and who are seeking careers in science. Meanwhile, our complex technological civilization needs every brilliant and creative young mind it can recruit into science. No doubt there are many reasons for this worrisome trend, but the so-called "science wars" may be partly responsible.

The worst threat of postmodernism is to the social and behavioral sciences, including psychology and psychoanalysis. On that point, I agree with Sokal and Bricmont (1998: 206f), who list three main negative effects: first, one can waste a lot of time reading and arguing against a difficult literature of pseudo-issues, which offers very few rewards. Second, because it is trendy, the authors of this literature serve as destructive role models for students and young colleagues, modeling obscurantism, shallow scholarship, poor reasoning, and intellectual dishonesty. Third, it cuts the ground from under those of us who are trying to apply our knowledge to the solution of the pressing social and political problems of our time.

Within psychoanalysis, it has a similarly destructive effect. As it happens, psychoanalysis was particularly vulnerable to postmodern attack, in considerable part because of some aspects of Freud's personality and work. Raised in an autocratic culture, he took it for granted that he had the right to dominate the movement he had created, enforcing subservience to his formulations of the theory and practice. Those who would not accept such terms were extruded, to form their own rival movements. Treating his theory as if it was a dogma, he rejected as inappropriate any attempts to introduce ordinary scientific methods and criteria for evaluating it.

In his naïf objectivism, Freud had declared, "We possess the truth," such as the notion of a universal, innate Oedipus complex. That created a setup for any relativist critique. He declared psychoanalysis to be a natural science; because most of his followers had never worked as scientists, it was easy for them to believe that, in the established sciences, the untenable assumption prevailed that the truth could be directly observed. Sooner or later, even those who remained loyal to his banner became restive, especially in the democratic culture of the United States. Hermeneutics and now social constructivism offer an escape from the rigidity, the dogmatism, the authoritarian culture of traditional Freudian institutes and societies, the formulaic coldness of technique, the overemphasis on the intrapsychic, and neglect of both the patient's sociocultural milieu and the realities of analyst–patient relationships. No wonder the rebellion took the extreme forms we see in many psychoanalytic writers under the influence of postmodernism.

As I have been arguing for over a decade (Holt 1989, 1992), psychoanalysis is in a time of crisis, faced by bolder and more effective criticisms of its theory, of its treatment methods' effectiveness, even attacks on the personal integrity of its founder. When many outsiders are challenging its claim to be a science, this is no time to concede the point by embracing hermeneutics. That move will only accelerate the abandonment of psychoanalysis for shorter, cheaper, trendier forms of psychotherapy that are more reimbursable by insurers. The road to becoming a legitimate science is not a short or easy one, but it is possible as well as urgent to take it. Possible, however, only if the confident and modish claims of postmodernism are firmly rejected.

What we should do about it

Obviously, I believe that we should resist, expose, and refute most of the efforts of postmodernists to lead us down counterproductive paths in our own disciplines. That includes most of what they have to say about philosophy and metaphysics, particularly epistemology. But we should also absorb and use what is good: the postmodernists' resistance to authoritarianism, fundamentalism, and other forms of dogmatism, and the contextual nature of facts.

Psychoanalysis has a regrettably destructive authoritarian heritage. As I have argued elsewhere, it can be traced to notable authoritarian trends in Freud's own personality as well as in the social milieu within which he grew up. It seemed only natural for his first followers to adopt attitudes and behavior toward him that may be called "authoritarian submission." Those included, notably and famously, respect for Freud's writings that goes as far as reverential adoration. Dissent within the movement was often treated by excommunication, or at the least the questioner was allowed to remain only on the condition of reanalysis of his "negative transference." Whether Freud's epigones rebelled and formed their own schools or stayed within the fold, for the most part they identified themselves with him and long after his death perpetuated undemocratic, hierarchical institutions – psychoanalytic societies and institutes.

The effect of his heritage on psychoanalytic treatment was often unfortunate. The approved technique was clinical, remote, and authoritative, which patients often experienced as cold. Much of the transference was uninterpreted because that part of analysts' own transference to their training analysts (submission) was not considered pathological or unrealistic.

Happily, however, there has been gradual change for the better. More deviation is tolerated without expulsion, and more analysts are recognizing and counteracting the authoritarianism of the past. To the extent that postmodern tendencies in the larger culture have helped this process, we should be thankful for it. But we should be careful not to let appropriate gratitude generalize into too sweeping acceptance of a certain class of psychoanalytic writers who seem to be much influenced by postmodernism. Typically, they emphasize what is good in it and explicitly reject radical relativism or idealist metaphysics. Nevertheless, apparently unaware of the contradiction, they quote authors whose ideas do have those metaphysical commitments.

One who does just that is Donnel Stern (1985), whom Irwin Hoffman acknowledges as a major influence. Stern says that postmodernism is responsible for the following list of influences:

> the current focus on the here-and-now aspects of transference and countertransference, a view of character as an active, world-building process, an increasing emphasis on the person's status as an active agent; the recognition of the immense contribution of the immediate interpersonal situation on any experience, even memory, that arises in the situation; the inaccuracy of the traditional concept of the analyst's neutrality; and the recognition that no single school of psychoanalysis holds the key to the truth.
>
> (Stern 1985: 204)

So far, so good, though I do not think anyone needs constructivism or hermeneutics to accept those sensible ideas. Moreover, Stern (1985: 206) says that he believes in realism of a fallibilist or transcendental type, for "constructivist epistemology does not require relativist ontology." And yet he begins the paper with an approving quotation of the following: ". . . any so-called reality is . . . an invention whose inventor is unaware of his act of invention, who considers it as something that exists independent of him" (Watzlawick 1984: 10). That clearly rejects realism, though Stern asserts his belief in a real world. He cannot have it both ways. I agree with Gillett (1998b), that postmodern writers are reluctant to make a clean break with "Controversial (metaphysical) Relativism," because their position, which they think of as radical, collapses to the endorsement of truisms. Thus, Stern's insistence that our sense data and ideas are related to reality in a complex and indirect way is simply what Gillett (1998a) calls "Non-Controversial Relativism." It does not require a break with the epistemology of the most sophisticated contemporary sciences.

In refreshing contrast to his colleagues and contemporaries who are under the spell of postmodernism, Sid Blatt wisely holds back from the temptation to generalize to the philosophical level. Psychologists and psychoanalysts everywhere would do well to follow his example, sticking to the level at which their training and experience qualifies them best to work, and leaving metaphysics to the professional philosophers. As to postmodernism, it has too little to offer to be worth the time and trouble needed if one is to extract the occasional kernel from confusing chaff.

References

Adams, H. (1918) *The Education of Henry Adams*, Boston, MA: Houghton Mifflin.

Boring, E. G. (1929; 2nd edn 1957) *A History of Experimental Psychology*, New York: Appleton-Century-Crofts.

Chase, A. (2000, June) Harvard and the making of the Unabomber, *Atlantic Monthly* 285(6): 41–65.

Chomsky, N. (2000) Contribution to symposium on postmodernism, retrieved March 23, 2001, from <http://www.zmag.org>.

Damasio, A. (1994) *Descartes' Error: emotion, reason, and the human brain*, New York: Putnam.

Ellenberger, H. F. (1970) *The Discovery of the Unconscious: the history and evolution of dynamic psychiatry*, New York: Basic Books.

Fishman, D. B. (1999) *The Case for Pragmatic Psychology*, New York: New York University Press.

Gillett, E. (1998a) 'Relativism and the social constructivist paradigm', *Philosophy, Psychology, and Psychiatry* 5: 37–48.

—— (1998b) 'Response to the commentaries', *Philosophy, Psychology, and Psychiatry* 5: 62–5.

Gould, S. J. (2000) 'Deconstructing the "Science Wars" by reconstructing an old mold', *Science*, 287: 253–61.

Holland, N. N. (1999) 'Deconstruction', *International Journal of Psycho-Analysis* 80: 153–62.

Holt, R. R. (1989) *Freud Reappraised: a fresh look at psychoanalytic theory*, New York: Guilford.

—— (1992) 'The contemporary crises of psychoanalysis', *Psychoanalysis and Contemporary Thought* 15: 375–403.

—— (2000) 'Case dismissed. Review of D. Fishman, The case for pragmatic psychology', *Contemporary Psychology* 45: 108–11.

Inkeles, A. (1983) *Exploring Individual Modernity*, New York: Columbia University Press.

Klein, G. S. (1970) *Perception, Motives, and Personality*, New York: Knopf.

Lovejoy, A. O. (1936) *The Great Chain of Being: a study of the history of an idea*, Cambridge, MA: Harvard University Press.

Lyotard, J.-F. (1989) *The Lyotard Reader*, Oxford, England, and New York: Basil Blackwell.

Mumford, L. (1967) *The Myth of the Machine: vol.1. technics and human development*, New York: Harcourt Brace Jovanovich.

—— (1970) *The Myth of the Machine: vol. 2. the pentagon of power*, New York: Harcourt Brace Jovanovich.

Nordenskiöld, E. (1928) *The History of Biology: a survey*, New York: Knopf.

Pepper, S. C. (1942) *World Hypotheses: a study in evidence*, Berkeley, CA, and Los Angeles: University of California Press.

Perry, W. G., Jr. (1970) *Forms of Intellectual and Ethical Development in the College Years: a scheme*, New York: Holt, Rinehart & Winston.

Singer, C. (1959) *A Short History of Scientific Ideas to 1900*, New York: Oxford University Press.

Snow, C. P. (1993) *The Two Cultures*, 2nd, enlarged edn, New York: Cambridge University Press.

Sokal, A. (1996) Transgressing the boundaries: toward a transformative hermeneutics of quantum gravity, *Social Text*, 46/47 (Spring/Summer): 217–52.

—— and Bricmont, J. (1998) *Fashionable Nonsense: postmodern intellectuals' abuse of science*, New York: Picador USA.

Stern, D. B. (1985) Some controversies regarding constructivism and psycho-analysis, *Contemporary Psychoanalysis* 21: 201–8.

'Think Tank; lofty ideas that may be losing altitude' (1997, November 1) *The New York Times*: B13.

Watzlawick, P. (ed. and introduction) (1984). 'The invented reality: How do we know what we believe we know?', in *Contributions to Constructivism*, New York: Norton.

Whitehead, A. N. (1925) *Science and the Modern World*, New York: Mentor Books, 1952.

Index

abandonment 8, 79, 92, 93, 251
Abrams, S. 201
abuse 109, 110
accommodation 31, 244
Ackerman, S. A. 82
actor effect 29
Adams, H. 292
adolescents 81, 82, 121
adoption 13, 51–2, 53
Adorno, T. W. 264–5, 267–8, 269
Adult Attachment Interview 11
affect naming 68
aggression 53, 262; introjective
    depression 93; narcissism 258
Alanen, Y. O. 108, 109, 118
Albert, M. 295
alien self 195, 197, 198, 200, 206, 207
alienation 11, 245, 247, 261, 262, 290
alter ego 259
Altmann, S. 24
American Psychoanalytic Association
    xvii, xviii, 6, 228
Amitay, O. A. 80–1, 82
amnesia 204
anaclitic personality 242, 245; as bound
    opposite to introjective personality
    244; defense mechanisms 122–3;
    depression xv, 8, 13, 92–3, 96, 97, 98;
    and greed 248, 249, 250; mode of
    treatment 120; "moving-toward"
    trend 251; narcissism 260–1; society
    as anaclitic 247; therapeutic change
    164; see also dependency; two-
    configurations model
analytic relationship 201–2, 298–9;
    representational change 203–4, 208;
    space within the 62, 63
analytic (therapeutic) dyad 30, 36

Andrusyna, T. 15, 213–21
anger xv, 93
anorexia 160
antifoundationalism 292
anxiety: disorders 77; gender
    incongruence 123, 124; object
    relations theory 231; objective 126;
    self-society dilemma 242
Anzieu, D. 59
Arnold, B. 146
Aronowitz, S. 264, 266–7, 268
Aronson, J. K. 145
arrogance 280–1
art 59–60
articulation 9, 140, 142, 159, 160
Aryan, M. 142
assimilation 244
associative freedom 230
attachment 8, 191; developmental model
    273–4; disorganized 195, 197;
    externalization of alien self 198; and
    religious faith 275–8, 279, 281, 282–3,
    284; styles of 79, 144, 146; see also
    relatedness
attachment theory 8, 9, 43, 191;
    cognitive-affective development 11;
    internal working models 44, 51;
    monotropy 50; parental
    representations 52
Auerbach, J. S. xviii, 1–19, 68, 75, 142,
    144, 145, 191, 195, 201
Austen Riggs Center 6, 7, 12, 118,
    121–5, 128, 131, 164
authoritarianism 298, 299–300
autobiographical data 157, 158
autobiographical memory 204–6
autocorrelation 31, 32
automatic thoughts 95, 97

autonomy: Beck's theory of depression
1, 95–6, 98; dependent mothers 82;
developmental model 274; introjective
depression 92, 93; Mutuality of
Autonomy scale 158, 164; religious
faith 281
Avery, R. R. 49

Bakhtin, M. 45
balance 243
Barber, J. P. 216
Barbour, C. 162
Bateman, A. 198
Bateson, G. 24, 110
BDI see Beck Depression Inventory
Beck, A. 1, 14, 93–5, 96–7, 98, 99
Beck Depression Inventory (BDI) 215,
217, 218, 219
Beck, S. xvi, 5
Beebe, B. 13, 23–42, 44
behavioral dialogue 31
Behrends, R. S. 191
Bein, E. 145
belief 200
Bell, R. Q. 26
Bender, D. S. 146
Benjamin, J. 265
Berman, W. 155
Berzofsky, M. 66
biological factors of schizophrenia
104–7, 174; see also neurobiology
Bion, W. R. 194, 195
Blass, R. B. 15, 191, 273–87
Blatt, E. xvi, 3–4, 59
Blatt, S. J. xiv–xvii, 1–2, 43, 213, 288,
300; art 59–60; attachment/
separateness developmental model
191, 273–4; biography of 2–7;
boundary disturbances 9, 138, 161–3;
cognitive distortions 80; critics of 85;
dependency and self-criticism 75–6,
84; depression 91, 92–3, 96, 97, 98, 99;
greed and society 247; intellectual
contributions of 7–12;
intersubjectivity 195; IQ and clinical
change 125; as mentor xviii, xix–xx,
167, 241–2, 255; narcissism 255, 260,
269–70; narratives 214; object
representations 47, 48, 54, 138–49,
155–61; personality and therapeutic
outcomes 12, 120, 131; psychosocial
treatment 14; reflective functioning

68; Riggs study 122, 123; Rorschach
method 14, 154–5, 163–4, 165–6;
schizophrenia 118; scientific method
222; spatial representations 59;
therapeutic change 201; two-
configurations model 13, 15, 242, 245,
248, 250, 252, 253; Vincent Foster
suicide 60; women and relational style
217
Bleuler, M. 118, 172, 173, 181
Block, J. 126
Block, J. H. 126
Bloom, L. 23–4
bodily actions 66–7
body image 59
body-self space 60, 63, 64
Bolgar, H. xvi
borderline personality organization:
boundary disturbances 9, 162, 163;
defense mechanisms 128; evocative
constancy disturbances 10, 13; object
representations 139, 140, 141, 159–61;
see also personality disorders
Bornstein, R. F. 141, 143
boundary constancy 10
boundary disturbances 9, 13, 138,
161–3
boundary representation 161–3
boundedness 58, 59, 62
Bowers, M. 104
Bowlby, J. 10, 50, 205
brain: functions 105, 106; hippocampal
damage 173; plasticity of 107; thought
disorder 173, 183
Brazelton, T. B. 28
Brenneis, C. B. 160
Bricmont, J. 289, 297, 298
Britton, R. 195, 200
Bromberg, P. 58
Bruner, J. S. 213
Bruno Klopfer Award xv, 7
Bucci, W. 34
Buchholz, E. 35
bulimia 145
Burns, B. 148
Bursten, B. 261

Cannon, W. B. 110
capitalism 290, 295
Cappella, J. N. 29
case study method 222–37
Cavell, M. 60, 65, 194

CCRT *see* Core Conflictual
  Relationship Theme
Chapman, J. P. 173, 182, 184
Chapman, L. J. 173, 182, 184
Chase, A. 289
children: abuse of 109, 110; adopted
  51–2, 53; affective understanding
  194–5; alien self 197; cognitive
  structures 156; defense mechanisms
  121; internalization 43, 45, 77, 123;
  maltreated 53; middle childhood 13,
  43–57; parent-child interactions 78–9,
  80–1; parental representations 46, 47,
  48, 49, 50–4; selfobject relationships
  258–9; *see also* infant research;
  mother-infant interaction; parents
Chomsky, N. 182, 295–6
Ciompi, L. 104, 109
CL *see* Conceptual Level scale
clinical change 200–1, 206–8;
  assessment of 225–6; IQ and
  defensive mechanisms 125, 128–30;
  Rorschach method 164–5; Thought
  Disorder Index 178; *see also*
  psychotherapy; therapeutic outcomes
Clyman, R. B. 204
Coe, J. E. 146
cognition: dependency/self-criticism 76,
  78–80; negative 93–5; *see also* mental
  representations
cognitive development 9–11, 13, 47,
  156
cognitive distortions 80, 93–4, 97
"cognitive morphology" 9–10
cognitive-affective schemas 97, 99
cognitive-behavioral approach 91–2,
  97–8, 137, 147
cognitive-dynamic approach 231–2,
  233
cognitive-representational approach 7,
  8, 9
Colarusso, C. A. 224
Coleman, M. J. 178
communication: dyadic systems view of
  13, 23–42; face-to-face 25;
  schizophrenics 179–80; social 23–4;
  vocal timing 32, 33; *see also* dialogue;
  language; verbalization
communism 292
community 275, 276, 283
Concept of the Object Scale (COS) 9,
  138–40, 145–7, 148, 159, 160–1

Conceptual Level (CL) scale 9, 47, 48,
  49, 50–1; assessment of object
  representations 140–1; attachment
  style 146; bulimic patients 145; orality
  143–4
conceptual-representational level 9, 47,
  140
concrete-perceptual level 9, 47, 140
conditioning 105, 106, 109, 110
confabulation 138, 162, 163, 177,
  180
conflict: cognitive distortion of
  dependent individuals 80; parental
  representations 49
consumerism 249
containment 202
contamination 138, 162, 163, 177
context: language 293; personality 243;
  psychoanalytic case studies 228; social
  243, 252, 261, 262, 297–8
control-mastery theory 229
Cook, B. 145
Coonerty, S. 144
cooperation 11
coordinated interpersonal timing
  31
Core Conflictual Relationship Theme
  (CCRT) 213–14, 215
corporate greed 255–6
Corson, E. O. 108
Corson, S. A. 108
COS *see* Concept of the Object Scale
countertransference 63, 198, 225; dyadic
  systems view 30; postmodernism 300;
  psychic space 66
Coyne, J. C. 76
Cramer, P. 14, 120–33, 142, 143
critical social theory 256, 257, 263–8,
  269
Crits-Cristoph, P. 44, 215
Crittenden, P. M. 205
Cruse, D. A. 180
cultural relativism 269, 289
culture: cross-cultural studies 65, 243;
  narcissism 256, 261–3, 268, 269;
  postmodernism 289
Curtis, J. T. 229
Cushman, P. 249

D-R Scale *see* Differentiation-
  Relatedness Scale
D'Afflitti, J. P. xv, 96, 141

Dahl, H. 230
Darwin, C. 291
DAS *see* Dysfunctional Attitude
  Scale
Daut, R. L. 182
declarative (explicit) memory
  204–5
deconstruction 293
defense mechanisms 14, 93, 120–33;
  clinical change 128–30; IQ and
  personality change 125, 126–8; object
  representations 142; Riggs study
  121–4, 125, 128, 131
denial 92, 93, 121, 122; gender
  incongruence 123, 124; IQ and
  clinical/personality change 126, 127,
  129, 130; object representations
  142
Dennett, D. C. 194
dependency: anaclitic depression xv, 8,
  92; cognitive distortions 80;
  developmental perspective 75–6;
  disturbed relationships 76–7; and
  greed 250; interpersonal implications
  82, 83; life span development 80–2;
  mental representations 78–9;
  motivational orientations 77–8;
  "moving-toward" trend 251;
  specificity hypothesis 14, 84;
  therapeutic change in patients 12;
  vulnerability to depression 83–5, 96;
  see also anaclitic personality;
  nurturance
depression 1, 91–103; anaclitic xv, 8, 13,
  92–3, 96, 97, 98; Beck Depression
  Inventory 215, 217, 218, 219; Beck's
  theory of 1, 93–6, 97, 98, 99;
  Conceptual Level scale 140, 141;
  dependency/self-criticism dichotomy
  76, 77; Depressive Experiences
  Questionnaire 8, 77, 96, 98, 141;
  introjective xv, 8, 13, 92–3, 96, 97, 98,
  145; Mr A's case 192, 193, 200; object
  representations 145, 160; parental
  representations 143; postpartum 79;
  relationship narratives 214, 217, 218;
  social support 79; specificity
  hypothesis 14; vulnerability to 76, 81,
  83–5, 91–3, 94, 95–7, 98–9; women
  217
Depressive Experiences Questionnaire
  (DEQ) 8, 77, 96, 98, 141

DEQ *see* Depressive Experiences
  Questionnaire
Derrida, J. 293
despair 280
desymbolization 66, 69
developmental models 201
developmental psychology 294
deviant verbalization 161, 162,
  174–5
diagnosis 145, 178
dialogic structure 44–5
dialogue 25, 44; behavioral 31; clinical
  vignettes 224; mutual 31
Diamond, D. 15, 142, 144, 165,
  255–72
diathesis-stress component 76, 77
Dickens, C. 257
Dietrich, D. R. 143
Dietrich Object Relations and Object
  Representations Scale 143
differentiation 9, 65, 140, 142, 159, 160,
  273–4
Differentiation-Relatedness (D-R) Scale
  142
Diguer, L. 15, 213–21
dopamine 104, 106, 107
dreams: object representations 146–7,
  157, 158; spatial representations
  59
drive theory 137, 223, 258, 260
Duncan, N. 79
dyadic systems 13, 23–42; bidirectional
  model of influence 25–30; emergent
  properties of the dyad 29–30, 44;
  historical background of 24–5; rules
  of regulation 30–5; stability of
  responsivity 28–9
dynamic interactionism 76, 77, 84
Dysfunctional Attitude Scale (DAS) 12,
  96, 97, 98
dysfunctional attitudes 94, 95, 97
dysphoria 76, 99

eating disorders 77
echo 31
economics 245–6
Edelson, M. 228
education 290
ego: boundary disturbances 162; critical
  social theory 263; defense mechanisms
  126–7; intelligence 120, 125;
  narcissism 258, 259, 260, 263, 265,

268; object relations 137;
schizophrenic patients 139; spatial
representation 59; *see also* self
ego psychology 157, 158, 159
egocentrism 269, 291
Elliott, R. 229, 234
Ellis, C. 4
Emde, R. N. 44
emotions: affective understanding
194–5; depressive schema 97;
representation of self-states 196
empathy 5, 33, 144, 202, 204
enactment 66, 70, 198
Engel, M. xvi, 5
Engelmann, T. C. 147
Enlightenment 289, 290, 295, 296
Erikson, E. H. 10, 11, 60, 274, 277
events paradigm 229
evidence-based medicine 194
evocative constancy 10, 13
Exner, J. E. Jr. 148, 165
expansion 58, 62
experimental infant research 26
explicit (declarative) memory 204–5
Extein, I. 104
external-iconic level 9, 47, 140
externalization 197–8, 206–7

fabulized combination 138, 162, 163,
176, 180
facial expression 32–3
Fairbairn, W. R. D. 137, 231, 232,
233
Fairweather scale 122, 130
Fairweather, T. 122
faith 15, 273–87
family: narcissism 262–3, 264; relatives
of schizophrenics 110, 112, 173–4; *see
also* parents
father: child representations of 50–1;
collapse of parental authority 264–5;
self-criticism 80–1; *see also* parents
Federn, P. 59
feminism 292, 295
fetus behaviour 28
Fishman, D. B. 234, 288, 289
Fiske, D. xvi
Fitzpatrick, D. A. 79
five-factor personality model 127–8
Fleck, S. 14, 104–19
Fonagy, P. 15, 68, 191–212, 226,
228

Ford, R. 118, 121, 125, 142,
145
formal thought disorder 172–87
formalism 293
Foster, V. 60
Fraiberg, S. 9
Frankfurt School 15, 263, 265
free association 230
Freedman, N. 13, 58–71
French, T. M. 105
Freud, A. 7, 9, 126
Freud, S. 92, 209, 256, 291;
authoritarian personality of 298, 299;
cases 222; drive theory 137; influence
on Blatt 4; internalization 155, 166;
mother-infant relation 50; narcissism
257, 263, 266; oedipal stage 11;
religion 273, 281–2; repression 204;
space 58
Fritsch, R. C. 140
Fromm, E. 247, 277
Fromm, E. xvi

Galley, D. J. 143
Gelman, W. xvii, 4
gender: anaclitic/introjective patients 93,
96, 122–3; gender incongruence
123–4; relationship episodes 216–17,
219–20; *see also* men; women
generativity 81–2
genetic influences on schizophrenia 108,
109, 110, 111, 174, 184–5
Gerber, J. D. 146
Gergely, G. 194–5
Gill, M. 154, 165, 174–5
Gillett, E. 300
God 147, 274–84
Goldman-Rakic, P. S. 105, 107
Gombrich, E. 7
Gould, S. J. 297–8
grandiose self 255, 258–9, 260, 261,
267
gratification 47, 156
greed 15, 245–52, 253, 255
Green, A. 257
Greenberg, J. 35
Grinker, R. Sr. xvi, 5
Grossman, K. E. 50
Grotstein, J. 58
Gruen, R. J. 144
guilt xv, 8, 231
Guthrie, G. 4

Habermas, J. 24
Haith, M. 26
Hampstead Child Therapy Clinic 7
Haracz, J. L. 104
Harder, D. W. 122
Harrison, A. 205
Hebrew University of Jerusalem xvi,
    7
Heck, S. A. 141–2, 147
heedlessness 247–8, 249, 250
Henry, W. xvi
hermeneutic single-case efficacy design
    234
hermeneutics 288, 291, 294, 298, 299,
    300
Herr, C. E. 144
Hilliard, R. B. 227, 229
Hobbes, T. 247
Hoffman, I. 300
holding environment 201
Holland, N. N. 292, 293
Holmes, T. H. 104
Holmstrom, R. W. 140
Holt, R. R. 15, 154, 288–302
Holzman, P. S. 14, 172–87
Homann, E. 75, 143
Horkheimer, M. 263–5, 267–8
Horney, K. 250–1, 252
Human Response Variable (HRV) 148
humanism 292
hysterical personality disorders 139

identification 121, 122; gender
    incongruence 123–4; IQ and clinical/
    personality change 127, 129, 130;
    narcissism 265; object representations
    142
identity: gender incongruence 123–4;
    maturation 13; mental states 194; self-
    definition 242, 245
illusion 282
implicit (procedural) memory 94, 204–5,
    206, 208
imprinting 107, 109
impulse control 126
incest 109
incorporation 123
individuation: dependent individuals 78;
    developmental model 273–4;
    Eriksonian model 11; object
    representations 144; therapeutic
    action 201; see also separation

infant research: dyadic regulation 27,
    31; mental representations 35,
    203–4; misattunement 206; neurotic
    patients 208; self-other
    differentiation 257; social exchange
    26; see also children; mother-infant
    interaction
inhibition 105–6, 109
insatiability 247–8, 249, 250, 251
insight 203
integration 9, 140, 142, 159, 160
intelligence 120, 124–31
intentional stance 194, 199
interaction chronometry 23, 27
interaction structures 31, 33–5, 44–5
interactionism 76, 77, 84
interactive regulation 27–8
internal working models 44, 50, 51, 79,
    205
internal-iconic level 9, 47, 140
internalization 77, 81, 123, 163, 166–7;
    boundaries 161; cognitive structures
    156; collapse of parental authority
    264, 265; dyadic rules 34; Freud 155,
    166; object relations theory 43; self-
    states 194, 195, 196; Vygotsky 45
interpersonal process: depression 76;
    mother-infant interactions 23, 31
interpersonal relationships: anaclitic
    patients 164; dependency/self-criticism
    dichotomy 82–3; depression 92, 93;
    early life experience influence on 76;
    internalization 45, 163; maturation
    13; object relations theory 137; object
    representations 138, 144, 155, 156,
    157; responsivity 29; therapeutic
    process 164; see also relatedness
interpersonal responsivity 28–9, 44–5
intersubjective shifts 192, 194–8, 200,
    206–7, 208
intersubjectivity 11, 45, 65, 69, 144, 195
intimacy 78, 79, 92, 93, 96
intrapsychic function 45
introjection 123
introjective personality 242, 245; as
    bound opposite to anaclitic
    personality 244; defense mechanisms
    122–3; depression xv, 8, 13, 92–3, 96,
    97, 98, 145; and greed 248, 249, 250;
    mode of treatment 12, 120; "moving-
    against/moving-away" trend 251;
    narcissism 260–1; society as

introjective 247; therapeutic change
164; *see also* self-definition; two-
configurations model
IQ 7, 124–31

Jacobson, E. 9
Jaffe, J. 13, 23–42
Jarmas, A. L. 145
Jewish Vocational Service (JVS) 4
Johnson, D. R. 145
Johnston, M. H. 173, 175
Jones, E. E. 229–30
Jones, J. W. 284
JVS *see* Jewish Vocational Service

Kandel, E. R. 105, 106
Kazak, A. E. 145
Kepecs, J. xvi
Kern, C. 147
Kernberg, O. 157, 205, 257–63, 264,
265, 268
Kety, S. S. 174
Khatri, N. 14, 91–103
Kierkegaard, S. 278–9, 280
Klein, M. 58, 137
knowledge 200
Koestner, R. 81
Kohut, H. 137, 192, 257–63, 264, 266–7,
268–9
Koós, O. 195
Korchin, S. xvi, 5, 6
Kraepelin, E. 172, 181
Kubie, L. S. 105–6

Lacan, J. 293
Lachmann, Frank 13, 23–42, 44
Lambert, L. M. 146–7
Langer, S. 68
language: deconstruction 293;
psycholinguistic approaches 182–3;
schizophrenic patients 110, 112;
structuralism 293; thought disorder
175, 179–80, 181–2; *see also*
communication; verbalization
Lapidus, L. B. 139, 144
Lasch, C. 261, 264–5, 267–8, 269
latent schizophrenics 173
learning 106, 107
Leckman, J. F. 106
Leichtman, M. 166
Leone, D. R. 143
Lerner, H. D. 14, 139, 140, 154–71

Lerner, P. 155, 165, 166
Levi, P. 54
Levi-Strauss, C. 293
Levy, K. N. xviii, 1–19, 75, 142, 144,
146, 191
Lewin, B. 59
libido 257, 258, 266
linkage studies 184–5
linking 69
literary criticism 293
Locke, J. 35
Loevinger, J. 126
Loewald, H. W. 203, 260
loneliness 92, 93, 146
loss 2–3, 8
Luborsky, L. 15, 44, 213–21
Luria, A. R. 106, 110
Lyons-Ruth, K. 205
Lyotard, J.-F. 293

McCann, L. 15, 222–37
MacLean, P. D. 108
Mahler, M. S. 9, 137, 157
Main, M. 11
malevolence 83, 159, 161, 164
mania 172–3, 180, 181
Marcuse, H. 264, 266, 267, 268
Maroudas, C. 97
Marschke-Tobier, K. 223
Marx, K. 247
Marziali, E. 141
materialism 249, 251, 290
Matthysse, S. 175–7
maturation 10, 11, 13, 48, 273
Mayes, L. C. 201
Mayman, M. 154, 157, 158
meaning: deconstruction 293; dialogical
structure 44
media images 256, 262
Meissner, W. W. 276, 279
memory 106, 107, 204–6; declarative
204–5; narratives 216; procedural
204–5, 206, 208
men: introjective patients 93, 96, 122–3;
relationship episodes 216–17
Menninger Clinic 5, 6, 174
Menninger Factor 1/2 scales 122, 129,
130
Menninger Psychotherapy Research
Project 12, 120
mental models 205, 206
mental processes 192, 199–200, 207–8

mental representations: Blatt's childhood experiences 3; changes in 192, 202–6, 207, 208; dependency/self-criticism 76, 78–80, 82–3; dyadic systems view 34; infant research 35; mediational tools 45; and mental processes 199; middle childhood 46, 47–53, 54; nodal points 10, 13; ORI coding technique 46; of parents 46, 47, 48, 49, 50–4; psychological testing 14; self-states 196; social cognition 97; spatialization 67; therapeutic process 14–15; see also object representations; self-representation

Messer, S. B. 15, 222–37
metacognitive skills 99
metaphysics 291–2, 297, 300, 301
Meyer, A. 104
middle childhood 13, 43–57
Mill, J. S. 35
Mitchell, S. 35
MOA see Mutuality of Autonomy scale
Modell, A. 34–5
modernism 289, 290, 291, 292, 293, 295
Mongrain, Myriam 14, 75–90
monotropy 50
mood 84, 99
moral relativism 289, 291
moral sentiments 246
Moran, G. S. 226, 228
Morgan, A. 205
mother: adopted children 51–2, 53; child representations of 50–1; dependency 82; dilution of maternal nurturance 264; self-criticism 80–1, 82; see also parents
mother-infant interaction 13, 23; bidirectional influences 25–7, 32–3; developmental models 201; dialogical reciprocity 44; dyadic rules 34, 36; emergent properties of the dyad 29; Freud 50; illusion 282; mutual regulation 27, 28, 31; responsivity 28–9; self-regulation 27–8; time series regression analysis 31–3; see also children; infant research
motivational orientations 76, 77–8
Mount Zion Psychotherapy Research Group 229, 231–3
Mountcastle, V. P. 106
movement response xv
multiple case depth research 234

Mumford, L. 292–3
Murray, H. A. 5, 289
mutual dialogues 31
mutual influence 24, 26
mutual regulation 27, 28, 30, 31, 34, 35
Mutuality of Autonomy (MOA) scale 158, 164
Myodovnick, E. 48

narcissism 15, 192, 194, 198, 255–72
narratives 15, 46, 200, 213–21
naturalistic infant research 26
need gratification 47, 156
negative cognition 93–5
neglect 93, 95, 197
Neonatal Assessment Scale 28
nervous system 106–7, 205
neurobiology 104, 111, 112
neurotic patients 140, 208
normal thinking 175
nurturance 77–8, 92, 93; and greed 248; maternal 264; see also dependency

object constancy 10, 13, 142
object relational space 63, 64, 68
object relations: assessment of 14, 157, 163; attachment 274; children 43; dialogical reciprocity 44; Human Response Variable 148; internalization 155; narcissism 259, 260, 262, 268, 269; and object representations 47, 48, 137, 139, 147, 158; parental representations 52; personality development 9; psychic equivalence 200; and the Rorschach 154–71; Rutgers Psychotherapy Research Group 231, 232–3; self and object constancy 10; spatialization 13
Object Relations Inventory (ORI) 1, 46–7, 49; see also Conceptual Level scale
object representations 11, 34–5, 36, 43–4, 137–53; assessment of 14, 138–43, 147–9, 156–65; boundary disturbances 138; concept of 155–6; depression 92; dialogical perspective 45–6; middle childhood 13, 46, 47–53, 54; narcissism 258; qualitative dimensions of 46–8, 49, 50–1, 140–1; representational change 202–6, 207,

208; structural dimensions of 46, 47, 49, 50–1, 140, 141; *see also* Conceptual Level scale; mental representations; object relations
oedipal stage 10, 11, 259, 264, 266
Ogden, T. 58
old age 82
Oleniuk, J. 141
olfactory cues 61
one-person psychology model 29, 30, 35–6, 65
O'Neill, R. M. 141
opiate dependence 160
orality 143–4
ORI *see* Object Relations Inventory
other: boundary disturbances 163; ORI procedure 46; representational change 203; self-other interactions 44, 205, 206, 257

paradoxical representation 160
paranoia 139, 173
parents: adopted children 51–2, 53; assessment of parental representations 140–1, 143–5, 147–8; child representations of 46, 47, 48, 49, 50–4; collapse of parental authority 264–5; dependent/self-critical representations of 79; parent-child interactions 78–9, 80–1; schizophrenic patients 112; self-absorption 195; selfobject relationships 258–9; *see also* family; father; mother
partner effect 29
partner preferences 78
PAS *see* Perceptual Aberration Scale
pathology *see* psychopathology
Pavlovian conditioning 105, 106
PCIS *see* Plan Compatibility of Intervention Scale
Peer Nomination Inventory 49
peer relationships 49–50
Penn Psychotherapy Project 214, 215
perception: internal working models 44; Rorschach method 165, 166
Perceptual Aberration Scale (PAS) 184
perfectionism 12, 96, 98; *see also* self-criticism
perfume 62
Perry, W. 294

personality: clinical change 164; defense mechanisms 125, 126–8, 130, 131; five-factor model 127–8; IQ and personality change 125, 126–8; narcissistic 258, 261–2, 265, 267; procedural memory influence on 204, 205; schizophrenia 111, 112; spatial representation 59; therapeutic treatment outcomes 12, 120, 131; two-configurations model 7, 8, 13, 242–53; vulnerability to depression 95, 96, 98; *see also* anaclitic personality; introjective personality; personality disorders
personality development 8, 9, 13; coevolution of neurophysiological organization 108–9; narcissism 260; object representations 137, 157; psychopathology 75
personality disorders 77, 199; defense mechanisms 124; narcissistic 260, 261, 263, 264, 265, 269; object representations 139; *see also* borderline personality organization; psychopathology
PFM *see* Plan Formulation Method
Piaget, J. 8, 9, 34, 156, 213, 244
Pincus, A. L. 141–2, 147
Pious, W. 6
Plan Compatibility of Intervention Scale (PCIS) 232–3
Plan Formulation Method (PFM) 231
Polka, S. K. xvi, 5
Porcerelli, J. H. 143
positivism 289
Posner, D. L. 146
post-traumatic syndromes 104, 108
postmodernism 15, 270, 288–302
poststructuralism 293
Powers, T. A. 81
PQS *see* Psychotherapy Process Q-set
pragmatic case study 234
pragmatism 288, 292
predictability of dyadic behavior 30
premorbid adjustment 139
preoedipal stage 10, 258, 259, 265, 266
pretend 199, 207
Priel, B. 13, 43–57, 82
primary object 201
procedural (implicit) memory 204–5, 206, 208

projection 121, 122, 197; gender incongruence 123, 124; IQ and clinical/personality change 126, 127, 128, 129, 130; object representations 142
prosocial behavior 49–50
protoconversation 31
prototypicality 177–8
psychic equivalence 199, 200, 207
psychic space 58–61, 65–6, 67, 69
psychic structure 28, 34, 36
psychoanalysis 4, 12, 15; assessment procedures 154; authoritarian nature of 298, 299–300; case study method 222–34; communication 23, 24; depression 92, 98; emergent dyadic properties 30; French school of 194; intrapsychic structures 155; introjective patients 120; narcissism 256–63, 267, 268–9; as narrative process 213; object representations 34–5, 137, 156; postmodernism threat to 15, 298–9; religion 281–4; self representations 34–5; social context 252; space 58, 59, 60, 64; therapeutic action 191–209; two-configurations model 243; see also object relations; psychodynamic approaches; psychotherapy
psychobiology 104
psychodynamic approaches 91–2, 98, 137, 147, 230–3; see also psychoanalysis
psycholinguistic approaches 182–3
psychological testing 6, 7, 14
psychopathology 7, 8, 9–10, 11, 13–14; anaclitic 92; boundary disturbances 162–3; critical social theory 263, 264; defense mechanisms 129, 130; object representations 160, 161; personality-centered approach 75, 85; see also borderline personality organization; personality disorders; psychotic patients; schizophrenia
psychosocial factors of schizophrenia 14, 104, 108, 109, 110–12, 118
psychotherapy 11–12, 14–15; cognitive-behavioral 97–8; narratives 15, 213–21; object representations 158; patient progress 231, 232, 233; process aims 194, 200, 207; psychodynamic 98, 230–3; single-case research 15,
226–30, 231, 233–4; supportive-expressive 120, 214, 219; therapeutic action 191–212; therapeutic process 163–5, 194, 200, 208, 231, 232; see also analytic relationship; clinical change; psychoanalysis; therapeutic outcomes
Psychotherapy Process Q-set (PQS) 229–30
psychotic patients: defense mechanisms 122, 124, 128; object representations 138, 140, 159–60; psychosis-prone individuals 184; thought disorder 180; see also personality disorders
Putnam, R. 247

qualitative analysis 227–9, 234
quantitative analysis 31, 142, 227, 229–30, 234
Quinlan, D. M. xv, 96, 141, 142, 145, 147

Rahe, R. H. 104
Rahner, K. 280
Rapaport, D. 5–6, 7, 137, 154, 157–8, 161, 165, 172, 174–5
rationalism 289, 291
rationality 295
Raulin, M. L. 184
REs see relationship episodes
realism 297, 300
reciprocal and compensatory influence 31
reciprocity 24, 31
recognition constancy 10
reflective function 62, 63, 68, 194, 195, 199–202, 203
regulation: dyadic rules of 30–5; mutual 27, 28, 30, 31, 34, 35; see also self-regulation
Reiser, M. F. 104
relatedness 8, 9, 11, 255, 273; analyst role 201–2; defense mechanisms 122; depression 92; Differentiation-Relatedness Scale 142; dyadic systems view of communication 34, 36; early life experiences 76; individual stability of responsivity 28–9; maturation 13; mutual regulation 31; narcissistic disorders 260–1; need for 245; psychopathology 75; psychotherapy 12; religion 282, 283–4; self-regulation

43; vulnerability to threats to 84; *see also* attachment; interpersonal relationships
relational knowing 44, 69
relationship effect 29
relationship episodes (REs) 213–14, 215–19
relativism 269, 288–9, 291, 294–5, 297, 300
reliability 225, 233
religious faith 15, 147, 273–87
replication 226, 227, 233
representational processes xv, 165–6, 202–6; *see also* mental representations; object representations; self-representation
repression 92, 93, 204
responsivity 28–9, 44–5
Riggs study 121–4, 125, 128, 131
Ritzler, B. 14, 59, 137–53, 160, 162
Rivlin-Beniaminy, N. 48
Rogers, C. xvi, 5
romantic partner preferences 78
Romanticism 291
Rorschach Comprehensive System 148
Rorschach, H. 165
Rorschach Inkblot Test xv, 1, 4, 5, 14, 154–71; defense mechanisms 122; object representations 138, 139, 140, 142, 144; ORI narratives 46; representational processes 165–6; suicidal patients 59; thought disorder 9, 174–81
Rorty, R. 289
Rosch, E. 177–8
Rosenbaum, A. L. 225
Rosenbaum, S. C. 146
Rosenberg, S. D. 142
Rosenblatt, B. 35, 44
Rosenfeld, H. 198
Rosenwald, A. xvi, 5
Rosenzweig, M. R. 107
Roth, D. 59
Rothstein, D. N. 146
Ruesch, J. 24
Rutgers Psychotherapy Research Group 230–3
Ryan, R. M. 49

the sacred 284
sadomasochism 223
St. John of the Cross 276

St. Peter, S. 140, 160
Sameroff, A. 33
Sampson, H. 229, 233
Sander, L. 25–6, 27
Sandler, J. 35, 44, 46
Santor, D. 14, 75–90
SAS *see* Sociotropy-Autonomy Scale
Saussure, F. de 293
Schafer, R. xvi, 6, 137, 154, 165, 174–5
Schaffer, C. E. xviii, 1–19
Scheflen, A. E. 104
schemas 44, 156, 244; dependent/self-critical parental representations 79; depressive cognitive 94–5, 96–7, 99; infant action 34
Schilder, P. 59
Schimek, J. 160
schizophrenia 9, 10, 104–19; boundary disturbances 9, 162, 163; diagnosis 145, 178; dreams 146–7; etiology of 14, 104, 174; language use 175, 179–80, 181–3; latent schizophrenics 173; object representations 137–8, 139, 140, 147, 160; paranoid/nonparanoid subtypes 13; thought disorder 14, 172–87; *see also* psychopathology
Schneider, K. J. 234
science 290, 291, 292, 293, 295, 296–8
scientific method 222, 228, 296, 297
SCORS *see* Social Cognition and Object Relations Scale
scripts 44, 205
SE therapy *see* supportive-expressive psychotherapy
Searles, H. 137–8
Segal, Z. V. 14, 84–5, 91–103
self: adopted children 52; alien 195, 197, 198, 200, 206, 207; boundary disturbances 163; constancy 10, 13; dependent attachment style 79; grandiose 255, 258–9, 260, 261, 267; limits of the 279, 280; mental self-states 194, 195, 196, 206; narcissism 257, 258, 260–1, 263, 264, 266, 268; object representations 43, 44; relationship structures 28; and religious faith 277, 278, 279–80, 284; self-critical attachment style 79; self-other interactions 44, 205, 206, 257; self-society dilemma 242; *see also* ego; self-representation

self-criticism 8, 12, 251; cognitive
distortions 80; developmental
perspective 75–6; disturbed
relationships 76–7; interpersonal
implications 82–3; life span
development 80–2; mental
representations 78–9; motivational
orientations 78; specificity hypothesis
14; vulnerability to depression 83–5,
96, 98; *see also* introjective personality
self-definition 8, 9, 11, 242, 255, 273;
anaclitic depression 93, 96; and greed
248, 250; introjective depression 93,
96; "moving-against/moving-away"
trend 251, 252; narcissistic disorders
260–1; need for 244, 245;
psychopathology 75; psychotherapy
12; *see also* introjective personality;
separateness
self-esteem: defense mechanisms 121,
123; grandiose self 259; introjective
depression xv; vulnerability to threats
to 84
self-interest 245–6
selfobject relationships 258–9; *see also*
children; parents
self-perception 48, 80
self-regulation: bidirectional model of
influence 25, 27–8; dyadic systems
view of communication 24, 36; infant
research 35; patterns of relatedness 43
self-representation 147, 156, 201;
childhood neglect/abuse 197; children
44, 46; depressive 99; dyadic systems
view 34–5, 36; narcissism 257, 258; *see
also* self
self-soothing 62, 63, 68, 69
sensorimotor-preoperational level 9, 47,
140
separateness 191, 273–4; patient-analyst
65; religious belief 278–81, 282–3,
284; *see also* self-definition
separation: anaclitic depression 8;
anxiety of dependent mothers 82;
Eriksonian model 11; need for 244;
object relations theory 231; object
representations 144; parental
representations 49; religious faith 277;
therapeutic action 201; *see also*
individuation
sexuality 262, 266
sexualization 223

Shahar, G. 82
Shapiro, D. A. 229
Shaver, P. R. 142, 144
Shenton, M. E. 183
Sherrington, C. 106
Shichman, S. 75, 80
sign approach 154
Silberschatz, G. 229
Singer, M. T. 108, 110
single-case research 15, 226–30, 231,
233–4
Smith, A. 245–6, 247, 248
Snow, C. P. 292
social cognition 43, 44, 76, 97
Social Cognition and Object Relations
Scale (SCORS) 143
social constructivism 288, 298, 300
social context 243, 252, 261, 262, 297–8
social exchange 26
social interaction 23, 24, 31, 76–7
social isolation 83
social referencing 201
social support 76, 77, 79, 82, 83, 84
social theory, critical 256, 257, 263–8,
269
socialism 292
Society for Personality Assessment xv, 7
sociotropy 1, 95, 96, 98
Sociotropy-Autonomy Scale (SAS) 96,
98
Sokal, A. 289, 297, 298
Solms, M. 204
space 13, 58–71; actuality of 58–9, 60,
65–6, 70; and art 59–60; body-self 60,
63, 64; generativity of 58, 59–60,
66–7; object relational 63, 64, 68;
physical 61–2, 63, 64, 65; potential 60,
64, 66; representational 58, 59, 67–9;
70; symbolizing 64, 65, 67, 69;
transitional 64, 281, 282
spatialization 13, 59, 60–1, 64–5, 66–9,
70
Spear, W. E. 139
specificity hypothesis 14, 84
Spence, D. P. 201, 228–9, 230
Spitz, R. 25, 44
splitting 53, 203
Spruiell, V. 260
Sroufe, L. A. 50
Stauffacher, J. C. 175
Stein, M. I. xiv–xvii, 5
Stern, D. N. 30, 34, 45, 205

Stern, D. B. 300
Stiles, W. B. 229
Strauss, J. S. 122
stress 76, 77, 84, 108
structuralism 293
substance abuse 77
Suess, G. J. 50
Sugarman, A. 162
suicidal patients 59
superego 8, 155, 258, 259, 263, 265
supportive-expressive (SE)
    psychotherapy 120, 214, 219
symbol formation 67–9
symbolization 65, 67–9; discursive 68;
    dynamic 68–9; incipient 68; verbal
    66–7
symbolizing space 64, 65, 67, 69
synchronization 31

Target, M. 15, 68, 191–212, 226
TAT see Thematic Apperception Test
Tavistock Centre 7
TDCRP see Treatment of Depression
    Collaborative Research Program
TDI see Thought Disorder Index
technology 290
Thematic Apperception Test (TAT) 121,
    127, 142–3, 154, 158
therapeutic action 191–212; see also
    psychotherapy
therapeutic outcomes 194, 200, 208;
    object representations 144–5, 146;
    personality relationship 12, 120, 131;
    relational narratives 218, 219, 220; see
    also clinical change; psychotherapy
therapeutic process 14–15, 163–5, 194,
    200, 208, 231, 232; see also
    psychotherapy
Thompson, R. 81
thought disorder 9, 14, 122, 138,
    172–87; see also schizophrenia
Thought Disorder Index (TDI) 174–5,
    176–7, 178–83, 184, 185
Tillich, P. 276, 277, 279
time-series regression (TSR) analysis 27,
    31–3
Titone, D. 182
Toohey, M. L. 108, 110
tracking 31
traditionalism 290
transactional approaches 29, 45
transcendence 276, 278, 283, 284

transference 208, 225, 230, 299; dyadic
    systems view 30, 36; postmodernism
    300; psychic space 66; reflective
    processes 201
transitional epistemology 63, 64
transitional objects 281, 282, 283
trauma 109, 110, 137
Treatment of Depression Collaborative
    Research Program (TDCRP) 12
triangulation 65
Tronick, E. 24, 30, 205
trust 275–6, 277, 278, 279, 281, 283–4
truth 292
TSR see time-series regression analysis
Turnbull, O. 204
twinship 259
two-configurations model 7, 8, 9, 13,
    242–5; and greed 245, 247, 248–50,
    252, 253; psychotherapeutic processes
    15; sociocultural phenomena 15; see
    also anaclitic personality; introjective
    personality
two-person psychology model 29, 35–6,
    228–9

uncertainty 200, 278–9
University of Michigan 157, 158–9
Urist, J. 158

validity 225, 233
verbal symbolization 66–7
verbalization 9, 161, 162, 174–5, 180–1,
    184; see also language
Viderman, S. 58
Viglione, D. J. Jr. 148
vocal timing 32, 33
Vuchetich, J. P. 184
vulnerability to depression 76, 81, 83–5,
    91–3, 94, 95–7, 98–9
Vygotsky, L. S. 24, 45

Wachtel, P. L. 2, 15, 241–54
Waddington, C. H. 10
Wallerstein, R. S. 12, 194
Warburg Institute of Renaissance
    Studies 7
Watkins, J. G. 175
Watson, J. 194–5
Watzlawick, P. 300
Wechsler Adult Intelligence Scale 125,
    127
Weiss, J. 229, 231, 233

Wepman, J. xvi
Werner, H. 8, 9, 156, 159
Westen, D. 143
Western New England Institute for
    Psychoanalysis (WNEIP) xvi, xvii, 6
White, M. D. 146
Wild, C. M. 138
Wilson, A. 163
Windholz, M. 229–30
Winnicott, D. W. 60, 64, 137, 273, 281,
    282, 283–4
wish fulfillment 281–2
WNEIP see Western New England
    Institute for Psychoanalysis

women: anaclitic patients 92–3, 96,
    122–3; dependency/self-criticism
    dichotomy 78; object representations
    146; relationship episodes 216–17,
    219–20
Wynne, L. C. 108, 110

Yale University xvi, 6, 157, 159–61,
    241

Zeanah, C. 34
Zelnick, L. 35
Zimet, C. xvi, 6
Zuroff, D. C. 14, 75–90

Printed and bound by CPI Group (UK) Ltd, Croydon, CR0 4YY

23/10/2024

01777671-0014